AI, Telemedicine, and Governance in Global Healthcare Transformation

Cong Sui
https://orcid.org/0009-0008-2657-2580

West Midlands Health Tech Innovation Accelerator, UK & University of Birmingham, UK & University College London, UK

Poshan Yu
https://orcid.org/0000-0003-1069-3675

Soochow University, China & European Business Institute, Luxembourg & Australian Studies Centre, Shanghai University, China

IGI Global
Scientific Publishing
Publishing Tomorrow's Research Today

Vice President of Editorial Melissa Wagner
Director of Acquisitions Mikaela Felty
Director of Book Development Jocelynn Hessler
Production Manager Mike Brehm
Cover Design Jose Rosado

Published in the United States of America by
IGI Global Scientific Publishing
701 East Chocolate Avenue
Hershey, PA, 17033, USA
Tel: 717-533-8845 | Fax: 717-533-7115
Website: https://www.igi-global.com E-mail: cust@igi-global.com

Library of Congress Cataloging-in-Publication Data

Names: Sui, Cong, 1986- editor | Yu, Poshan editor
Title: AI, telemedicine, and governance in global healthcare transformation / edited by Cong Sui and Poshan Yu.
Description: Hershey, PA : IGI Global Scientific Publishing, [2026 | Includes bibliographical references and index. | Summary: "This book explores the effects of AI and telemedicine technologies on global healthcare delivery, patient care, and medical decision-making. It examines the ethical, legal, and governance challenges associated with digital healthcare, including data privacy, accessibility, equity, regulation, and the responsible use of emerging technologies"-- Provided by publisher.
Identifiers: LCCN 2026028477 (print) | LCCN 2026028478 (ebook) | ISBN 9798260022382 hardcover | ISBN 9798260022399 paperback | ISBN 9798260022405 ebook
Subjects: LCSH: Artificial intelligence--Medical applications | Telecommunication in medicine | Medical informatics
Classification: LCC R859.7.A78 A48 2027 (print) | LCC R859.7.A78 (ebook)
LC record available at https://lccn.loc.gov/2026028477
LC ebook record available at https://lccn.loc.gov/2026028478

British Cataloguing in Publication Data
A Cataloguing in Publication record for this book is available from the British Library.

Table of Contents

Foreword xii

Preface xiv

Chapter 1
Digital Technology Adoption Challenges in Primary Healthcare: An Empirical Study and the NASSS Framework 1
Rajan Punitharajah, Brunel University of London, UK
Julie Davies, Brunel University of London, UK
Sheikh Mateen Ellahi, Elm Tree Medical Centre, UK

Chapter 2
The Benefits of Generative AI for Global Health Partnerships: From Fragmentation to Cohesion 39
Cong Sui, University of Birmingham, UK & University College London, UK
Dimitrios Kalogeropoulos, Global Health and Digital Innovation Foundation, UK

Chapter 3
Overview of Telemedicine in Central Africa, Specifically in Democratic Republic of Congo 75
Samuel Kajama Tshikuta, Coppin State University, USA
A. K. Sharadhi, University of Arizona, USA

Chapter 4
Strengthening Telemedicine and Remote Patient Monitoring in Nigeria With Artificial Intelligence 103
Basil Osayin Daudu, Kogi State Univerisity, Nigeria
Esther Besty Anaiye, National Open University of Nigeria, Nigeria

Chapter 5
Enablers and Barriers to Digital Transformation of Integrated Care Systems (ICS) Across NHS England 133
Han Liew, National University Hospital, Singapore
Abdul M. Seckam, Healthcare Business Solutions, UK
Marzena Nieroda, University College London, UK

Chapter 6
Effect of Digital Mental Health Technology on Mental Healthcare Accessibility in Sub-Saharan Africa: A Systematic Review 169
Dede Atsu Kobla Latey, The London School of Economics and Political Science, UK
Robert Lubajo, WHO Regional Office for Africa, South Sudan

Chapter 7
Mapping Online Patient Narratives in China's Private Healthcare: A Semantic Network Approach 207
Yufeng Xue, Southern Medical University, China & ISCTE, University Institute of Lisbon, Portugal
Ana Brochado, Universidade Aberta, Portugal & Dinâmia'CET-Iscte, Portugal

Chapter 8
Analysis of Ethical Issues in Medical Decision-Making Driven by Artificial Intelligence and Governance Strategies: Focusing on the Diversified Governance Network With Multi-Stakeholder Collaboration 241
Poshan Yu, Soochow University, China & European Business Institute, Luxembourg & Australian Studies Centre, Shanghai University, China
Yiheng Chen, Independent Researcher, China
Chandra Lukita, Universitas Catur Insan Cendekia, Indonesia

Chapter 9
Ethical Frameworks for AI-Driven Medical Innovations: Balancing Progress and Patient Welfare 273
Poshan Yu, Soochow University, China & European Business Institute, Luxembourg & Australian Studies Centre, Shanghai University, China
Xinyuan Jiang, Independent Researcher, China
Chandra Lukita, Universitas Catur Insan Cendekia, Indonesia

Chapter 10
The Regulatory Challenges From the Intersection of AI and Blockchain Technology in Healthcare: A Case Study of BurstIQ 307
Eleftheria Panagiotopoulou, University College London, UK
Mohan P. M. Mishra, FinJuris, UAE

Compilation of References 351

About the Contributors 423

Index 433

Detailed Table of Contents

Foreword xii

Preface xiv

Chapter 1
Digital Technology Adoption Challenges in Primary Healthcare: An Empirical Study and the NASSS Framework 1
Rajan Punitharajah, Brunel University of London, UK
Julie Davies, Brunel University of London, UK
Sheikh Mateen Ellahi, Elm Tree Medical Centre, UK

Globally, rising healthcare costs and workforce pressures highlight the need for digital transformation in primary care. This chapter explores adoption challenges of digital technologies, including AI, robotics, and automation, through the lens of the NASSS framework. Drawing on literature, case studies, and empirical research with UK practitioners, we examine enablers and barriers to implementation, spanning ethical, regulatory, and cultural dimensions. We distinguish between backend efficiencies and frontline clinical applications, highlighting both opportunities and resistance. Findings underscore the importance of governance, training, and co-design to bridge the strategy implementation gap and ensure equitable, sustainable, and value-based healthcare delivery.

Chapter 2
The Benefits of Generative AI for Global Health Partnerships: From Fragmentation to Cohesion 39
Cong Sui, University of Birmingham, UK & University College London, UK
Dimitrios Kalogeropoulos, Global Health and Digital Innovation Foundation, UK

Global health partnerships (GHPs) remain fragmented, unco-ordinated and donor-driven. GHPs lack a coherent framework for their entire lifecycle, making a universal solution impossible. As a case in point, Global Health & Digital Innovation Foundation (GHDIF) is leveraging generative AI (GAI) to build a connected digital platform in global health to address the issues, though its specific mechanisms for benefit remain unclear. This study identifies key aspects where GAI can enhance GHPs by applying a Partnership Analysis Framework and a literature review of sources like PubMed and Web of Science. Findings indicate GAI's potential in four areas: analyzing contextual factors and prerequisites, structuring projects, monitoring processes and performance, and measuring outcomes and stakeholder value. Supported by evidence, the review recommends GHDIF establish a coherent ontology, build partnership standards, and cooperate with the UN. As the first paper to demonstrate how GAI can benefit GHPs, this chapter provides a foundational roadmap for integration.

Chapter 3
Overview of Telemedicine in Central Africa, Specifically in Democratic Republic of Congo 75
Samuel Kajama Tshikuta, Coppin State University, USA
A. K. Sharadhi, University of Arizona, USA

Technology through telemedicine makes it possible to conduct efficient interventions that contribute to narrowing health inequalities conditioned by various geopolitical aspects. Most central African countries, including the Democratic Republic (DR) of Congo, experience a shortage of healthcare professionals, especially in rural regions. This is caused by the non-advancement of technology, poor infrastructure, electricity outages, and the limited number of graduate students enrolling in medical institutions. To minimize this impact, telemedicine is used and implemented in some areas to facilitate easy access to healthcare. Even though telemedicine was booming during COVID-19, there are still areas of imbalance, especially in central African countries. The purpose of this research is to bring more insight into the complete adoption of telemedicine in DR Congo healthcare systems.

Chapter 4
Strengthening Telemedicine and Remote Patient Monitoring in Nigeria With Artificial Intelligence 103
Basil Osayin Daudu, Kogi State Univerisity, Nigeria
Esther Besty Anaiye, National Open University of Nigeria, Nigeria

The advancement of telemedicine empowers healthcare providers to treat patients remotely via telecommunication technology, thus bridging the healthcare gap for patients in remote regions of Nigeria. As such, the objectives of the chapter are to: (i) assess the compliance of Nigerian healthcare providers with telemedicine and remote patient monitoring practices, (ii) evaluate the proficiency of Nigerian healthcare providers in utilizing telemedicine practices, and (iii) retrieve patient opinions on telemedicine and remote monitoring services that Nigerian healthcare providers offer. The methodology used in this chapter primarily involves quantitative analysis. The collected data were analyzed critically and descriptively using tools such as chi-square. Based on the research findings, there is a need for the government to intensify telemedicine practices and invest more in artificial intelligence as a facilitator of telemedicine and a solution to the challenges hindering its implementation in Nigeria.

Chapter 5
Enablers and Barriers to Digital Transformation of Integrated Care Systems (ICS) Across NHS England 133
Han Liew, National University Hospital, Singapore
Abdul M. Seckam, Healthcare Business Solutions, UK
Marzena Nieroda, University College London, UK

NHS England is shifting toward digital health technologies (DHT) to enhance care delivery, supported by both intrapreneurs and entrepreneurs. However, digital health companies face a key challenge: "no evidence, no implementation vs. no implementation, no evidence." The Health and Care Bill introduced 42 Integrated Care Systems (ICSs) to lead digital transformation, though barriers such as financial constraints, fragmented infrastructure, and leadership gaps persist. This scoping review analyzed 23 studies to identify enablers and barriers from digital health companies' perspectives, using the Service-Dominant logic and DEDHI framework. Findings were categorized across micro (patients, clinicians), meso (organisations, providers), and macro (policymakers) levels. The study highlights the need for stakeholder collaboration, investment, and regulatory clarity to scale DHT adoption within ICSs.

Chapter 6
Effect of Digital Mental Health Technology on Mental Healthcare Accessibility in Sub-Saharan Africa: A Systematic Review 169
Dede Atsu Kobla Latey, The London School of Economics and Political Science, UK
Robert Lubajo, WHO Regional Office for Africa, South Sudan

Mental health conditions are a growing public health concern in sub-Saharan Africa (SSA), where access to care remains severely limited due to shortages of professionals, infrastructure gaps, stigma, and urban-rural disparities. Digital mental health interventions have emerged as promising tools to bridge these gaps. However, the extent to which these technologies influence access to mental healthcare in SSA has not been systematically examined. A systematic review of peer-reviewed literature published between January 2000 and June 2025 was conducted to understand digital mental health technologies and their impact on mental healthcare accessibility in Sub Saharan Africa using Levesque et al.'s healthcare access framework, which conceptualizes access across five dimensions. The dimension of Acceptability emerged as the most frequently addressed access dimension. Availability and accommodation were also commonly discussed. Affordability and approachability were less frequently studied Surprisingly, only a few studies explored the dimension of appropriateness.

Chapter 7
Mapping Online Patient Narratives in China's Private Healthcare: A Semantic Network Approach 207
Yufeng Xue, Southern Medical University, China & ISCTE, University Institute of Lisbon, Portugal
Ana Brochado, Universidade Aberta, Portugal & Dinâmia'CET-Iscte, Portugal

This study sought to identify the main dimensions of narratives shared online by consumers of physical examination services provided by a private hospital in China, as well as the main themes associated with clients' satisfaction and unsatisfaction. The research relied on secondary data (satisfaction ratings and Web reviews). Content analyses were conducted with Leximancer and Regional Operations Support Team Content Mining software. The reviews cover all phases of patients' experiences. The main dimensions of physical examination services are linked with the themes of staff attitude, medical check-up, hospital environment, price, procedure, and consultation. Satisfied patients are more likely to share narratives about core services (imedical check-ups, procedures, and examinations), while unsatisfied clients focus on staff attitudes and prices. The findings add to the knowledge about physical examinations' service quality dimensions and confirm the usefulness of online review content analysis to healthcare management practitioners and researchers.

Chapter 8
Analysis of Ethical Issues in Medical Decision-Making Driven by Artificial Intelligence and Governance Strategies: Focusing on the Diversified Governance Network With Multi-Stakeholder Collaboration 241
Poshan Yu, Soochow University, China & European Business Institute, Luxembourg & Australian Studies Centre, Shanghai University, China
Yiheng Chen, Independent Researcher, China
Chandra Lukita, Universitas Catur Insan Cendekia, Indonesia

With the growing complexity of global health challenges, the demand for efficient medical services is rising. AI in medical decision-making brings new opportunities but also ethical concerns. This study analyzes research trends in AI-medicine, explores ethical issues in AI-driven medical decision-making, and proposes solutions. Based on stakeholder theory, it shows patients face privacy risks, hospitals have liability issues, and the government struggles with regulation. A multi-stakeholder collaborative governance model is suggested to address these. Using Citespace, the research pinpoints key areas to guide future studies.

Chapter 9
Ethical Frameworks for AI-Driven Medical Innovations: Balancing Progress and Patient Welfare 273
Poshan Yu, Soochow University, China & European Business Institute, Luxembourg & Australian Studies Centre, Shanghai University, China
Xinyuan Jiang, Independent Researcher, China
Chandra Lukita, Universitas Catur Insan Cendekia, Indonesia

The integration of AI in healthcare brings innovation but also ethical challenges. Using Citespace for bibliometric analysis of 2010 - 2025 literature from WoS and CNKI, the study identifies thematic hotspots and knowledge gaps in tech-related ethics for medicine. Western research emphasizes algorithmic fairness, while Eastern work focuses on ethical governance. Seven key gaps exist, including lack of cross-cultural harmonization. The study proposes ethical guidelines like participatory validation and culturally adaptive governance. Comparing regional policies shows the need to embed ethics in AI design. A triadic framework integrating technical, ethical, and clinical aspects offers strategies to balance AI's potential with patient well-being.

Chapter 10
The Regulatory Challenges From the Intersection of AI and Blockchain Technology in Healthcare: A Case Study of BurstIQ 307
Eleftheria Panagiotopoulou, University College London, UK
Mohan P. M. Mishra, FinJuris, UAE

Artificial intelligence (AI) and blockchain convergence is a paradigm shift in the current delivery of healthcare services, essentially changing how medical information is processed, secured, and used in any clinical setting around the globe. The once optional intersection is progressively becoming a necessity to build scalable, ethical, patient-centric digital health systems. This chapter uses a qualitative methodology – focusing on the case study of BurstIQ – to examine the regulatory challenges that arise from this convergence. The findings reveal that AI-blockchain systems introduce an unprecedented level of regulatory complexity that current frameworks are ill-equipped to deal with. The incorporation process demands trust in the systems, construction compliance, and stakeholders' active involvement. This chapter proposes a unified governance paradigm in which AI-blockchain is regulated as interconnected architectures, prioritising privacy-preserving and compliant infrastructure that allows innovation while maintaining existing regulatory relationships.

Compilation of References 351

About the Contributors 423

Index 433

Foreword

The global health landscape is undergoing a profound period of transformation. Across health systems worldwide, pressures arising from demographic change, workforce shortages, rising chronic disease burden, and persistent inequities are converging with rapid advances in artificial intelligence, telemedicine, and digital health technologies. Increasingly, healthcare systems are moving beyond isolated digital initiatives towards more interconnected and data-driven models of care delivery, where digital platforms, remote monitoring, and AI-enabled decision support are becoming embedded within everyday clinical and operational practice.

At the same time, this transition exposes significant challenges. Many health systems continue to operate through fragmented infrastructures, siloed governance arrangements, and uneven digital maturity. While technological capability is advancing rapidly, questions surrounding interoperability, accountability, workforce readiness, patient safety, and ethical governance remain central. The challenge is therefore not simply how to digitise healthcare, but how to ensure that digital transformation contributes to more coordinated, equitable, resilient, and learning-oriented health systems.

These themes are increasingly visible across global policy and practice discussions. Artificial intelligence and telemedicine offer unprecedented opportunities to improve access to care, strengthen continuity across care pathways, support real-time system learning, and enhance population health management. However, technology alone cannot resolve structural fragmentation or weak institutional coordination. Sustainable transformation requires governance frameworks, operational models, and collaborative ecosystems capable of aligning innovation with public-interest outcomes and patient-centred care.

It is within this context that AI, Telemedicine, and Governance in Global Healthcare Transformation, edited by Dr Cong Sui and Dr Poshan Yu, makes a timely and important contribution. Drawing upon interdisciplinary perspectives spanning digital innovation, global health, governance, and healthcare systems transformation, the volume brings together a broad range of international experiences and analytical approaches examining how emerging technologies are reshaping healthcare delivery across diverse settings.

The book addresses both the opportunities and the complexities associated with digital transformation in healthcare. Early chapters examine the adoption of digital technologies in primary healthcare through frameworks such as NASSS, highlighting organisational, cultural, ethical, and workforce-related barriers to implementation. The volume also explores how generative AI may strengthen global health partnerships by improving coordination, monitoring, and collaboration across increasingly complex healthcare ecosystems.

Several contributions provide important regional perspectives on telemedicine adoption and digital health implementation within low-resource settings, including analyses from the Democratic Republic of Congo, Nigeria, and Sub-Saharan Africa. These chapters illustrate how digital technologies may help address healthcare access gaps while also revealing the infrastructural, regulatory, and workforce constraints that continue to shape implementation realities.

The volume further examines digital transformation within NHS England's Integrated Care Systems, identifying both enabling factors and persistent operational barriers influencing system integration. Additional chapters investigate digital mental health accessibility, patient-generated narratives within China's private healthcare sector, and the evolving relationship between patient experience, digital engagement, and service quality.

Importantly, the book also engages directly with the ethical and governance dimensions of AI-enabled healthcare. Contributions examining multi-stakeholder governance frameworks, ethical approaches to AI-driven medical innovation, and the regulatory implications of combining AI with blockchain technologies highlight the growing importance of adaptive governance models capable of balancing innovation, accountability, privacy, and patient welfare.

Collectively, these chapters demonstrate that digital transformation in healthcare is not solely a technical undertaking. It is equally an organisational, regulatory, and societal challenge requiring coordination across institutions, professions, and sectors. The value of this volume lies in its ability to bring together these interconnected dimensions within a single multidisciplinary discussion.

As health systems continue to navigate rapid technological change, books such as this play an important role in supporting dialogue across policy, research, clinical practice, and innovation communities. By examining digital transformation through both global and context-specific perspectives, this volume contributes meaningfully to ongoing conversations surrounding the future of healthcare governance, patient safety, and learning health systems in an increasingly interconnected world.

Dimitrios Kalogeropoulos
Global Health & Digital Innovation Foundation, London, UK

Preface

INTRODUCTION

The rapid convergence of artificial intelligence (AI), telemedicine, and digital governance is reshaping healthcare systems across the globe in unprecedented ways. From remote diagnostics and predictive analytics to digital mental health interventions and blockchain-enabled medical infrastructures, healthcare is undergoing a transformation that extends beyond technology itself. These developments are redefining how healthcare is delivered, regulated, experienced, and governed across diverse social, economic, and geopolitical contexts, while simultaneously shaping emerging digital cultures within healthcare systems. As editors, we believe that this transformation demands not only technical innovation but also interdisciplinary reflection, ethical accountability, and inclusive global collaboration.

This edited volume, *AI, Telemedicine, and Governance in Global Healthcare Transformation*, was conceived in response to the growing need for critical scholarship that bridges emerging technologies with healthcare policy, governance frameworks, implementation realities, and patient-centered care.

While digital health innovations continue to accelerate, major disparities remain in infrastructure, access, regulation, digital literacy, and institutional readiness across regions. The chapters collected in this book collectively explore these tensions and opportunities, offering perspectives from researchers, healthcare and practitioners, non-governmental organizations (NGOs), and private sector stakeholders working across Europe, Africa, Asia, and beyond.

The book brings together multidisciplinary contributions that investigate how AI, and telemedicine, digital governance, and evolving digital cultures are influencing healthcare ecosystems at multiple levels, including clinical decision-making, healthcare accessibility, stakeholder engagement, organizational readiness, global health partnerships, integrated care systems, mental health services, patient narratives, ethical governance, and regulatory frameworks. The contributors engage with both theoretical and applied dimensions of healthcare transformation, emphasizing the importance of equitable implementation, responsible governance, and sustainable innovation. Through empirical studies, systematic reviews, case analyses, and conceptual frameworks, this volume seeks to contribute meaningfully to ongoing global conversations surrounding the future of healthcare in the digital era.

A defining strength of this collection lies in its international and interdisciplinary scope. The contributors examine healthcare transformation across high-income and low-resource settings, highlighting how contextual realities shape technological adoption and governance strategies. The volume particularly foregrounds issues of inclusion, ethics, accessibility, digital culture, and regulatory coordination, recognizing that digital healthcare solutions cannot succeed without trust, digital readiness, accountability, stakeholder engagement, and culturally adaptive implementation strategies. In doing so, the book moves beyond technological optimism and instead presents a balanced examination of both opportunities and limitations associated with AI-enabled healthcare transformation.

The COVID-19 pandemic accelerated the adoption of telemedicine and digital healthcare technologies worldwide, revealing both the resilience and fragility of healthcare systems. Yet, the post-pandemic landscape has also demonstrated that sustainable digital transformation requires more than emergency implementation. It requires long-term governance models, interoperable infrastructures, ethical safeguards, culturally adaptive policies, and collaborative ecosystems capable of addressing evolving healthcare challenges. The chapters in this book therefore not only examine technological advancements but also interrogate the institutional, ethical, and policy environments necessary to support them responsibly.

As editors, we hope this volume serves as a valuable resource for researchers, healthcare professionals, policymakers, technology developers, postgraduate students, and global health practitioners interested in understanding the complex intersections between AI, telemedicine, and healthcare governance. We also hope that the insights presented here will inspire further interdisciplinary collaboration and evidence-based policymaking aimed at building more accessible, ethical, and resilient healthcare systems worldwide.

CHAPTER OVERVIEW

Chapter 1, "Digital Technology Adoption Challenges in Primary Healthcare: An Empirical Study and the NASSS Framework," investigates the barriers and enablers associated with implementing digital technologies in primary healthcare. Drawing upon the NASSS framework, the chapter examines technological, organizational, ethical, and cultural dimensions influencing adoption, while emphasizing the role of governance, co-design, and workforce readiness in ensuring sustainable implementation.

Chapter 2, "The Benefits of Generative AI for Global Health Partnerships: From Fragmentation to Cohesion," explores how generative AI can strengthen global health partnerships by improving coordination, project structuring, monitoring, and outcome evaluation. The chapter proposes a foundational roadmap for integrating generative AI into partnership ecosystems while highlighting the importance of ontology development, standardization, and international collaboration.

Chapter 3, "Overview of Telemedicine in Central Africa, Specifically in Democratic Republic of Congo: Telemedicine in DR Congo," provides an important regional perspective on telemedicine adoption within Central Africa. Focusing on the Democratic Republic of Congo, the chapter examines healthcare inequalities, infrastructural limitations, and workforce shortages while discussing how telemedicine can improve healthcare accessibility in underserved regions.

Chapter 4, "Strengthening Telemedicine and Remote Patient Monitoring in Nigeria With Artificial Intelligence," analyzes the adoption of telemedicine and AI-enabled remote patient monitoring in Nigeria. Through quantitative analysis, the authors assess provider compliance, technological proficiency, and patient perceptions, while identifying key policy and investment priorities needed to expand digital healthcare services.

Chapter 5, "Enablers and Barriers to Digital Transformation to Integrated Care Systems (ICS) across NHS England," examines the transition toward digital health technologies within NHS England's Integrated Care Systems. The chapter identifies implementation barriers and enablers from the perspective of digital health companies and highlights the importance of stakeholder collaboration, regulatory clarity, and infrastructure investment.

Chapter 6, "Effect of Digital Mental Health Technology on Mental Healthcare Accessibility in Sub-Saharan Africa: A Systematic Review," presents a systematic review of digital mental health interventions across Sub-Saharan Africa. Using Levesque et al.'s healthcare access framework, the chapter evaluates how digital technologies influence dimensions of accessibility, acceptability, affordability, and appropriateness within mental healthcare systems.

Chapter 7, "Mapping Online Patient Narratives in China's Private Healthcare: A Semantic Network Approach," explores patient-generated online narratives related to private healthcare services in China. Through semantic network and content analysis, the chapter identifies key themes shaping patient satisfaction and dissatisfaction, offering important insights into healthcare service quality and digital patient engagement.

Chapter 8, "Analysis of Ethical Issues in Medical Decision-Making Driven by Artificial Intelligence and Governance Strategies: Focusing on the Diversified Governance Network with Multi-Stakeholder Collaboration," examines ethical concerns surrounding AI-driven medical decision-making. Grounded in stakeholder theory, the chapter proposes a collaborative governance framework involving patients, hospitals, governments, and technology stakeholders to address emerging ethical and regulatory challenges.

Chapter 9, "Ethical Frameworks for AI-Driven Medical Innovations -- Balancing Progress and Patient Welfare," investigates global ethical debates concerning AI-enabled healthcare innovations through bibliometric analysis and comparative policy examination. The chapter develops a triadic framework integrating technical, ethical, and clinical considerations to support culturally adaptive and patient-centered AI governance.

Chapter 10, "The Regulatory Challenges from the Intersection of AI and Blockchain Technology in Healthcare: A Case Study of BurstIQ," analyzes the regulatory complexities associated with converging AI and blockchain technologies in healthcare systems. Using the BurstIQ case study, the chapter proposes a unified governance paradigm capable of supporting privacy-preserving, interoperable, and compliant healthcare infrastructures while fostering innovation.

CONCLUSION

Collectively, these chapters provide a comprehensive exploration of contemporary healthcare transformation shaped by AI, telemedicine, digital platforms, and governance innovation. While the contexts and methodologies vary, a common theme emerges throughout the volume: technological advancement alone is insufficient without ethical stewardship, inclusive governance, stakeholder collaboration, and sustainable implementation strategies. The contributions in this book therefore illuminate both the promise and the complexity of digitally transformed healthcare systems.

In closing, we extend our sincere appreciation to all contributing authors for their scholarly dedication, intellectual rigor, and collaborative spirit in bringing this volume to fruition. We are equally grateful to the reviewers, editorial teams, and institutional partners whose support and expertise have contributed significantly to the development of this work. Their collective efforts reflect the interdisciplinary and international cooperation necessary to advance healthcare innovation responsibly.

Finally, we hope this book encourages continued dialogue, research, and policy development at the intersection of AI, telemedicine, and healthcare governance. As healthcare systems worldwide continue to evolve amid rapid technological change, the need for ethical, inclusive, and globally informed approaches has never been greater. It is our aspiration that this volume will contribute to shaping future healthcare ecosystems that are not only technologically advanced, but also equitable, accountable, and centered on human well-being.

Cong Sui
West Midlands Health Tech Innovation Accelerator, UK & University of Birmingham, UK & University College London, UK

Poshan Yu
Soochow University, China & European Business Institute, Luxembourg & Australian Studies Centre, Shanghai University, China

Chapter 1
Digital Technology Adoption Challenges in Primary Healthcare: An Empirical Study and the NASSS Framework

Rajan Punitharajah
http://orcid.org/0009-0004-2499-1619
Brunel University of London, UK

Julie Davies
http://orcid.org/0000-0002-6875-3100
Brunel University of London, UK

Sheikh Mateen Ellahi
http://orcid.org/0009-0001-2286-4999
Elm Tree Medical Centre, UK

ABSTRACT

Globally, rising healthcare costs and workforce pressures highlight the need for digital transformation in primary care. This chapter explores adoption challenges of digital technologies, including AI, robotics, and automation, through the lens of the NASSS framework. Drawing on literature, case studies, and empirical research with UK practitioners, we examine enablers and barriers to implementation, spanning ethical, regulatory, and cultural dimensions. We distinguish between backend efficiencies and frontline clinical applications, highlighting both opportunities and

DOI: 10.4018/979-8-2600-2238-2.ch001

resistance. Findings underscore the importance of governance, training, and co-design to bridge the strategy implementation gap and ensure equitable, sustainable, and value-based healthcare delivery.

INTRODUCTION

Globally, the burdens of national and personal expenditure on healthcare are growing. This can be mitigated by greater expenditure on primary care (Hou et al., 2022). Public policy to drive a left shift from acute to primary, community and home care to improve access is increasingly promoting AI-enabled approaches. However, the adoption of digital health technology in primary care is challenging with gaps between strategy and implementation (Terry et al., 2022). Yet national prosperity and productivity in developed and developing countries depend on population health well-being and the use of technology to relieve disease and costs burdens and to improve prevention, diagnosis and treatment outside acute hospital settings using appropriate digital solutions that overcome health inequalities (Geracitano et al., 2024).

This chapter focuses on the challenges in adopting digital technologies in primary care. Drawing on literature reviews, theoretical frameworks and case studies, the co-authors (an AI specialist, General Practitioner (GP) partner and university professor) illustrate how healthcare digital technology can be implemented in different countries to support policies for universal access and value-based healthcare delivery for complex populations. Specifically, the authors discuss benefits, challenges, and ethical implications based on a survey and interviewees with practitioners and experts in UK primary healthcare.

DEFINING HEALTHCARE TECHNOLOGIES

The integration of digital technologies into healthcare, particularly in primary care settings, represents a significant innovation that is transforming how medical services are delivered to patients. For example, robotic services in healthcare encompass a wide range of technologies designed to assist in diagnosis, treatment, surgery, patient management, healthcare professionals, and administrative tasks.

A PwC (2024) report on *Essential Eight Technologies for Health Services: AI Leads Investment Priorities* included a survey that asked where companies planned to prioritise investment in emerging technologies over the next 12 months. The results listed artificial intelligence (77%), followed by the Internet of Things (43%), augmented reality (30%), virtual reality (29%), and advanced robotics (25%). This report provides evidence that, despite the rise of AI, advanced robotics remains significant in healthcare services. However, there is an opportunity for AI and robotics services to work together. This projection indicates a growing demand for robotics in the healthcare sector, particularly in the era of AI advancements.

Primary care digital technologies can be considered in two main areas: backend technologies (administrative efficiency) and frontend technologies (clinical support). Table 1 provides examples.

Table 1. Case examples

No.	Examples of Back End Technologies	Cases	Benefits
1.	Health tech 1, JifffJaff, GP Automate	Blood filing	Saves clinicians' time, faster responses to patients.
2.	As above, Tortus	Coding letters	Saves non-clinical/administration time.
3.	AI scribe companies – Syntax, Heidi	Generating letters	Saves clinical time, better coding of notes, clarity of documentation.
No.	**Front End Technologies**	**Cases**	**Benefits**
1.	Accurx, anima, many other companies	Chest pain	Reduces time on administration, more concise patient information without calling patients, improved access for patients.

Source: authors

OVERVIEW OF DRIVING AND RESTRAINING FORCES FOR CHANGE

This chapter examines global challenges in adopting digital health technology, including robotics, AI and other key leading healthcare digital technologies to improve access to primary care for patients in underserved or remote areas. It focuses on the driving and restraining forces, benefits, ethical issues, and impacts for patients, healthcare professionals, and other stakeholders. With workforce shortages, lengthy wait times, ageing populations and comorbidities driving demand, digital technologies can improve patient throughput and efficiency as well as the quality of life for citizens and healthcare workers. Based on a narrative literature view, Figure 1 summarises key enablers and barriers to implementing digital technology in primary care.

Figure 1. Force field analysis of digital technology adoption in primary healthcare

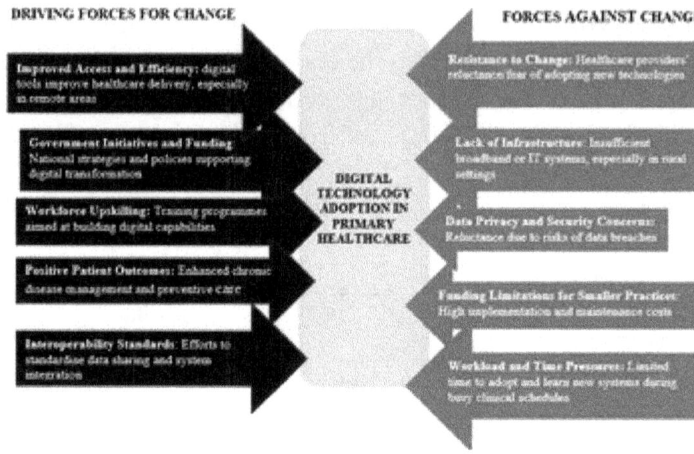

(Lewin, 1951)

Key enablers include the promise of reducing inequalities, improving access and efficiencies as well as patient outcomes, government policies and the need to establish interoperability standards. Key sources of resistance to digital health technology adoption in primary healthcare comprise fear and reluctance, inadequate infrastructure, concerns about data breaches, a lack of funding for implementation and maintenance and the huge workloads and lack of time that healthcare practitioners experience which result in limited or no bandwidth to devote their energy to technology adoption despite the return on investment.

THE NASSS FRAMEWORK

To conceptualise our perspectives, the authors draw on the NASSS framework in Table 2 to highlight key considerations when adopting technology in primary care. This provides an understanding of contingencies, front and back end processes to support value-based healthcare, key stakeholders and organisational factors as well as ecosystems and the need to embed and adapt technology. This is a useful checklist to anticipate and identify pain points and overcome resistance through dialogue and collaboration.

Table 2. NASSS framework applied to technology adoption in primary care (Greenhalgh et al., 2018, p. 3)

1. Condition
• Increasing life expectancy adds pressure on services, particularly for elderly care. • Growing backlog in treatment and screening due to resource shortages.
2. Technology: Technology in Primary Healthcare Includes Front End / Back End Function Processes
• Robotics, AI offer automation of tasks, improved diagnostics, and potential for reduced waiting times. • High capital costs, training needs, and integration with outdated infrastructure are major barriers. • Concerns about diagnostic accuracy and need for continuous updates and post-surveillance. • Maximise the full potential of existing technology.
3. Value Proposition
• Perceived long-term cost savings through reduced chronic illness burden and increased efficiency. • Ethical and psychological concerns over loss of human touch, especially among older patients. • Industry experts emphasise selecting experienced vendors and co-design approaches with regulators with view of healthcare staff and patient centric.
4. Adopters
• Internal: GPs and nurses fear job losses, lack of training, and cultural resistance. • External: Older patients express distrust, discomfort with tech, and psychological anxiety. • Clinicians may face steep learning curves, patients' scepticism about AI diagnoses. Variable readiness among user groups. • Younger generations more receptive. Generational differences play a key role.
5. Organisation
• NHS faces structural issues: staff shortages, high burnout, and digital underuse. • Successful implementation needs strong leadership, change management, and integration with workflows. • Larger practices better positioned for scalable innovation.
6. Wider System
• Regulatory complexities (e.g., GDPR, MHRS, CE marking) challenge adoption. • Need for governance on data safety, liability, and AI transparency. • Government support and fast-track policies (like those used during COVID-19) are viewed as necessary.
7. Embedding and Adaptation
• Transition viewed as long-term (5–10 YEARS) with hybrid models seen as most viable. • Need for iterative deployment, starting with younger, tech-savvy demographics. • On-going training, trust-building, and ethical clarity are essential for sustainability.

The Context of the NHS in England

According to the King's Fund (2024), the National Health Service *(*NHS*)* in England employs approximately 1.34 million full-time equivalent staff (as of February 2024) and it is one of the world's largest employers. As of March 2024, there were 100,700 vacancies in the NHS including 8,800 medical professionals and 31,300 nursing staff. The Darzi (2024, p. 3) report on the NHS in England stated that "A&E is in an awful state" and that "GPs are seeing more patients than ever before, but with the number of fully qualified GPs relative to the population falling, waiting times are rising, and patient satisfaction is at its lowest ever level." In response, the British Prime Minister Sir Keir Starmer highlighted three key priorities, "First, moving from an analogue to a digital NHS. Second, we've got to shift more care from hospitals to communities. Third, we've got to be much bolder in moving from sickness to prevention" (Limb, 2024).

Current NHS policy in England is, therefore, encouraging data-empowered health ecosystems (Li et al., 2025) and enhanced digital access to primary care service provision using "digital facilitation" (Abel et al., 2024). GP practices in England are now using telephone systems with voice recognition technology for automatic transcriptions and quick triage (NHS England, 2025). A new GP contract is modernising general practice by requiring GP surgeries to establish systems for patients to request appointments on-line during working hours which frees up phones for those who are most in need and who cannot access digital services. It avoids the 8am rush for appointments established in the NHS England (2023) *Delivery plan for recovering access to primary care.*

RESEARCH STUDY

This chapter's insights into technology adoption in primary care are based on a narrative review of academic literature, reports and news media. These inform our empirical research that comprises a survey, semi-structured qualitative interviews and case study. Our central research question is: what are the enablers and barriers for technology adoption in primary care?

The narrative literature review included 25 academic articles, 12 sources for secondary research and eight market trend reports from Duke Health, IBM, IQVIA, McKinsey & Company, PwC, and The Economist. Additionally, the authors considered social news from reputable channels like BBC and newspapers such as the Financial Times. Conducting secondary research through journals, case studies, and newspapers provides valuable insights.

Ethics was approved for the study by the first author's university and a pilot survey was conducted to ensure questions resonated with response. The survey used multiple-choice answers for all 19 questions to maximise responses. A convenience sample of 25 healthcare professionals completed the survey – these are referred to as group 1 in the comments presented in the findings. Multiple-choice surveys provide structured, objective data for thematic analysis. The sample of five industry experts interviewed comprised one senior vice president (SVP) and one vice president (VP) in the pharmaceutical industry, both with over 20 years' experience in digital transformation; a senior partner from Tata Consultancy Services, also with over 20 years' experience, a Group CEO of a company that operates primary healthcare services nationally in the UK, and a GP management consultant. The interviewees are referred to as group 2. The first author asked each interviewee a range of six questions, including a single open-ended question that allowed them to provide detailed responses. This approach facilitated the analysis in a descriptive summary of direct quotes from participants' feedback.

FINDINGS

Twenty-five healthcare professionals participated in an on-line survey over 49 days between January and February 2025. The survey contained 19 questions. The sample included 32% qualified GPs, 20% GP trainees, 16% consultants, 12% specialist medical doctors in other fields such as psychiatry, 8% nurses, 4% hospital specialist trainees, 4% hospital doctors and 4% other. Their experiences varied, for example, 68% had been in their current role for less than five years, 16% for 5–10 years, 12% for 10–15 years, and 4% for over 20 years. Only 12% of participants had used robotics services in primary care. The purpose of sharing the survey results is to highlight selected responses that are most relevant to the questions.

Benefits of Adopting Digital Health Technologies in Primary Care

Group 1 UK healthcare primary care/NHS professionals responded to the question: How do you think robotics service will affect the economic structure of the healthcare system, especially in the UK where budget limitations are a concern?

In this group, 84% agreed that high upfront capital investment, maintenance and upgrade costs, and training and upskilling expenses will significantly impact costs. Most survey respondents believed that there is high upfront capital investment in purchasing robots, on-going maintenance, and upgrades to existing equipment and computers to ensure all the equipment, and computers are integrated. Secondly, they noted that training and upskilling healthcare professionals will require investment. Training and upskilling will play a key role, not just training to focus on the use of robotics but also additional regulated training to ensure healthcare professionals can work safely and service patients as well as report issues of any errors or incorrect information. The respondents also commented on the importance of additional investment for continuous training.

Another question in the survey asked: What are the economic key benefits to healthcare systems in using robotic services. Responses were grouped into two themes.

72% agreed that the impact of technology on patient throughput and service capacity would increase the number of patients treated, reduce recovery times and lead to faster diagnosis and treatment. 60% agreed about the long-term economic benefits such as reducing the costs of chronic cases by providing more accurate diagnoses faster. Most participants felt that patient throughput would increase due to improved efficiency. However, 28% of participants expressed scepticism while 40% believed in long-term economic benefits. Some individuals commented that so much ill health is vague, complicated and psychological, therefore, the authors must observe how digital services will work in practice for particular demographics, i.e., older people or the younger generation, and for particular illnesses.

The third question asked which departments would be most suitable for the safe deployment of digital/robotic services in primary care. Responses focused on:

Remote monitoring, enhanced imaging analysis, automating administrative tasks and robotics-assisted surgeries, X-ray department and blood tests.

The fourth question asked how the integration of digital/robotic services into healthcare in the UK has affected the overall structure of healthcare delivery. Common themes mentioned in the answers referred to automated routing tasks, reduced waiting, and reduced surgery time.

The fifth question asked respondents about the top three factors they believed influenced patients' acceptance of digital/robotic services. The top three factors identified were: "*reduced waiting times, diagnostic accuracy, and rapid diagnosis.*"

Another question focused on key benefits for the integration of digital/robotic services into healthcare in the UK that affect the overall structure of healthcare delivery. 72% agreed automated routing of tasks would be beneficial. 4% disagreed and 24% were neutral. 68% of the group believed technology would reduce waiting times, while 4% disagreed and 28% remained neutral.

A further question asked: Based on your experience in primary care in the UK and the evolution of technology, how long do you think the transition to digital/robotics services in healthcare will take from a hybrid model?

38% of the participants thought it will take 10 years. 27% suggested five years while 18% are unsure and the other 18% believe it is not possible."

Another question focused on recommendations for implementing robotics services in general within primary care.

56% recommended a mixed approach of automation where possible and a hybrid approach in high-risk areas and 12% recommended a hybrid approach with robots and GPs working together. 12% believe in full automation following a pilot study and scaling up.

When asked about the future, some believe in full automation, others advocate a hybrid model of robots and humans working together in high-risk areas, or consistently hybrid.

Group 2 industry expert interviewee responses to the question: What are your top three recommendations for assisting external solution providers for successfully implementing technology in a regulated environment?

You would not get a company like Meta to implement robotic services in healthcare due to the lack of experience and Meta trend of loose regulation.

It is important to have a selection process to select technology provided for implementation with some key criteria such as experience in robotics service implementation in healthcare, experience in co-development, thinking about patients who are impacted by healthcare professionals.

In most cases, the evolution of technology is too fast and industry standards and regulations are behind.

The above response is quite clear. Within a regulated environment, it is essential to have the right technology partner, one that is highly specific to the technology and has a strong track record of implementation experience. Additionally, the partner should be willing to co-design the solution with the customer. For example, if a service is implemented to administer patients' blood intake within primary care, a technology partner with prior experience in similar implementations within a primary care setting is necessary. This ensures that the design and training processes are effectively incorporated across all settings.

During his interview, the GP management consultant emphasized digital technologies have a critical role in reducing administrative burdens and supporting clinical decision making. This can be considered in two main areas: (i) back end technologies for administrative efficiency and (ii) front end technologies for clinical support.

Digital transformation in healthcare can significantly boost operational efficiency by automating routine administrative tasks such as referral processing, appointment scheduling, and reviewing blood test results. By taking on these time-consuming duties, automation frees up clinicians to focus more on complex, value-added patient care. This increase in productivity is particularly vital in the face of workforce shortages, helping healthcare systems do more with limited personnel.

The following five themes emerged from our dataset:

1. **Improved Patient Care**: Optimising roles within care teams supported by digital tools enhances the system's overall capacity to provide timely and effective care. Importantly, these tools are designed to assist rather than replace clinical decision-making, allowing healthcare professionals to make better-informed judgments while preserving their autonomy and expertise in patient care.
2. **Workforce Well-being**: Time-saving technologies can contribute positively to clinician well-being by reducing burnout and enabling better work-life balance. When routine workload is minimised, professionals have more flexibility, which supports career sustainability and opens pathways for portfolio careers roles

that combine clinical duties with other areas such as research, education, or innovation.

3. **Implementation Strategy:** Successful digital implementation relies on thorough planning, including readiness assessments that align workflows with the existing skill sets of staff. Initially selecting Robotic Process Automation (RPA) over more complex AI systems can prove strategic in easing integration within NHS structures, allowing smoother, lower-risk entry into digital operations.
4. **Training and Adoption**: Effective adoption is underpinned by strong leadership, a focus on digital safety, and a commitment to designing systems around patient needs. Robust change management strategies are particularly important for encouraging adoption among older adults and less tech-savvy users, ensuring that digital transformation is inclusive and widely accepted.
5. **Innovation and Scalability**: Larger healthcare practices provide fertile ground for testing and scaling innovative, data-driven solutions. These environments allow for more rapid iteration and feedback loops. Additionally, collaboration across multiple practices enhances access to resources and enables personalised care models, making digital healthcare more effective and equitable.

Challenges in Adopting Digital Health Technologies in Primary Care

Group 1 responses of UK primary care and NHS professionals

44% of the survey participants believed that individuals aged 70+ and older may encounter challenges when using robotic services. Additionally, 32% of the same group think people between the ages of 50 and 60 will struggle with these services. Participants' responses highlighted that older individuals may not adapt easily to digital services for several reasons. These include the lack of face-to-face interaction, which might have an emotional impact, issues with trust, and concerns about using technology. Within the older group, they would need empathy and clear two-way communications to feel secure in the diagnosis of their illness.

Group 1 of UK healthcare primary care/NHS professional responded to the question: What challenges do healthcare facilities face in terms of infrastructure when implementing robotic service technologies?

84% agreed that equipment is the key challenge. 72% agreed that the interface with existing equipment is the key challenge. 72% believed that maintenance is a key challenge. There is a general belief that some existing equipment is outdated and that it may not be easy to integrate this with new technology. Additionally, the interface between new robotics and existing equipment presents a key challenge, potentially leading to dysfunctional technology which could impact both patients and healthcare professionals.

The next question related to how patients will respond to services in the following areas: robots as receptionists, frontline nurses, providing remote monitoring, personalised rehabilitation, selected routine operations, robotic-assisted surgeries, and in X-ray departments.

Respondents talked about high concerns in terms of psychological acceptance and trust. They pointed out that healthcare services are highly personal and sensitive, and that patients are generally nervous about health issues with concerns such as: "*Is my diagnosis correct*?" or "*How can I trust the information, decision, or action taken by a robot*?" Simple human interactions, such as a healthcare professional holding a patient's hand, making eye contact, and delivering good or bad news with empathy, play a crucial role in reassuring patients and guiding them through the next steps. Humans often believe they have a "sixth sense" which robots lack, making trust a significant factor in the acceptance of robotics in healthcare operations.

The final question focused on top three concerns related to robotic services. The responses were:

25% patient safety,12% existing it digital platform maturity low, 12% cost.

Group 2 industry experts responded to this question: What patterns do you see related to AI/robotic services adaptation challenges in your industry?

Respondents noted trends in the lack of use case for IT versus business concerns. They believed that AI strategy needs to be part of corporate strategy, i.e. with clear KPIs required at executive level. Service value creation was regarded as crucial in a vision of robotic services solutions with a need to communication the key benefits to a service outcome using technology. For example, from an operational perspective these include efficiency and productivity.

Group 2 Industry experts responded to the question: When considering robotics service and automation from a technological perspective, do you believe age will be a significant factor? Their comments noted that in healthcare, often there is the fear of losing the human touch, the social contact element that AI/ robotics could replace. A survey in a medical centre for self-checking showed that people prefer the assurance of a check-in with a receptionist instead of a screen interface. The age of patients is viewed as a challenge.

Group 2 industry experts discussed the challenges they face related to technology implementation in their services:

Key highlights include culture awareness, sponsorship from leadership, impact on external and internal stakeholders, upskilling and training.

In summary, industry experts believe successful transformation is overwhelming. Especially in a highly regulated environment, it is important to identify and map all key stakeholders, suppliers and technology partners internally and externally. It is also vital to address skill gaps early and continuously.

Group 1 Responses to the question: What do you anticipate in terms of changes in the regulatory structure of policies as robotics services become more common in healthcare?

Responses mentioned the common theme of Software, medical devices, UK AI regulation and continuous monitoring and post surveillance. Significant responses among participants focused on changes in software medical devices. These devices need thorough integration and testing, necessitating strong governance for safe use. Most participants support continuous monitoring and post-surveillance to ensure proper reporting and corrective action if robotic services provide incorrect information or behaviour.

Group 2 Industry experts responded to the question: What are your top three pieces of advice for preparing internal stakeholders for technology adaptation in a regulated environment?

Key takeaways included the "Need to separate internal/external stakeholder requirements for major transformation projects (i.e. Internal stakeholders like GP, nurses and external regulation bodies, external compliance, vendor for technology). Secondly, advice was given to work with quality and regulation and co-build solutions following inspiring examples from the COVID-19 vaccine programme. Finally, responses stressed the need for working groups to address fear, trust and benefits.

During his interview, the GP Management Consultant highlighted several challenges that hinder digital adoption, including limited funding, insufficient time allocated for staff training, regulatory complexity, and underuse of existing technologies. These barriers can slow down transformation efforts and reduce the return on digital investments if not proactively addressed.

The following emerged in the interviews as key themes:

1. **Workload Concerns**: Technology must deliver measurable benefits without becoming an added burden to clinicians. Any digital solution introduced should streamline work rather than complicate it and must clearly demonstrate value to gain the trust and buy-in of healthcare professionals.
2. **Regulatory Complexity**: Digital health initiatives must comply with regulations such as GDPR, NHS-specific standards, and cybersecurity protocols. Meeting these requirements involves substantial upfront investment in legal, technical, and organizational resources, which can slow down implementation and add to the cost.
3. **Cultural and Organisational Readiness:** Beyond technical readiness, successful digital adoption depends heavily on cultural acceptance and strong change leadership. Organisations must foster a culture of openness to innovation, supported by champions who can lead digital transformation efforts from within.

The respondents' sentiments resonated with the experiences of the third co-author who is a partner in his own GP practice, Elm Tree Medical Centre in Thornaby in Northeast England. He has found the adoption of digital triage to be a complex journey. Initially, system integration issues arose, as the existing IT infrastructure struggled to support the application programming interface (API) required for seamless engagement with the new digital system. This hindered the smooth rollout and efficiency of the technology. Additionally, there were cultural hurdles in adapting to digital triage as some staff were hesitant about the transition, leading to resistance to change. Training required everyone to be up to speed with the new system. This entailed substantial time and costs, further complicating the adoption process. Balancing these challenges while ensuring patient care remains is a delicate task.

ETHICAL ISSUES

Group 1 professionals responded to the question: What are the top three challenges for healthcare professionals? The responses indicated:

24% trust, 22% technological anxiety and 20% regulatory.

Group 1 responded to the question: What are the top three challenges for patients?

28% technological anxiety, 24% trust, 14% data protection.

To summarise, diagnostic accuracy directly affects patient outcomes. Incorrect results can alter the healthcare professional-patient relationship. New regulations will require more frequent training and updates. Misuse of data poses risks to both patient and professional privacy.

Group 2 industry experts addressed the main challenges patients may face. The most common theme they highlighted was: "Effective management of change, ease of use, trust and security." There is a correlation between the responses from the Group 1 healthcare professionals and Group 2 industry experts regarding concerns about robotics adaptation. These concerns include trust, technological anxiety, and ease of use.

A Group 2 industry expert responded to the question: What are the lessons learned from automation adaptation training and people's fears about automation or robot service AI in a regulated healthcare environment?

The expert asserted:

Automation often reduces organisational headcount so resistance is primarily based on a fear of job losses. It is, therefore, important to emphasise how staff will have more time to add value.

People in healthcare often fear losing the human touch, the social contact element that AI could replace – a survey in a medical centre about self-checking showed that people prefer the assurance of a check-in with a receptionist rather than a screen interface.

Output from automation is only as good as the quality of data input.

Overall, it is critical to involve healthcare professionals who are affected by the changes and to ensure high quality data for patient safety.

A Group 2 industry expert responded to the question on providing advice about change management strategy:

Change management strategy should always start with the WHY, why should AI and robotics be introduced, what will they achieve? What's the do nothing option? What will the user gain and lose? Often AI and robotics are presented as a "worker" who never tires, sleeps or takes a holiday and so threatens job security.

Once the storytelling is set (business case for change), it is important to demonstrate the capability of the tool to generate buy-in, curiosity and interest.

The most challenging issue is technology anxiety. If the user is not at the centre of the design of the tool and implementation, the technology is likely to fail.

AI and robotics require the right training and set-up. If the person doing the training or set up does not adhere to certain rules, the outcome may vary and miss the mark.

To summarise the above responses, proper change management, understanding of the user experience, addressing technology anxiety, and ensuring adequate training are essential for successful outcomes to adopt technological solutions in primary care. To introduce AI and robotics effectively, change agents need to start with a clear reason for adaptation, highlight benefits, and provide appropriate and continuous support for healthcare professionals. It is vital to build a strong business case and demonstrate the value of tools to gain buy-in. It is also necessary to focus on overcoming technology anxiety and past failures and to prioritise user experience. Finally, it is necessary to provide proper training and follow guidelines to achieve desired results without threatening individuals' livelihoods.

During his interview, the GP management consultant highlighted equity in access as a key concern. It is vital to ensure that digital tools do not widen the digital divide in healthcare access. Older adults and those less comfortable with technology may find digital interfaces challenging so alternative solutions like telephone support must remain available to maintain inclusivity and fairness in care delivery (e.g., Husain and Greenhalgh, 2025).

DISCUSSION

This mixed methods study sheds light on how healthcare professionals in primary care and the NHS view robotic services adaptation and provides insights from industry experts. The discussion focuses on benefits, challenges and ethical issues. Findings highlight the importance of addressing social factors for internal and external stakeholders, adhering to legal requirements, and considering ethical concerns for the successful adaptation of robotic services in primary care. This incorporates survey and interview responses, literature reviews, and reports from reputable organisations.

According to the report published by McKinsey Global Institute (Bradley et al., 2024), depending on the pace of robotics solutions adaptation, 40% of physical work done by people could be automated in less than 20 years. Maynou et al. (2022) states that after the introduction of the da Vinci Robot, there was a rapid adaptation of robots within NHS England. The use of robotic surgery for radical prostatectomy increased from 5% in 2006 to 88% of all prostatectomies performed within the English NHS in 2018.

Keyue and Qiongfang (2024) reported China's first AI hospital town debuts, revolutionising healthcare with AI. The concept of an AI hospital town presents numerous advantages, notably in medical education and healthcare delivery. It offers a risk-free environment where medical students can practice on virtual patients, boosting diagnostic and treatment proficiency. AI doctors demonstrate remarkable efficiency by managing tens of thousands of cases in a short time span and exhibit high accuracy in medical exams. Furthermore, such systems could make healthcare more affordable and accessible while aiding in pandemic preparedness through simulations. The technology also holds promise for advancing telemedicine by enabling virtual doctors to treat real patients remotely.

- **Enhanced training**: AI hospital town allows medical students to safely practice diagnosis and treatment on virtual patients, improving skills without real-world risk.
- **Efficiency and scalability**: AI doctors can treat 10,000 patients in days, compared to two years for human doctors.
- **High accuracy**: AI agents achieved a 93.06% success rate on medical exams for respiratory diseases.
- **Cost-effective healthcare**: Potential to provide affordable, accessible, and high-quality healthcare services at scale.
- **Pandemic preparedness**: AI simulations can model the spread and control of infectious diseases.
- **Telemedicine potential**: Real patients could one day be treated by virtual doctors, enhancing remote care delivery.

The study by Frishammar et al. (2023) was conducted in association with an HDP provider in Sweden that developed DHP technology for primary care. The study noted that digital support provides faster help for easier problems or recurring errors, such as prescription renewal and mitigating risks of waiting in a healthcare centre with sick people. Another example examined a high density population urban city mainly during the winter season to explore how digital technologies can help. Ijiga et al. (2024) found that technological innovations mitigate wider health challenges in New York City (NYC) in dense urban settings during winter. The integration of technology in the city's infrastructure and health systems showed significant potential in enhancing quality of life and addressing various public health challenges. The study examined Smart New York City, how information, telecommunication, mobile technology, and artificial intelligence (AI) were integrated into NYC's infrastructure. The study surveyed 425 NYC residents and found that 96% experience positive effects on their quality of life from using smart technology. According to Ijiga et al. (2024), the specific technologies used to address winter health challenges in New York City included:

- **Electronic Health Records in Correctional Facilities:** EHR enabled efficient tracking of patient health data, timely access to medical records, and better co-ordination of care, which is essential in a confined and densely populated environment.
- **EHR Tool for COVID-19 Management:** The tools offered decision-making support, accounting for the lack of clinical knowledge and operational challenges during patient surges.
- **Precision Public Health for COVID-19:** Using data on a high-risk population and neighbourhood factors, health authorities can better target interventions such as vaccination campaigns and resource allocation during winter. Targeted approach is crucial in densely populated urban areas like NYC.

The above technologies demonstrate NYC's commitment to leveraging innovative solutions to address health challenges. While the review specifically focuses on NYC, the findings and conclusions drawn may not be universally applicable to other urban settings with different socio-economic, cultural, and environmental contexts. The unique characteristics of NYC, including its infrastructure, population density, and climate, influence the applicability of the reviewed technological innovations.

The survey of healthcare professionals indicated which departments would be safest for implementing robotic services in several areas. This suggests there is recognition among healthcare professionals that robotics services could be safely introduced into primary care settings. Industry experts believe that robotics services could help address the rising population, increasing elderly care demands, and staffing shortages in UK primary care. Qureshi and Syed (2014) reported a study which indicated that by 2050, one in four people in the UK will be aged 65 or older.

The key takeaway is that the design and implementation of robotics services must address all stakeholder requirements rather than focusing solely on theoretical benefits. This includes determining regulatory body requirements for adapting robotics services, which must be highly specific to the area where robotics will be deployed and integrated into co-design efforts.

Depending on the deployment area within primary care, it is essential to ensure that during a pilot or trial phase a human assistant is available to support patients, answer concerns, and help individuals operate the robotic system. One proposal suggested by an industry expert is to first deploy robotics services to younger generations before expanding to all age groups, as younger individuals tend to be more technologically adept and could assist their family members, acting as indirect promoters of the service.

From an internal stakeholder perspective, healthcare professionals must understand decision-making processes. A human-centric approach that enhances users' understanding of how AI outputs are generated can boost confidence and adaptation. For example, helping doctors understand why AI models behave in certain ways builds trust. Elendu et al. (2023) note that responsibility in cases of AI or robotics errors is challenging. Therefore, it is essential to establish clear governance structures, roles, and responsibilities.

Based on surveys, interviews, and studies, robotic services have the potential to improve healthcare service delivery efficiency through remote monitoring, health-related reminders, and increased diagnostic accuracy. Industry experts acknowledge that while introducing robotic services may initially increase workload, once they become integrated and routine, the workload – especially for healthcare professionals – will decrease. According to Blease et al. (2019), many GPs report high levels of burnout, stress, and concerns about unsafe workload issues that could be alleviated with technology.

Healthcare professionals strongly believe that integrating robotics services into UK healthcare will be beneficial, particularly in automating routine tasks, reducing waiting times, and assisting with surgeries. Papadopoulos et al. (2020) conducted a study involving 420 participants (including 73% older adults, 2% informal carers, and 31% formal caregivers and staff) across six European countries (Austria, France, Israel, Netherlands, and the UK) and Australia, Canada, Japan, and the USA found that enjoyment and engagement were crucial factors in interacting with social assistive humanoid robotics (SAHR). In 10 trials, 83% of participants highly valued their experience, with engagement and enjoyment being strongly linked to the personalisation of services. According to Holland et al. (2021), service robots can relieve pressure on healthcare staff by assisting with daily activities, allowing them to focus on higher-priority tasks. According to Buck et al. (2022), in diagnostic efficiency, a radiologist may handle 60 diagnostic findings per day, whereas AI could work continuously and deliver 180–200 findings daily, significantly benefiting patients.

Healthcare professionals also agree that the top three factors that will increase the acceptance of robotics services are reduced waiting times, diagnostic accuracy, and rapid diagnosis. The UK Prime Minister (PM) talked about an experience where AI helped diagnose a complex blood clot case, pinpointing it in less than three minutes. The PM went on to say that AI is not the future – it is the present in Britain, changing lives, turbocharging growth, and radically improving public services (GOV.UK, 2025).

Vallès-Peris et al. (2021) conducted in-depth interviews with patients hospitalized with COVID-19 in Catalonia (Spain), aged between 58 and 83 years. None of the patients had interacted with any robotics systems, but the study aimed to collect public discourse on the benefits of robotics in hospitals. One of the questions asked was: *Can you imagine a hospital where you would receive the same care and be treated in the same way, but fully robotic?* A patient explained how he used the internet to book a COVID-19 vaccine and avoid long queues, illustrating the benefits of technology. Vallès-Peris et al. (2021) illustrated in the context of the COVID-19 pandemic experience how patients accepted and positively valued the automation of care because it relieved caregivers' burden.

Despite growing enthusiasm for digital health worldwide, widespread adoption remains elusive, particularly outside well-resourced healthcare systems. While the promise of technology is immense, the path to real-world integration is obstructed by a number of persistent barriers. Drawing from comparative experiences in the UK, India, and Nigeria, this section explores the critical impediments to adoption and how they manifest differently across diverse healthcare contexts.

Infrastructure forms the foundation upon which digital health must be built. In high-income countries such as the UK, this typically means stable internet access, reliable electricity, and interoperable digital platforms. Yet even within the NHS, challenges exist which include fragmented systems between trusts and regions, inconsistent data sharing, and concerns around cybersecurity. All hinder seamless adoption (Horn and Kerasidou, 2020).

In contrast, infrastructural limitations in countries like Nigeria and India are far more basic. In many Nigerian public health facilities, frequent power cuts and unreliable internet access can make even simple digital tools unusable (Chukwu et al., 2022). Rural health centres in India often operate with minimal technological support, frequently lacking computers, let alone cloud-based systems or telemedicine infrastructure (Kumar and Ganesh, 2024). This infrastructural fragility makes it difficult to scale successful projects or sustain innovation over time. Until these foundational gaps are addressed, digital health will remain limited to urban centres, reinforcing the very inequities it aims to reduce.

The UK Government's *AI Opportunities Action Plan* (Department for Science, Innovation and Technology, 2025) emphasized opportunities for AI to support growth and productivity with tangible benefits for UK citizens. In this context, expectations for the development of AI and robotics have received new impetus. In the context of primary care and the NHS, the UK government has shown it is ambitious to leverage AI to increase efficiency and save lives. It must learn lessons from the COVID-19 pandemic (Vallès-Peris et al., 2021) when governments globally implemented unprecedented policies with limited information to reduce infection rates.

Governance plays a crucial role in either enabling or hindering digital health adoption. In the UK, while data protection legislation such as the General Data Protection Regulation (GDPR) safeguards patient information, it also introduces a level of complexity that can deter smaller innovators (Savirimuthu, 2020). Nevertheless, the presence of clear policy frameworks at least provides a roadmap for adoption, scale, and evaluation.

In contrast, both India (Soni and Kumari, 2025) and Nigeria (Ubalaeze, 2025) are still in the process of establishing strong digital health governance. India's National Digital Health Mission represents a significant step forward, but regulation and enforcement remain inconsistent. In Nigeria, data privacy legislation is still evolving, leaving both providers and patients uncertain about how their data is stored, accessed, or shared. In such contexts, mistrust of digital platforms can undermine adoption, particularly when systems are introduced by external organisations without deep local engagement.

In the view of Elendu et al. (2023), patients must be informed about the role of AI and robotics, including instances where these technologies are making decisions. During an interview, an industry expert stressed that the two key components of robotic system design are regulatory and legal requirements, as well as a patient-centric approach. Survey results indicate that patients experience technological anxiety, particularly regarding trust and data protection. Like healthcare professionals, these concerns must be addressed by applying existing laws such as GDPR to ensure data protection and transparency in data sharing.

All robotic medical devices must undergo clearance from the Medicines and Healthcare Products Regulatory Agency (MHRS).

According to Steil et al. (2019), doctors are legally required to act following professional standards, explaining all relevant circumstances to patients so they can provide fully informed consent. When using robotic systems in operating theatres, fully tested systems must be employed. Additionally, doctors must inform patients if they are using robotic-assisted methods instead of traditional procedures. These steps, when integrated into the patient journey, help build confidence and trust in robotic services, ensuring patients feel they have options.

Several existing and evolving regulations protect both patients and healthcare professionals:

- In 2023, the UK published the *AI Regulation White Paper*, reaffirming its *sector-led regulations* introduced in 2018 while adding broader *cross-sector principles* applicable to all AI organisations. According to Gikay (2024), the UK's approach contrasts with the EU AI Act, which makes a strong effort to address AI risks but may inadvertently leave out certain use cases. Additionally, the EU AI Act's rigid classification of AI applications could slow innovation. In contrast, the UK's *incremental, sector-based* approach allows for tailored regulations in industries such as pharmaceuticals and FMCG while maintaining safeguards.
- Chapter 2, Section 5 of the *Classification of the Medical Devices Regulation and Safety 2002* categorises medical devices from Class I to Class III (lowest to highest risk). Therefore, primary care must strictly adhere to regulations governing quality control, safety standards, licensing, reporting, documentation, medical oversight, conformity assessment, CE marking, and post-market surveillance.
- The *Consumer Rights Act* raises challenges for AI applications in healthcare, particularly in areas such as:
    - **Service quality**: Ensuring AI reliability and efficiency
    - **Clear and accurate information**: Providing transparent details on AI success rates and limitations
    - **Fair terms and conditions**: Preventing unfair advantages for patients and ambiguous contractual wording
    - **Unlawful data processing**: Ensuring compliance with legal frameworks

According to the Copyright, Designs and Patents Act 1988 (UK), s 9(3), copyright and authorship protection apply to "the person by whom the arrangements necessary for the creation of the work are undertaken." This could extend to software code used in AI models (Selvadurai and Matulionyte, 2020). However, the scope of such protection remains an ongoing debate, posing challenges for healthcare as AI and robotics continue to evolve.

Although digital health tools are often promoted as cost-saving in the long term, the initial investment required can be prohibitive, especially in under-resourced settings. In the UK, health systems can absorb upfront costs and conduct structured procurement processes. However, in Nigeria and India, even the cost of basic smartphones or internet access can be a significant obstacle for frontline staff and patients (Shekoni et al., 2024). Donor-funded pilot programmes frequently introduce advanced technologies without sustainable financial plans, resulting in systems that falter once funding is withdrawn.

There is often a misalignment between who pays and who benefits. A private clinic may bear the cost of implementing a digital system, while the broader health system benefits from efficiencies. Without clear incentives to support equitable investment, adoption is likely to be inconsistent.

Frishammar et al's (2023) study was conducted in association with HDP, a provider in Sweden which develops DHP technology for primary care. The elderly often lag behind in digital maturity (i.e., hands-on experience of using digital technology) compared with younger generations, who often experience digital products from a very early age. A new digital service impacted on the distribution of public resources. Non-users were afraid of technical problems or of making mistakes.

In the Indonesian context, Afrizal et al. (2019) noted that the public health system is decentralised. Strategies are designed to increase health coverage and for health information system to allow for organisational decision making, however, the adoption of electronic records among public health care organisations in Indonesia is low. Afrizal et al. (2019) highlight key obstacles that can occur during primary health care information system (PHCIS) implementation. These include workload problems with limited time allocations during clinical sessions, human resource shortages and inadequate information technology competencies. There are also infrastructure issues such as the availability of the internet, computers, and electricity. Additionally, there is a lack of training in IT for healthcare staff, as well as high employee turnover, which create barriers in PHCIS adoption. Table 3 indicates challenges in adopting technology in different healthcare systems globally, especially related to internet access and a lack of IT training, planning and project management. Deep cuts in USAID (Mbah et al., 2025) will make AI-enabled challenges ever more pressing in delivering community healthcare.

Table 3. Comparative overview of primary health care information system adoption barriers in developed and developing countries (Afrizal et al., 2019)

Barriers	Brazil	Sub-Saharan Africa	Tanzania	India	Malaysia	USA
Internet access						
Computer availability						
Availability of IT team/unit						
Electricity supply						
Infrequent IT use						
Users' computer skills						

continued on following page

Table 3. Continued

Barriers	Brazil	Sub-Saharan Africa	Tanzania	India	Malaysia	USA
Internet access						
Workload						
Employee turnover						
Lack of IT training						
Resistance to change						
Budget constraints						
Security						
Lack of planning, project management						
Lack of financial incentives						
Lack of technology support						
Loss of productivity						
Lack of functions, not meeting practice needs						
Lack of system maintenance						

To patients and healthcare professionals. For the adaptation of Robotics Services to be successfully implemented and evolve, it's important to have policymakers support and pass the laws to govern robotics services in primary care. More guard rails will bring security, protection, and safety to patients and healthcare professionals as well as better adaptation across all patients and healthcare professionals.

According to healthcare professionals, challenges related to technology implementation include cultural awareness, leadership sponsorship, and workforce training for upskilling. AI and robotics are set to revolutionise many fields. The World Economic Forum's *Future of Jobs Report* lists leadership and social influence as top skills that AI will not replace but will transform (Zahidi, 2023). Peifer et al. (2022) introduced four main aspects where AI will transform leadership: strategy, qualifications and competencies, culture, and human-AI interactions. With leadership responsibilities shifting, the skills required to lead AI-driven organisations will change. Watson et al. (2021) argue that leaders must become tech-savvy, capable of identifying high-quality data to make informed decisions, while also developing strong interpersonal and adaptable leadership skills.

A consistent barrier to digital health adoption lies within the very people the systems are designed to support healthcare professionals. In the UK, the introduction of digital tools such as electronic health records, artificial intelligence triage systems, and remote monitoring platforms has often been met with caution. Clinicians have expressed concern about increased administrative burden, loss of patient connection, or lack of time to learn new systems (Zhou et al., 2022). These concerns are not unfounded; poorly designed interfaces and insufficient integration into clinical workflows can, paradoxically, increase workload rather than reduce it.

In lower-income countries like India and Nigeria, resistance is compounded by low levels of digital literacy, limited training, and minimal professional support (Maikomo et al., 2021). For many clinicians in these contexts, particularly those in rural or underserved areas, technology can appear unfamiliar, unreliable, or even threatening. Without concerted efforts to co-design tools with healthcare workers and embed them meaningfully into clinical routines, resistance is likely to persist. Cultural considerations also play a role (Sindakis and Showkat, 2024) as in hierarchical health systems, junior staff may be reluctant to adopt or recommend digital tools without senior endorsement.

The response of healthcare professionals to digital tools also varies widely. In the UK, clinicians are supported by continuous professional development, structured governance, and peer support that enable more confident adoption. Even when challenges arise, they do so within a relatively well supported ecosystem.

By contrast, many clinicians in India and Nigeria work in overstretched settings with limited institutional backing. Digital tools that require additional time or training without immediate benefits are often pushed aside. Moreover, hierarchical systems and fragmented public-private structures can limit the ability of individuals to drive change. However, when digital systems are co-created with frontline teams and reflect their real priorities (such as decision support for community health workers) uptake and sustainability improve.

Patients are not passive recipients of digital health; they are active participants whose perceptions shape success. In the UK, digital tools such as online appointment booking, symptom checkers, and wearable health devices are becoming increasingly mainstream. However, digital exclusion remains a concern, particularly for older adults, people from disadvantaged backgrounds, or those with limited digital access.

In contrast, patients in rural parts of Nigeria and India may approach digital interventions with uncertainty or mistrust. Lack of exposure, language barriers, and misinformation can all hinder uptake. That said, when tools are simple, relevant to local needs, and delivered through trusted healthcare workers, they are often embraced. For example, mobile based maternal health programmes in Nigeria have significantly improved antenatal care attendance when introduced by community health teams (Bowser et al., 2018).

Healthcare professionals believe that older individuals may not easily adapt to robotics services due to the lack of face-to-face discussions with doctors. Empathy and communication are crucial aspects of human interaction, reinforcing the belief that technology cannot substitute for humans in providing compassionate care, according to (Blease et al., 2019).

During interviews, industry experts emphasized this concern, stating, *"My dad and mum will struggle to use robotics services and will not trust them."* One expert further claimed, *"My children, or the Gen Z generation, will be open to and may even prefer interacting with robots over humans."* According to Vallès-Peris et al. (2021), citizens generally place high value on face-to-face relationships with others, including doctors, nurses, and hospital staff.

Healthcare professionals also raised significant concerns about psychological acceptance, trust, and safety, which align with the concerns of industry experts. They argued that patients would need reassurance if robotics systems were used to diagnose their illnesses and prescribe medication. Questions arise such as: *How can they trust that the medicine is correct? What happens if the robotics system provides the wrong medication? What happens if a robotic system is used for surgery and stops working due to a power outage?* These are fundamental concerns that patients are likely to have.

Humans often believe they have a "sixth sense" that robots lack. As a result, trust will play a crucial role in patient decisions regarding robotics-assisted operations. Psychological factors are also a major concern. Every patient suffering from a disease or illness is already mentally affected by their health condition, its impact, and their family's well-being. This is normal human nature. If healthcare services are replaced by robotics – such as replacing a human receptionist in a GP centre – this could impact the patient journey from the very beginning. A patient who is already nervous or mentally distressed may struggle to book a follow-up appointment if they are unable to provide the correct inputs to the robotic receptionist, leading to further frustration and distress.

Vallès-Peris et al. (2021) argue that it is essential to identify ethical concerns and potential detrimental side effects of robotics adaptation. This includes aligning robotics integration with current societal challenges and ensuring ethical acceptability, social desirability, and long-term sustainability. Maynou et al. (2022) noted that the first da Vinci robot – the earliest form of a surgical robot – was classified as a medical device and only required clearance from the Medicines and Healthcare Products Regulatory Agency (MHRS) regarding its safety and specific purpose. It was first introduced into the NHS at St Thomas' NHS Foundation Trust in 2004.

Healthcare professionals are clear that as robotic services become more common in healthcare, regulators and existing laws will play a major role. One of the industry experts strongly emphasised during an interview that in a regulated environment, it is crucial to work closely with regulatory bodies and authorities to develop solutions. Ensuring that all criteria are met from the very beginning of a project as part of the design, testing, and establishing clear key performance indicators is essential to tracking mandatory requirements across all regulatory bodies. Elendu et al. (2023) claim that it is necessary to balance innovation with patient safety and establish interoperability standards to ensure that AI and robotic systems integrate seamlessly with existing healthcare infrastructure.

From the survey with healthcare professionals and interviews with industry experts, common themes emerged: trust, data privacy and protection, compliance, psychological acceptance, and patient safety. Kyrarini et al. (2021) contend that the law must provide guidance not only on safety but also on data protection, responsibility, transparency, autonomy, and dignity. As robots and AI advance rapidly, lawmakers must prioritise filling legal gaps. A key takeaway from an industry expert is that, in a regulated environment, it is important to identify and address gaps by working with regulatory bodies. As one expert noted, *"Technology will always outpace existing law."* In the case of AI and robotics advancements, time and resources are needed to work proactively and anticipate guardrails.

There are two dimensions to addressing these issues – one concerning internal stakeholders, including healthcare professionals, and the other concerning external stakeholders, such as patients. Key concerns include trust, data privacy, data protection, safety, and psychological assurance.

The IBM Institute for Business Value *Experts Insights* report found that the healthcare industry experiences the highest cost per data breach, averaging $10.10 million per incident (Kessem, 2022). Data privacy and security breaches are a top concern for 53% of enterprise architects, while security and governance remain the most challenging aspects of data engineering for engineers. High-quality data are essential for robotic services and influence behaviour, actions, and decisions. It is imperative to use accurate training data and maintain robust security measures to safeguard patient and healthcare professional data.

Elendu et al. (2023) argue that protecting patient data is crucial as AI and robotics generate vast amounts of sensitive information. Ensuring data privacy and security is paramount, as any breach could have severe consequences for patient trust and data integrity. Furthermore, responsible data handling practices must be adapted for collecting, storing, and utilising patient information.

Elendu et al. (2023) also stress the importance of enhancing accessibility to ensure AI and robotics services reach underserved or remote populations, addressing geographic disparities in healthcare. Ethical concerns arise for vulnerable populations who lack access to technology and digital literacy. Additionally, AI algorithms trained on biased datasets may exacerbate healthcare inequalities, while the digital divide disproportionately affects marginalised communities. Strategies must be implemented to bridge this gap and ensure equal access. Most of the cases relate to disparities, and digital dived are more frequent in the United States, it is important to learn from Westworld experience and apply measures, part design, and tests to ensure robotics services are available for everyone and considering all scenarios relate to ethical background, religions, age, sex, demography with the right set of data. It's also important to be transparent with patients if a robotics service is only available for kidney rare disease scanning for males over age 60 and in the London area. It is important to share the information with the patient and the reason behind it to build trust and confidence and share future road maps.

Obermeyer et al. (2019) explored the implications of AI-based predictions for patients. Their findings revealed that data collection is not proportionate between Black and White patients and that poorer individuals face significant barriers to accessing healthcare. Geographic and socioeconomic factors influence AI scores, making it essential to prevent biases when implementing robotic services in primary care. This example is again from the United States and in the United Kingdom, it must identify the gap that requires incremental reform. Local policies or codes of practice should be implemented. To ensure the consistent protection of civil liberty, a national policy that regulates the Robotics Service, is very specific to the service robotics will provide.

The use of robotics in primary care raises ethical concerns, particularly regarding diagnostic accuracy and its impact on patient outcomes. Incorrect results can affect healthcare relationships and necessitate upskilling among professionals. Additionally, new regulations will require frequent training. Data misuse poses risks to both patient and professional privacy, with survey results indicating significant concerns about data protection. Industry leaders have highlighted security as a key factor, with one expert stating, "The automation output is only as good as the quality of the data," emphasising the risk of biased results.

During an interview with an industry expert, a key concern was raised: *"Automation often resonates as reducing FTE sizing in an organisation, so resistance is primarily a fear of losing a job."* According to Holland et al. (2021), one of the major challenges in service robotics adaptation is acceptance, as professionals worry that robots will replace human workers. Implementing a change management programme with training opportunities can help healthcare professionals gain confidence, adapt to new technologies, and identify skill gaps. While job roles may evolve, robotics adaptation does not signify the end of healthcare professions.

An industry expert emphasised the importance of understanding *why* AI or robotics are introduced, what it aims to achieve, and how it benefits healthcare professionals. Demonstrating the tool's capabilities can foster engagement, curiosity, and trust.

Elendu et al. (2023) suggest that changing roles and job displacement will lead to the redefinition of responsibilities for healthcare professionals. Automating specific tasks may raise concerns about job security, making it essential to implement ethical considerations that ensure a smooth transition, including retraining opportunities for affected individuals.

According to Steil et al. (2019), the introduction of robotics in surgical settings significantly alters professional roles, team interactions, and communication, shifting dynamics towards human-machine collaboration. A key concern is accountability – who is responsible if an issue arises in robotic-assisted surgeries? Clearly defined roles, responsibilities, and regulatory frameworks are essential.

A white paper by Parker et al. (2024) recommends implementing monitoring and surveillance measures post-pilot to collect user feedback on AI performance and concerns. Establishing governance processes will reassure healthcare professionals, ensuring that if robotic systems malfunction, a structured feedback mechanism is in place. Like all technologies, AI and robotics require continuous updates, and drawing parallels with traditional software upgrades can help professionals adapt more seamlessly.

Industry experts highlight that AI and robotics require the right training and setup. If the training process does not adhere to specific protocols, outcomes may be inconsistent. Elendu et al. (2023) emphasized ethical considerations for healthcare professionals working with AI and robotics include professional responsibility in understanding and appropriately using these systems, ensuring patient safety, and remaining vigilant against system errors or biases. Continuous education is essential, with ethical frameworks promoting ongoing training to help healthcare professionals stay up to date with AI and robotics advancements and maintain competency. Low et al. (2021) conducted in-depth semi-structured interviews with 20 participants aged 50–65. Older adults in Singapore still prefer face-to-face interaction with healthcare professionals and may perceive technology as unnecessary or do not have the means to use it. Concerns include affordability of applications, devices, privacy and data protections and demographic digital divides

RECOMMENDATIONS

Finally, the authors recommend that primary digital healthcare policies and practices account for stakeholder management and strong governance; learn from previous technology adaptation within primary care and across the NHS; benchmark globally and expand existing robotic services. It is vital to consider different age groups; select the right technology integration partner; create a pool of health care professional champions; engage with the public; and invest in appropriate and regular training and change management.

1. **Stakeholder Management and Strong Governance; Learn from Previous Technology Adaptation within Primary Care and Across Healthcare Ecosystems**: Conduct a lessons-learned workshop focused on historical tech-

nology adaptation challenges in primary healthcare, such as the COVID-19 track and trace process. This will help identify obstacles faced in the past and other existing obstacles so that appropriate practices can be applied.

2. **Global Benchmarking:** Invest time to visit other countries globally that exemplify advances in digital services adaptation in primary care and learn from their successes and challenges.
3. **Expand Existing Digital Health and Robotic Services in Primary Care**: Leverage resources and processes to extend collaborations with other fields to support primary care.
4. **Consider Different Age Groups:** Understand patient demographics, especially age groups, when deploying services. Begin with younger patients and ensure human support is accessible for areas that affect all age groups during the first 12 months. Gradually reduce human assistance as digital services in primary care gain traction.
5. **Select the Right Technology Integration Partner**: Carefully choose a technology integration partner who very specifically implements digital/robotic services in the regulated healthcare environment.
6. **Create a Pool of Health Care Professional Champions**: Identify healthcare professionals with experience in using digital/robotics services as champions within primary care. These champions can train others to contribute to implementing change management processes.
7. **Public Engagement and Incentivisation:** Similar to medical trials, involve the public in design and testing phases to gather feedback. Additionally, appoint a public ambassador to champion services post-implementation, assisting with change management processes.
8. **Investment in Training and Change Management:** Invest in on-going training. This requires effective communications with employees and integrating their feedback. Constructive engagement underpins a solid foundation for implementing effective digital/robotic services adaptation across primary care.

CONCLUSION

In summary, barriers to digital health adoption are more than simply technological, they are deeply human, institutional, and systemic as Figure 1 and Table 1 have indicated. Without addressing the complex interplay of infrastructure, workload, psychological barriers, health professionals' training, policy, economics, and trust (Borges do Nascimento et al., 2023), even the most innovative solutions risk failing to achieve their intended impact to reap the benefits of digital technology in primary healthcare.

Comparing experiences from the UK, India, and Nigeria reveals a common lesson: the future of digital health will depend not only on what is built, but how, where, and with whom it is built. Survey analysis provides insights into ways healthcare professionals think about the robotic services adaptation in primary care. While they recognise the benefits, they also highlight concerns related to costs, social implications, and ethical considerations. Industry experts were able to share their perspectives on lessons learned, trends in the market and key focus points. The adaptation of digital technologies in primary care globally represents a significant shift in healthcare, with several benefits, including increased patient flow, enhanced service capacity, faster diagnoses and treatments, and reduced recovery times. However, concerns remain regarding trust, safety, data protection, bias, and technological anxiety among both patients and healthcare professionals.

The COVID-19 experience offered valuable lessons globally that can help governments, primary care providers, and the NHS as well as other national health ecosystems gain confidence in adapting robotic services. During the COVID-19 pandemic, regulators, healthcare professionals, scientists, private equity, civil servants and the government worked together to accelerate the production of vaccines globally and the UK championed the rollout of the first vaccines in Europe. A similar co-ordinated effort should be made for adopting digital and robotics services in primary care, especially given on-going crises in the NHS, which faces staff shortages, increasing demand, an ageing population, and a shortage of resources. The abolition of NHS England (Crisp, 2025) and financial and performance deficits with long waiting lists (Limiri, 2025) and concerns about productivity during austerity present a perfect storm for change with immense pressures. While digital technologies will not solve every problem within the healthcare field, their introduction will increase the workload for healthcare professionals due to high investment costs and the need for extensive change management for internal healthcare professionals and patients.

The transformation journey in a regulated environment is complex and requires careful navigation. Implementing robotic services necessitates early collaboration with regulators to ensure legal and safety compliance, as well as data protection from early in the project phases i.e., design, build and test phases to safeguard patients, healthcare professionals and technology. Strong ethical and governance frameworks ensure responsible and fair use of digital health technologies in primary care to address the social and moral implications for patients and healthcare providers. Other factors, such as economics, technology, and politics play a crucial role in the successful adaptation. However, our research indicates that addressing concerns, anxiety, and biases is vital to building confidence among healthcare professionals and patients. For successful integration of digital technologies globally, social, legal, and ethical factors must also be prioritised. These factors ensure that proper regulations are in place, diagnoses are accurate, and that there is a clear process for reporting issues. Additionally, factors such as patient age groups, geographical location, and change management processes including training, clear role definitions, and responsibilities in the new work environment s are essential for smooth adaptation. Crises can present enormous opportunities in primary care using AI (Greenhalgh et al., 2025) to make the right decisions with limited resources.

Finally, the authors recommend further research using longitudinal and ethnographic studies with community participatory action research and international comparisons in developed and developing economies to understand the challenges for primary healthcare providers in adopting digital technologies. In particular, the authors would welcome intersectional studies and opportunities for co-designing innovative solutions with female coders and data analysts to reduce algorithmic biases (Sasseville et al., 2025). It is vital to understand the technology strategy implementation divide and culturally sensitive human factors using relevant tools to complement and extend the NASSS framework in different primary care settings (Greenhalgh et al., 2018; Papoutsi and Greenhalgh, 2024).

REFERENCES

Abel, G., Atherton, H., Sussex, J., Akter, N., Aminu, A. Q., Bak, W., Bryce, C., Clark, C. E., Cockcroft, E., Evans, H., Gkousis, E., Jenkins, G., Jenkinson, C., Khan, N., Lambert, J., Leach, B., Marriott, C., Newbould, J., Parkinson, S., & Campbell, J. L. (2024). Current experience and future potential of facilitating access to digital NHS primary care services in England: The Di-Facto mixed-methods study. *Health and Social Care Delivery Research, 12*(32), 1–197. DOI: 10.3310/JKYT5803 PMID: 39324475

Afrizal, S. H., Handayani, P. W., Hidayanto, A. N., Eryando, T., Budiharsana, M., & Martha, E. (2019). Barriers and challenges to primary health care information system (PHCIS) adoption from health management perspective: A qualitative study. *Informatics in Medicine Unlocked, 17*, 100198. Advance online publication. DOI: 10.1016/j.imu.2019.100198

Blease, C., Kaptchuk, T. J., Bernstein, M. H., Mandl, K. D., Halamka, J. D., & DesRoches, C. M. (2019). Artificial intelligence and the future of primary care: Exploratory qualitative study of UK general practitioners' views. *Journal of Medical Internet Research, 21*(3), e12802. DOI: 10.2196/12802 PMID: 30892270

Borges do Nascimento, I. J., Abdulazeem, H., Vasanthan, L. T., Martinez, E. Z., Zucoloto, M. L., Østengaard, L., Azzopardi-Muscat, N., Zapata, T., & Novillo-Ortiz, D. (2023). Barriers and facilitators to utilizing digital health technologies by healthcare professionals. *NPJ Digital Medicine, 6*(1), 161. DOI: 10.1038/s41746-023-00899-4 PMID: 37723240

Bowser, D. M., Shepard, D. S., Nandakumar, A., Okunogbe, A., Morrill, T., Halasa-Rappel, Y., & Oluwayemisi, E. (2018). Cost effectiveness of mobile health for antenatal care and facility births in Nigeria. *Annals of Global Health, 84*(4), 592–602. DOI: 10.29024/aogh.2364 PMID: 30779506

Buck, C., Doctor, E., Hennrich, J., Jöhnk, J., & Eymann, T. (2022). General practitioners' attitudes toward artificial intelligence–enabled systems: Interview study. *Journal of Medical Internet Research, 24*(1), e28916. DOI: 10.2196/28916 PMID: 35084342

Chukwu, E., Garg, L., Foday, E., Konomanyi, A., Wright, R., & Smart, F. (2022). Electricity, computing hardware, and internet infrastructures in health facilities in Sierra Leone: Field mapping study. *JMIR Medical Informatics, 10*(2), e30040. DOI: 10.2196/30040 PMID: 35113026

Crisp, N. (2025). Abolishing NHS England: Risks and opportunities. *BMJ (Clinical Research Ed.), 388*, r553. Advance online publication. DOI: 10.1136/bmj.r553 PMID: 40101921

Darzi, A. (2024). *Independent investigation of the NHS in England*. UK Department of Health and Social Care, November 15. www.gov.uk/government/publications/independent-investigation-of-the-nhs-in-england

Department for Science, Innovation and Technology. (2025). *AI opportunities action plan*. GOV.UK. January 13.

Economist Impact. (2024). *Unlocking enterprise AI: Opportunities and strategies*, November 22.

Elendu, C., Amaechi, D. C., Elendu, T. C., Jingwa, K. A., Okoye, O. K., Okah, M. J., & Alimi, H. A. (2023). Ethical implications of AI and robotics in healthcare. *Revista de Medicina (São Paulo), 102*(50), e36671. DOI: 10.1097/MD.0000000000036671 PMID: 38115340

Frishammar, J., Essén, A., Bergström, F., & Ekman, T. (2023). Digital health platforms for the elderly? Key adoption and usage barriers and ways to address them. *Technological Forecasting and Social Change, 189*, 122319. Advance online publication. DOI: 10.1016/j.techfore.2023.122319

Geracitano, J., Barron, L., McSwain, D., & Khairat, S. (2024). How is digital health suitability measured for communities? A systematic review. *Digital Health, 10*, 20552076241288316. Advance online publication. DOI: 10.1177/20552076241288316 PMID: 39398896

Gikay, A. A. (2024). Risks, innovation, and adaptability in the UK's incrementalism versus the European Union's comprehensive artificial intelligence regulation. *International Journal of Law and Information Technology, 32*(1), eaae013. https://ssrn.com/abstract=4700121. DOI: 10.1093/ijlit/eaae013

GOV.UK. (2025). *PM speech on AI opportunities action plan*. January 13.

Greenhalgh, S., Guo, L., & Yeowell, G. (2025). 'In the midst of every crisis, lies great opportunity': Perceptions of the future use of artificial intelligence in the UK NHS primary care. *Musculoskeletal Care, 23*(2), e70092. DOI: 10.1002/msc.70092 PMID: 40238189

Greenhalgh, T., Wherton, J., Papoutsi, C., Lynch, J., Hughes, G., A'Court, C., Hinder, S., Procter, R., & Shaw, S. (2018). Analysing the role of complexity in explaining the fortunes of technology programmes: Empirical application of the NASSS framework. *BMC Medicine, 16*(1), 1–15. DOI: 10.1186/s12916-018-1050-6 PMID: 29754584

Holland, J., Kingston, L., McCarthy, C., Armstrong, E., O'Dwyer, P., Merz, F., & McConnell, M. (2021). Service robots in the healthcare sector. *Robotics (Basel, Switzerland), 10*(1), 1–47. DOI: 10.3390/robotics10010047

Horn, R., & Kerasidou, A. (2020). Sharing whilst caring: Solidarity and public trust in a data-driven healthcare system. *BMC Medical Ethics, 21*(1), 1–7. DOI: 10.1186/s12910-020-00553-8 PMID: 33143692

Hou, X., Liu, L., & Cain, J. (2022). Can higher spending on primary healthcare mitigate the impact of ageing and non-communicable diseases on health expenditure? *BMJ Global Health, 7*(12), e010513. Advance online publication. DOI: 10.1136/bmjgh-2022-010513 PMID: 36564087

Husain, L., & Greenhalgh, T. (2025). Examining intersectionality and barriers to the uptake of video consultations among older adults from disadvantaged backgrounds with limited English proficiency: Qualitative narrative interview study. *Journal of Medical Internet Research, 27*, e65690. Advance online publication. DOI: 10.2196/65690 PMID: 39761566

Ijiga, A. C., Peace, A. E., Idoko, I. P., Ezebuka, C. I., Harry, K. D., Ukatu, I. E., & Agbo, D. O. (2024). Technological innovations in mitigating winter health challenges in New York City, USA. *International Journal of Science and Research Archive, 11*(1), 535–551. DOI: 10.30574/ijsra.2024.11.1.0078

Kessem, L. (2022). *Healthcare breaches costliest for 12 years running, hit new $10.1M record high*. August 17. IBM.

Keyue, X., & Qiongfang, D. (2024). COVID-19 epidemic at low level but may rise during Spring Festival: National Health Commission. *Global Times (Beijing, China).*

Kumar, M. S., & Ganesh, D. (2024). Improving telemedicine through IoT and cloud computing: Opportunities and challenges. *Advances in Engineering and Intelligence Systems, 3*(3), 123–135. DOI: 10.22034/aeis.2024.474171.1217

Kyrarini, M., Lygerakis, F., Rajavenkatanarayanan, A., Sevastopoulos, C., Nambiappan, H. R., Chaitanya, K. K., Babu, A. R., Mathew, J., & Makedon, F. (2021). A survey of robots in healthcare. *Technologies, 9*(1), 8. DOI: 10.3390/technologies9010008

Li, L., Back, E., Lee, S., Shipley, R., Mapitse, N., Elbe, S., Smallman, M., Wilson, J., Yasin, I., Rees, G., Gordon, B., Murray, V., Roberts, S. L., Cupani, A., & Kostkova, P. (2025). Balancing risks and opportunities: Data-empowered-health ecosystems. *Journal of Medical Internet Research, 27*, e57237. DOI: 10.2196/57237 PMID: 40132190

Limb, M. (2024). PM says NHS must “reform or die” following damning report into state of the service. *BMJ (Clinical Research Ed.)*, q2001. Advance online publication. DOI: 10.1136/bmj.q2001 PMID: 39266245

Limiri, D. M. (2025). The impact of long wait times on patient health outcomes: The growing NHS crisis. *Journal of Public Health*, *3*. Advance online publication. DOI: 10.70389/PJPH.100020

Low, S. T., Sakhardande, P. G., Lai, Y. F., Long, A. D., & Kaur-Gill, S. (2021). Attitudes and perceptions toward healthcare technology adoption among older adults in Singapore: A qualitative study. *Frontiers in Public Health*, *9*, 588590. Advance online publication. DOI: 10.3389/fpubh.2021.588590 PMID: 33659232

Maikomo, J. M., Targema, T. S., & Obun-Andy, M. K. (2021). COVID-19 and the new normal in developing societies: An appraisal of Nigerians’ adaptation to digital life in public and private spheres. *Journal of Developing Societies*, *37*(3), 246–274. DOI: 10.1177/0169796X21996830

Maynou Pujolràs, L., Pearson, G., McGuire, A., & Serra-Sastre, V. (2022). The diffusion of robotic surgery: Examining technology use in the English NHS. *Health Policy (Amsterdam)*, *126*(4), 325–336. DOI: 10.1016/j.healthpol.2022.02.007 PMID: 35307200

Mbah, R. E., Hardgrave, C. M., Mbah, D. E., Nutt, A., & Russell, J. G. (2025). The impact of USAID budget cuts on global development initiatives: A review of challenges, responses, and implications. *Advances in Social Sciences Research Journal*, *12*(04), 219–232. Advance online publication. DOI: 10.14738/assrj.1204.18681

NHS England. (2023). *Delivery plan for recovering access to primary care*. NHS England.

NHS England. (2025). *GP practices embrace technology to improve patient access and provide choice*. April 24.

Obermeyer, Z., Powers, B., Vogeli, C., & Mullainathan, S. (2019). Dissecting racial bias in an algorithm used to manage the health of populations. *Science*, *366*(6464), 447–453. DOI: 10.1126/science.aax2342 PMID: 31649194

Papadopoulos, I., Koulouglioti, C., Lazzarino, R., & Ali, S. (2020). Enablers and barriers to the implementation of socially assistive humanoid robots in health and social care: A systematic review. *BMJ Open*, *10*(1), e033096. DOI: 10.1136/bmjopen-2019-033096 PMID: 31924639

Papadopoulos, I., Koulouglioti, C., Lazzarino, R., & Ali, S. (2020). Enablers and barriers to the implementation of socially assistive humanoid robots in health and social care: A systematic review. *BMJ Open, 10*(1), e033096. DOI: 10.1136/bmjopen-2019-033096 PMID: 31924639

Papoutsi, C., & Greenhalgh, T. (2024). Innovation, improvement, and implementation–conceptual frameworks for thinking through complex change. In *eHealth research theory and development* (pp. 220–236). Routledge. DOI: 10.4324/9781003302049-15

Parker, V. J., Economou, N. J., Health, D., & Silcox, C. (2024.). *White Paper. AI governance in health systems. Aligning innovation, accountability, and trust*. Margolis Institute for Health Policy, Duke Health.

Peifer, Y., Jeske, T., & Hille, S. (2022). Artificial intelligence and its impact on leaders and leadership. *Procedia Computer Science, 200*, 1024–1030. https://doi .org/ rights and contentDOI: 10.1016/j.procs.2022.01.301Get

PwC. (2024). *Essential eight technologies for health services: AI leads investment priorities*. PwC, August 19.

Qureshi, M. O., & Syed, R. S. (2014). The impact of robotics on employment and motivation of employees in the service sector, with special reference to health care. *Safety and Health at Work, 5*(4), 198–202. DOI: 10.1016/j.shaw.2014.07.003 PMID: 25516812

Sasseville, M., Ouellet, S., Rhéaume, C., Sahlia, M., Couture, V., Després, P., Paquette, J.-S., Darmon, D., Bergeron, F., & Gagnon, M. P. (2025). Bias Mitigation in Primary Health Care Artificial Intelligence Models: Scoping Review. *Journal of Medical Internet Research, 27*, e60269. Advance online publication. DOI: 10.2196/60269 PMID: 39773888

Savirimuthu, J. (2020). The GDPR, AI and the NHS code of conduct for data-driven health and care technology. In *Health data privacy under the GDPR* (pp. 133–156). Routledge., DOI: 10.4324/9780429022241-10

Selvadurai, N., & Matulionyte, R. (2020). Reconsidering creativity: Copyright protection for works generated using artificial intelligence. *Journal of Intellectual Property Law & Practice, 15*(7), 536–543. DOI: 10.1093/jiplp/jpaa062

Shekoni, O., Iversen, S., Diaz, G. J., Aune, A., Ubuane, P. O., Imam, Z., & André, B. (2024). Healthcare workers' perceptions about the use of mobile health technologies in public health facilities in Lagos, Nigeria. *SAGE Open Medicine, 12*, 20503121231224568. DOI: 10.1177/20503121231224568 PMID: 38347851

Sindakis, S., & Showkat, G. (2024). The digital revolution in India: Bridging the gap in rural technology adoption. *Journal of Innovation and Entrepreneurship, 13*(1), 29. DOI: 10.1186/s13731-024-00380-w

Soni, P. K., & Kumari, U. (2025). Revitalizing Health Governance: Charting a Resilient Path for India's Future. In *Intersecting realities of health resilience and governance in India: Emerging domestic and global perspectives* (pp. 55–73). Springer Nature Singapore.

Steil, J., Finas, D., Beck, S., Manzeschke, A., & Haux, R. (2019). Robotic systems in operating theaters: New forms of team–machine interaction in health care. *Methods of Information in Medicine, 58*(1), E14–E25. DOI: 10.1055/s-0039-1692465 PMID: 31342471

Terry, A. L., Kueper, J. K., Beleno, R., Brown, J. B., Cejic, S., Dang, J., Leger, D., McKay, S., Meredith, L., Pinto, A. D., Ryan, B. L., Stewart, M., Zwarenstein, M., & Lizotte, D. J. (2022). Is primary health care ready for artificial intelligence? What do primary health care stakeholders say? *BMC Medical Informatics and Decision Making, 22*(1), 237. DOI: 10.1186/s12911-022-01984-6 PMID: 36085203

The King's Fund. (2024). *Key facts and figures about the NHS.* The King's Fund, June 25.

Ubalaeze, S. (2025). The impact of digital transformation on healthcare delivery in Nigeria: Challenges and recommendations. *International Journal of Research and Scientific Innovation, 11*(15), 498–509.

Vallès-Peris, N., Barat-Auleda, O., & Domènech, M. (2021). Robots in healthcare? What patients say. *International Journal of Environmental Research and Public Health, 18*(18), 9933. Advance online publication. DOI: 10.3390/ijerph18189933 PMID: 34574861

Watson, G. J., Desouza, K. C., Ribiere, V. M., & Lindič, J. (2021). Will AI ever sit at the C-suite table? The future of senior leadership. *Business Horizons, 64*(4), 465–474. DOI: 10.1016/j.bushor.2021.02.011

Zahidi, S. (2023). *Future of jobs report*, April 30. World Economic Forum. https://www.weforum.org/publications/the-future-of-jobs-report-2023/digest/

Zhou, A. Y., Zghebi, S. S., Hodkinson, A., Hann, M., Grigoroglou, C., Ashcroft, D. M., Esmail, A., Chew-Graham, C. A., Payne, R., Little, P., Lusignan, S., Cherachi-Sohi, S., Spooner, S., Zhou, A. K., Kontopantelis, E., & Panagioti, M. (2022). Investigating the links between diagnostic uncertainty, emotional exhaustion, and turnover intention in General Practitioners working in the United Kingdom. *Frontiers in Psychiatry*, *13*, 936067. DOI: 10.3389/fpsyt.2022.936067 PMID: 35958644

Chapter 2
The Benefits of Generative AI for Global Health Partnerships:
From Fragmentation to Cohesion

Cong Sui
http://orcid.org/0009-0008-2657-2580
University of Birmingham, UK & University College London, UK

Dimitrios Kalogeropoulos
Global Health and Digital Innovation Foundation, UK

ABSTRACT

Global health partnerships (GHPs) remain fragmented, unco-ordinated and donor-driven. GHPs lack a coherent framework for their entire lifecycle, making a universal solution impossible. As a case in point, Global Health & Digital Innovation Foundation (GHDIF) is leveraging generative AI (GAI) to build a connected digital platform in global health to address the issues, though its specific mechanisms for benefit remain unclear. This study identifies key aspects where GAI can enhance GHPs by applying a Partnership Analysis Framework and a literature review of sources like PubMed and Web of Science. Findings indicate GAI's potential in four areas: analyzing contextual factors and prerequisites, structuring projects, monitoring processes and performance, and measuring outcomes and stakeholder value. Supported by evidence, the review recommends GHDIF establish a coherent ontology, build partnership standards, and cooperate with the UN. As the first paper to demonstrate how GAI can benefit GHPs, this chapter provides a foundational roadmap for integration.

DOI: 10.4018/979-8-2600-2238-2.ch002

1. INTRODUCTION

1.1 Public-Private Partnerships

Public-private partnerships (PPPs) have been widely applied in many areas with less change and uncertainty, such as various public infrastructures, energy, education, etc. (Li & Akintoye, 2003). There are a variety of partners containing public-private partnership, public-private mix, public-private workplace partnership and public-NGO partnership (Joudyian et al., 2021), to work together, share the information and gather together their diverse complementary capabilities under an integrated inter-institutional partnership model. The success of the partnerships models requires a transparent relationship, mutual commitment and an effective approach to evaluate and monitor the performance outcomes among different partners as well as a sustainable financial support (Joudyian et al., 2021). Plenty of challenges for the above partnerships are categorised into five areas: 1) insufficient knowledge and educated talents (Bourgeois et al., 2014; Gidado & Ejembi, 2009; Silow-Carroll, 2008); 2) lack of strategic vision and commitment in management (Lönnroth et al., 2004; Newell et al., 2005; Rangan et al., 2004; Ullah et al., 2012; World Health Organization, 1978; Zafar Ullah et al., 2006); 3) short of trust and capacity as well as disparities in ownership and power in human resources (Ganguly et al., 2014; Ramiah & Reich, 2006; Sheikh et al., 2006; Zafar Ullah et al., 2006); 4) unsustainable, inadequate and insecure funding sources (Engel & van Lente, 2014; Mudyarabikwa & Regmi, 2016; Uplekar, 2016) and 5) inadequate standardisation, defined indicators, monitoring and documentation systems in technological support (Ahmed & Nisar, 2010; Engel & van Lente, 2014; Imtiaz et al., 2017; Mudyarabikwa & Regmi, 2016; Rangan et al., 2004).

1.2 Global Health Partnerships

The emergence of PPPs in global health started in the 1990s, driven by the neo-liberal ideologies (Babacan, 2020). Public health sectors need private corporates to provide healthcare products, as they do not produce products. The global health partnerships (GHPs) involve multilateral stakeholders, containing recipient government, healthcare provider, life science company, etc. Different partners have different objectives, some of which are conflicted. For instance, the international organisations such as United Nations care more about whether the collaboration followed their core ethical principles, including beneficence, nonmaleficence, autonomy and equity (World Health Organization, 1999). They consider more about the outcome in the wider global health system. On the contrary, the for-profit industries aim to maximise their profits. They focus on the interventions to address a single disease

(Stuckler et al., 2011). The core value of GHPs sometimes is diluted by the private partners. A notable example is Coca-Cola Company lobbying for soda taxes from Save the Children (Freedhoff & Hébert, 2011).

The ubiquity of digitalisation in healthcare sectors is another driven factor promoting the PPPs in global health, resulting from the wide deployment of digital devices and their increasing amounts of users. Vast amounts of digital data are mostly stored and owned by private sectors, which are very difficult for public sectors to access (Breuer et al., 2020). The asymmetry in data creates a huge barrier for public sectors who have know-how, to gain access to the data. For the companies who own the data, however, do not know how to use it (World Economic Forum, 2023). The information asymmetry drives the formation of partnerships between public and private sectors. It will allow the data to yield greater impact on health outcomes. The demand for PPPs and their potential global health impacts are plotted in Figure 1.

Figure 1. Prioritising AI use matrix: Demand for PPPs vs their potential global health impacts

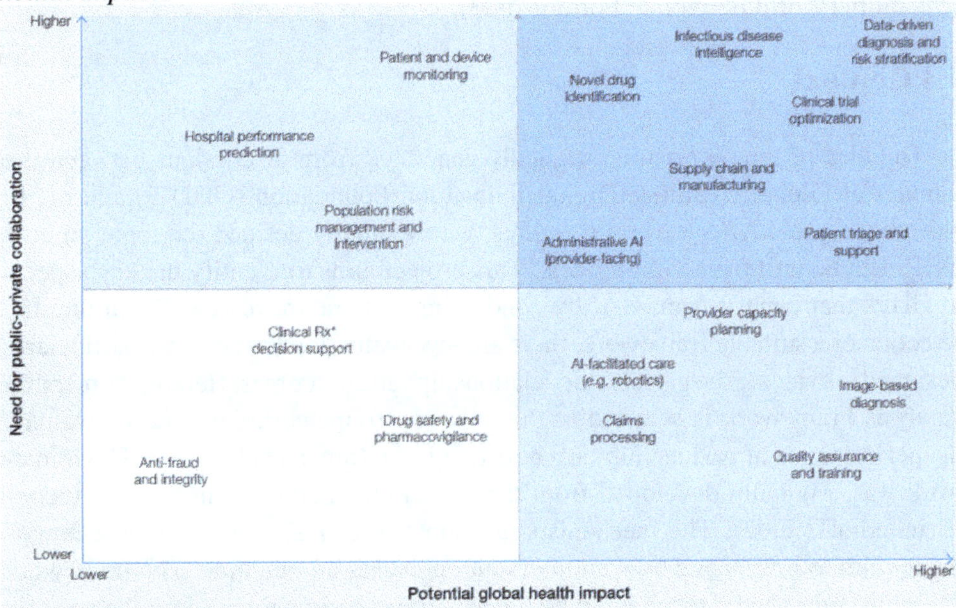

(World Economic Forum, 2023).

1.3 Generative Artificial Intelligence

Generative artificial intelligence (GAI) or large language models (LLMs) as a kind of machine learning is capable to generate synthetic data in various format, such as text, image, audio, video or code. These capabilities enable GAI or LLMs to flexibly fit into different models and various new tasks (Morley et al., 2023). For instance, OpenAI Chat Generative Pre-training Transformer (ChatGPT) and Google Bard are deemed a technological renaissance with huge potential (Health-Europe, 2023). Stanford University exploited GAI in synthetic clinical trials and biomedical research to accelerate their speed of commercialisation (Goth Itoi, 2022). Philips plans to utilise cloud-based generative AI to offer support in accurate diagnoses and the automation of administration tasks across various medical domains (modalities) (World Economic Forum, 2023). However, to the best of my knowledge there is no study on the application of GAI in global health, particularly the PPPs in global health, due to the highly unexpected danger of AI (Federspiel et al., 2023; Tredinnick & Laybats, 2023). Take global mental health as an example, the application of GAI or LLMs is urgently needed to reduce the massive shortage of workforce (van Heerden et al., 2023). On the other hand, the deployment of digital tools in healthcare sectors calls for the sustained PPPs, which need to be built on three foundational rules, namely useable and representative data, low-friction adoptability and easy scalability (World Economic Forum, 2023).

1.4 Context

The idea of the report was originally generated from discussions between the founder of Global Health & Digital Innovation Foundation (GHDIF) and me in November 2022. After several meetings, we eventually defined the topic on how GHPs can benefit from GAI models. This project aims to identify the key aspects in GHPs that benefit from GAI by conducting a literature review. Regarding the selection of a suitable framework, there are few evaluation frameworks particularly designed to evaluate the partnership relationships and outcomes. Herein, Partnership Analysis Framework is selected as the only one framework designed to evaluate the performance of partnership on a holistic view (Kamya et al., 2017). The framework was originally developed from the causal chain analysis in systems theory (Brinkerhoff, 2002). The mechanistic accounts of causality as a "middle-range" theory aim to investigate how an intervention causes an outcome. The framework is highly contextual dependent, which needs to be designed based on the specific indicator for each case (Charles & McNulty, 1999). The supporting evidence is thus demonstrated under this framework.

The structure of the report is shown in Figure 2. It starts from the determination of the key issues of PPPs in global health, followed by how the values of GHPs are diverted from the core ethical principles of WHO and public sectors. There are various reasons causing this issue. The key reason is attributed to the lack of necessary standards and norms to connect the whole GHP process. It calls for the establishment of a connected digital ecosystem in global health to solve the problem. The findings of how GHPs can benefit from the integrated digital system using GAI models are summarised in four aspects: (1) contextual factors and partnership prerequisites analysis, (2) structuring PPP projects, (3) partnership process & performance monitoring and (4) measurement of partnership outcome and value for stakeholders. Finally, three recommendations are proposed.

Figure 2. Report overview

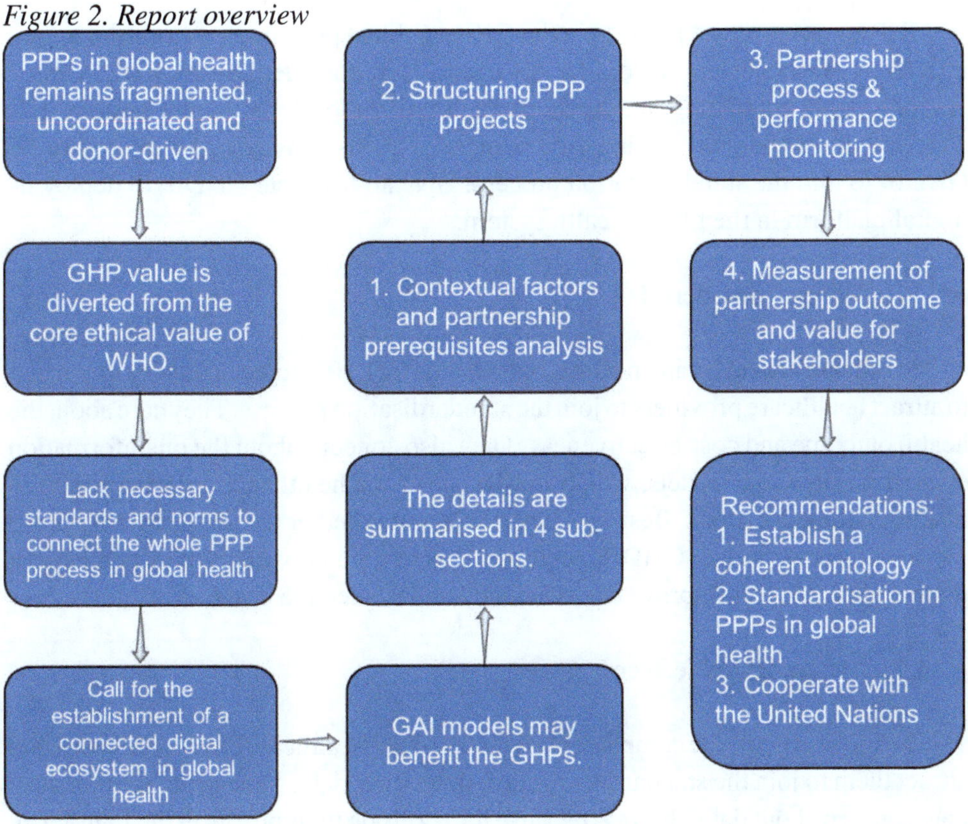

1.5 Stakeholder Analysis

Stakeholder Analysis for GHDIF

The stakeholders of GHDIF are analysed below and summarised in Table 1.

- Government

It is essential for GHDIF to get the permission from local government, when GHDIF intends to enter a new country. The government care about whether the project can improve health outcome and cost-effectiveness of the local healthcare system. The government is also concerned about whether their demand can be addressed properly in the GHPs. The data privacy is another issue of concern.

- GHP agency

GHP agencies play a key role in the GHPs. Ethical principles, sustainability and efficiency are important factors for the agencies to consider. For example, United Nations (UN) are setting standards and norms in the global health system. UN concerns about the risk of using GAI models or LLMs. It is a good opportunity for GHDIF to join the standardisation process. UN can facilitate GHDIF to deploy its digital platform in the global health system.

- Healthcare providers

Healthcare providers are the data source of the GHDIF project. It is very important to attract healthcare providers to join the standardisation process. They care about the health outcome and cost-effectiveness. They also concern about the misinformation created by the GAI models, which may mislead the healthcare professionals into making wrong decisions. Besides, they care about whether the platform can relieve the workforce shortage. GHDIF needs to demonstrate how the project can benefit them and how it can improve the efficiency and reduce the costs.

- Life science/MedTech companies

The for-profit private companies hold most of the healthcare data. It is essential to attract them to join the standardisation and share their data. Most private companies may concern about data-sharing, because it may erode their profits in the long-term.

- Digital platform and potential competitors

There are some existing digital platforms utilising the GAI models, such as ChatGPT and Google Bard. They have very different market positioning. They concern about data-ownership and their market shares. They are actually potential collaborators if GHDIF can show clear different market targeting. To the best of my knowledge, there are currently no competitors in digital platforms targeting the broad global health system.

- Patients

Patients are the end-users of the healthcare products. They may concern about the data privacy and misinformation created by GAI models. They may refuse to share their data with the platform.

- Owners and shareholders

Shareholders wish the company to achieve a long-term growth. The owners concern more about their freedom to make decisions. Besides, transparency and governance are important factors for them to consider.

- Investors

The financial performance is their top priority to concern, as they are expecting to get a good return on investment. They also concern about the risk control.

Table 1. Stakeholder analysis matrix for GHDIF

Stakeholder	Impact (how much does the project impact them)	Influence (how much influence do they have over the project)	What is important to the stakeholder	How could the stakeholder contribute to the project	How could the stakeholder block the project	Strategy for engaging the stakeholder
Government	High	High	Health outcome, cost-effectiveness, sustainability and their voice.	Support the deployment of the GHDIF platform in their healthcare system.	Legally prohibit the project	1.Put their interests at the center place; 2.Take local legal system into considerations.
GHP agency	High	High	Efficiency, core ethical principles and sustainability	Contribute to the standardisation.	Against the deployment of the project	1.Show the benefit to them; 2.Minimise their concerns by collaborating with them.
Healthcare provider	High	Medium	Health outcome and cost-effectiveness	1.Share their data; 2.Contribute to the standardisation.	1.Do not use the platform; 2.Do not share their data.	1.Show the benefit to them; 2.Take their concerns into consideration for the standardisation process; 3.Liaise with UN to build the global health standard.
Life science /MedTech companies	Medium	High	Profit	1.Share their data; 2.Contribute to the standardisation.	1.Do not use the platform; 2.Do not share their data.	1.Find the benefit to them; 2.Liaise with UN to build the global health standard.
Digital platform	Medium	High	Data ownership	1.Share data 2.Collaboration	Stop collaborating with GHDIF	1.Clear regulation 2.Risk-sharing
Patients	High	Medium	Data privacy; bias; misinformation & wrong decision.	Share their data	Do not share their data	1.Enhance information privacy and security; 2. Ethical considerations and bias detection.
Owners and shareholders	N/A	High	Long-term growth of the company; independent decision-making	Regulate and manage the operation of company	Have conflicting opinions	Align the goals of owners and shareholders.
Investors	Medium	Medium	ROI; risk management	Provide funding	Withdraw investment	Find some ways to ensure the profit.
Competitors	N/A	N/A	N/A	N/A	N/A	N/A

The GHPs involve various stakeholders containing government, technology part, healthcare providers, payers, etc. The stakeholders are highly complicated, and they vary case by case as is shown in Table 2. For the diagnosis and risk identification, many stakeholders can benefit from the utilisation of AI. The power asymmetry is not very serious. Whereas, for the infectious disease, government plays the dominant role in the prediction and control of the disease spread, following by the global health agency, whose role is to liaise with various partners. Regarding the clinical trials, private industry plays a more central role in the partnership.

Table 2. GHP matrix for three different areas

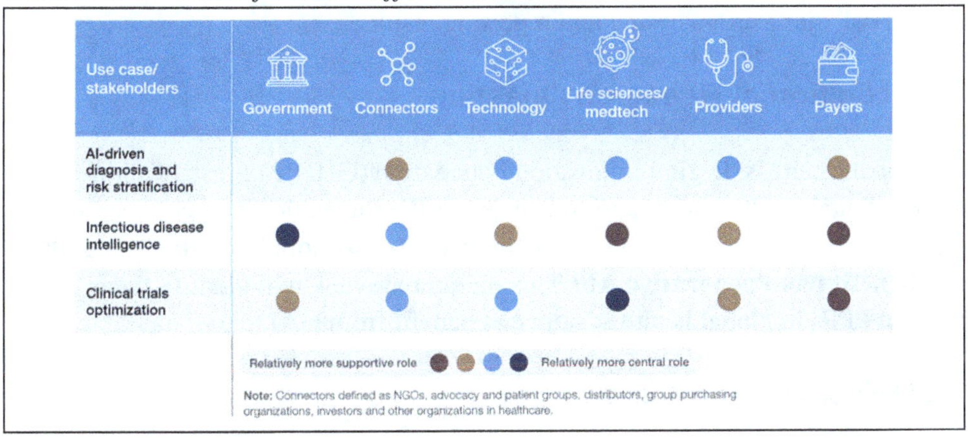

(World Economic Forum, 2023)

1.6 Problem Statement

PPPs are mainly popular in the traditional areas with less change and uncertainty (Ross & Yan, 2020), particularly focusing on a specific service or technology (Simcik Arese, 2018). However, PPPs are less capable to cope with the complex or dynamic situation, such as a new city/country based in a highly dynamic environment (Simcik Arese, 2018). The PPPs in global health exert plenty of issues, resulting in our fragmented, unco-ordinated and donor-driven GHPs. For example, conflicting goals among different partners, high institutional complexity and contextual shifts make a "one-size-fits-all" solution impossible to adopt. The GHPs are still lacking necessary standards and norms to connect the whole GHP process based on a coherent framework.

GHDIF is building a connected digital platform in global health exploiting the GAI models or LLMs, and GHDIF proposes that the platform ecosystem may support GHPs. However, there is no publication demonstrating how GHPs can benefit from the GAI models. There is a pressing need to do a literature review on the topic.

2. METHODOLOGY

This literature review is conducted based on the methodological framework of scoping review reported by Arksey & O'Malley (2005) and further improved by Levac et al. (2010). It contains 5 steps: (1) confirming the key question, (2) searching the relevant publications, (3) publication selection, (4) extracting/charting the data and (5) collating, summarising and reporting results.

2.1 Definition of Research Question

Global Health & Digital Innovation Foundation (GHDIF) is establishing a connected digital health ecosystem to accelerate the innovation and collaboration in global health. The key question is **in what aspects the global health partnerships can benefit from generative AI?** This literature review will identify the main aspects of PPPs in global health system can benefit from GAI.

2.2 Objectives and Aims

The above research question is separated into the four below sub-questions:

(1) how GAI can help analyse the contextual factors and partnership prerequisites;
(2) identify the ways that GAI can assist on structuring PPP projects;
(3) how the partnership practices, process and performance monitoring can benefit from GAI;
(4) how measurement of partnership outcome will be empowered by GAI.

The four sub-questions are formulated by the Partnership Analysis Framework in Figure 3a, which is selected as the only one framework designed to evaluate the performance of partnership on a holistic view (Kamya et al., 2017). The framework was originally developed from the causal chain analysis in systems theory as shown in Figure 3b (Brinkerhoff, 2002). The framework is further designed based on the specific indicator for each case, as it is highly contextual dependent (Charles & McNulty, 1999).

Figure 3. (a) Partnership Analysis Framework (Kamya et al., 2017); (b) Traditional causal chain theory (Brinkerhoff, 2002).

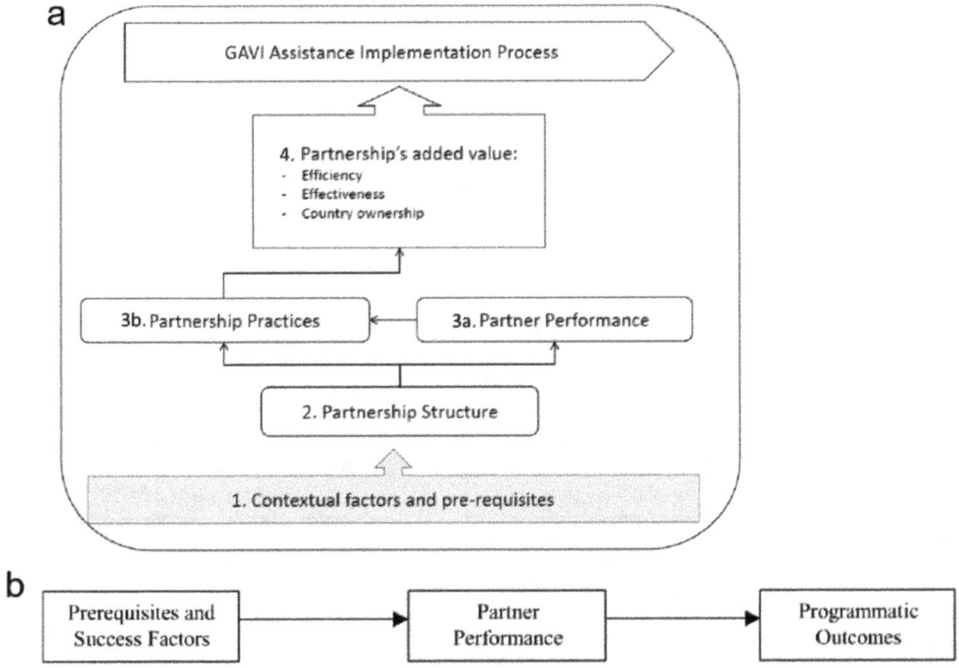

The benefits that GAI can bring will be summarised in the above 4 categories, namely contextual factors and partnership prerequisites, structuring PPP projects, partnership process & performance monitoring and the measurement of partnership outcome and value for stakeholders. Step 3a and 3b are merged into one sub-question.

2.3 Identification of Relevant Publications

Data Source

The relevant publications are selected by searching various data sources, including PubMed, Google Scholar and Web of Science.

Search Terms

The publication search contains 4 steps (Figure 4). The initial step combines the search terms from 3 concepts: public private partnership (PPP), generative artificial intelligence and global health. Each concept has multiple search terms as is shown in Table 3.

Figure 4. Flowchart of the literature review

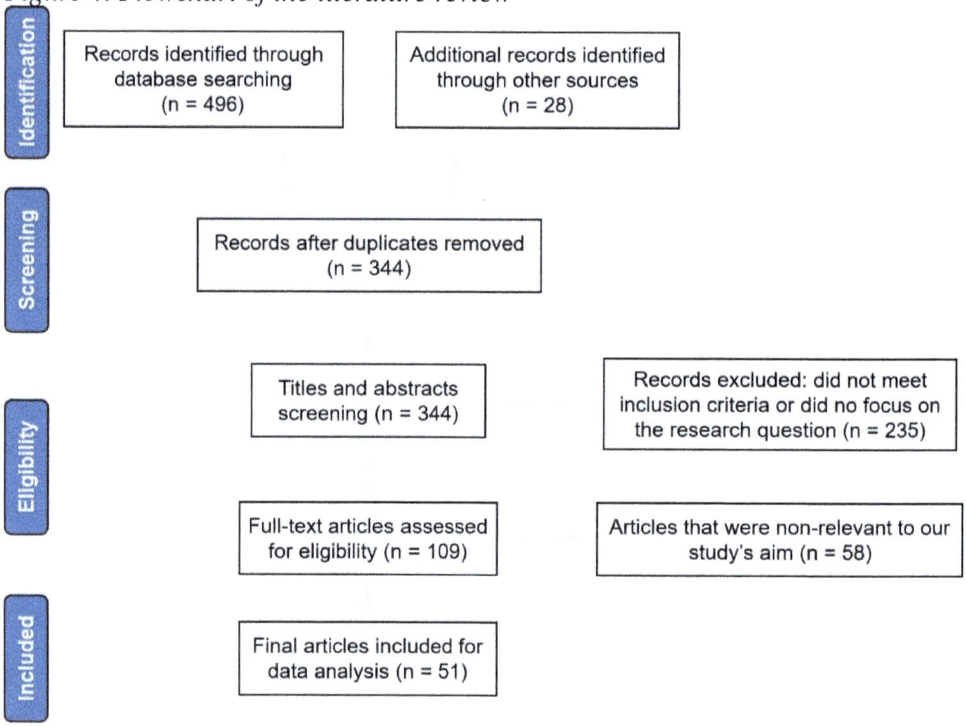

Table 3. Search terms

Search	Search terms
#1	"Public private partnership (PPP)" OR "Global public private partnership"
#2	"Global health" OR "International health"
#3	"Generative artificial intelligence" OR "Generative AI" OR "Generative adversarial networks" OR "Connected digital health" OR "Conversational AI" OR "Explainable AI" OR "Large language model (LLM)" OR "Chatbox" OR "ChatGPT"
#4	#1 AND #2 OR #1 AND #3 OR #1 AND #2 AND #3

2.4 Publication Selection

Publications were initially selected based on whether the studies reported the association among the 3 listed concepts in Table 3, namely PPP, GAI and global health. The research was conducted for "Title and abstract" in PubMed and Web of Science, as well as "Title" in Google Scholar. Only English written publications were included. No time constraints were set. The initial search delivered 496 papers, plus 28 additional papers obtained from other sources. After removing duplicates, 344 records remained. The publications were selected by 2 screening steps: (1) screening the title and abstract of above records, and (2) screening the full paper. The criteria were applied here: (1) the articles do not focus on public-private partnership (PPP) were discarded as "*off topic*"; (2) the records only focus on PPP, without discussing its relationship with global health or generative AI (GAI) were rejected as "*off scope*"; (3) the papers only touched the phenomenon involved in the PPP, but did not delve into the theory or practice of the association between PPP and global health or GAI. These records were retracted as "*off focus*". After the first level of screening, 109 publications were selected. After screening the full paper, 51 publications were included in the literature review.

2.5 Extracting the Data

All the 51 identified publications were read carefully, and the relevant information discussing the associations between "PPP and global health" or "PPP and GAI" was extracted. The key information related to the topic was summarised in Table 4 in Section 3.

2.6 Collating, Summarising and Reporting Results

The extracted information was collated, summarised and reorganised to answer the identified question. The findings were demonstrated using the Partnership Analysis Framework.

3. RESULTS

The identified 51 publications are summarised in a chronological sequence (Table 4). The key aspects in public-private partnerships (PPPs) in global health that can benefit from generative AI (GAI) are summarised below. How the whole process of PPPs can benefit from GAI is demonstrated at the beginning and followed by the four aspects of potential benefits, including (3.1) contextual factors and partnership prerequisites analysis, (3.2) structuring PPP projects, (3.3) partnership process & performance monitoring and (3.4) measurement of partnership outcome and value for stakeholders.

Table 4. Summary of key literature (n=51)

Author-year	Title	Relevant findings
Olliario (1997)	Will the fight against tropical diseases benefit from orphan drug status?	Serious competition among industry partners increases the opportunity costs.
Frost & Reich (1998)	Mectizan donation program: Origins, experiences, and relationships with co-ordinating bodies for onchocerciasis control	Representation in GHP may lack of neutral standpoint due to their funding source.
Tarabusi & Vickery (1998)	Globalization in the pharmaceutical industry, part I.	Serious competition among industry partners increases the opportunity costs.
Tarabusi & Vickery (1998)	Globalization in the pharmaceutical industry, part II.	Serious competition among industry partners increases the opportunity costs.
Dailami & Klein (1998)	Government support to private infrastructure projects in emerging markets	Public sectors need to attract the funds from private sector to relieve their financial pressure.
Buse & Walt (2000)	Global public-private partnerships: part I-a new development in health? Bulletin of the World Health organization.	The interagency competition significantly undermines the effectiveness of the GHP.
Buse & Walt (2000)	Global public-private partnerships: part II-what are the health issues for global governance?	1. The voice of weak partners and poor recipient countries is ignored; 2. Standardised guidelines that align public sector with the private industry are still under construction; 3. Building a connected digital ecosystem can help the UN regain a central role in the international policy-making; 4. Information asymmetry between public sectors and private industries is an issue in GHPs. 5. Legitimate representation, accountability and competence of PPP project are three key aspects to analyse in advance.
Casper (2004)	Updated discussion paper on the core business model of a mature global fund. in ninth board meeting of the Global Fund,	Poor alignment among different partners leads to plenty of repetitive work and waste.
Wildlife Conservation Society (2004)	One World, One Health: building interdisciplinary bridges to health in a globalized world.	Establishing a holistic approach to preventing epidemic / epizootic disease and for maintaining ecosystem integrity for the benefit of humans, their domesticated animals, and the foundational biodiversity that supports us all.
Kumar & Prasad (2004)	Public-private partnerships in urban infrastructure	It is impossible to directly transfer the findings of PPPs from one country to the others.
Caines et al. (2004)	Assessing the impact of global health partnerships	Private corporate and large global health foundations make a strong voice in the committee.

continued on following page

Table 4. Continued

Author-year	Title	Relevant findings
Jamali (2004)	Success and failure mechanisms of public private partnerships (PPPs) in developing countries: Insights from the Lebanese context	The GHPs require continuous setting standards and monitoring the whole PPP process.
Paris Declaration (2005)	Paris declaration on aid effectiveness: Ownership, harmonisation, alignment, results and mutual accountability.	Lack of harmonisation in the partnership procedures has delayed the GHP progress.
Conway et al. (2006)	Building better partnerships for global health	Limited domestic resources were diverted from national priorities, resulting in the national macroeconomic instability.
Bloomfield (2006)	The challenging business of long-term public-private partnerships: Reflections on local experience	PPP in global health requires highly complicated long-term contracts and multi-stage collaboration based in various institutionalised backgrounds.
Ruger (2009)	Global health governance and the World Bank	1. GHPs remain fragmented, unco-ordinated and donor-driven. 2. The value of GHP is thus diverted from the core value of WHO.
Steijn et al. (2011)	Public private partnerships: Added value by organizational form or management?	The efficient network management and monitoring exerts a significant impact on the PPP performance.
Stuckler et al. (2011)	Global health philanthropy and institutional relationships: how should conflicts of interest be addressed?	1. The conflicted goals and power-asymmetries made the GHPs significantly driven by private industries; 2. GHP narrowly targets a specific issue, rather than the wider global healthcare system
Ruckert & Labonté (2014)	Public-private partnerships (PPPs) in global health: the good, the bad and the ugly.	Both health determinants and the social determinants of health need to be considered for GHPs.
Boardman et al. (2015)	Comparative analyses of infrastructure public-private partnerships	Some relevant information is not accessible. This is deemed as a significant drawback in the healthcare PPPs.
Santandrea et al. (2016)	Value for money in UK healthcare public-private partnerships: A fragility perspective	Value for Money is a factor used in the assessment of PPP outcomes.
Wang et al. (2018)	Public-private partnership in Public Administration discipline: a literature review	1. The role of each partner may shift over time; 2. Efficiency and effectiveness are significant factors to evaluate PPP projects. 3. Beyond the technical indicators, governance is also considered as important factors.
Muinga et al. (2020)	Digital health Systems in Kenyan Public Hospitals: a mixed-methods survey	Many healthcare projects implementations are restricted by short of funds, due to the lack of trusts and no data-sharing policies.

continued on following page

Table 4. Continued

Author-year	Title	Relevant findings
Ross & Yan (2020)	Comparing public-private partnerships and traditional public procurement: Efficiency vs. flexibility	PPPs are popular in the traditional areas with less change and uncertainty.
Glukhikh et al. (2021)	Systems Engineering Methodology for Designing Digital Public-Private Partnership Platforms	The benefits of building an integrated digital platform: 1. Prevent overvalued capital and corruption schemes; 2. Avoid conflicting goals among partners; 3. Promote the communications among stakeholders; 4. Improve the efficiency and effectiveness of the implementation of healthcare projects; 5. Assist in goal alignments among stakeholders.
Kanabar et al. (2023)	The AI Revolution in Project Management: Elevating Productivity with Generative AI	Details how GAI can be directly applied to various stages of the project lifecycle and boost productivity.
Kar et al. (2023)	Unravelling the impact of generative artificial intelligence (GAI) in industrial applications: A review of scientific and grey literature	Maps the impact, themes, and challenges of GAI across a wide range of industries.
World Bank (2023)	Digital-in-Health: Unlocking the Value for Everyone	Definition of the structuring of PPP project.
World Bank Group (2023)	Structuring PPP Projects	Definition of the structuring of PPP project.
Akkem et al. (2024)	A comprehensive review of synthetic data generation in smart farming by using variational autoencoder and generative adversarial network	GAI can generate synthetic data based on the existing data; GAN present a powerful solution to data scarcity in agriculture.
Bainey, K. (2024)	AI-driven project management: Harnessing the power of artificial intelligence and ChatGPT to achieve peak productivity and success	GAI can facilitate the project monitoring and management. GAI can automate routine tasks, assist in risk identification and mitigation, optimise resource allocation, and improve stakeholder communication through automated and personalised updates.
de Haan et al. (2024)	Unstructured data research in business: Toward a structured approach	GAI can synthesise vast amounts of unstructured data from diverse sources, moving beyond ad-hoc analysis to a standardised process.
Hao et al. (2024)	Transforming assessment: The impacts and implications of large language models and generative AI	The role of GAI in assessment and measurement.
Khan et al. (2024)	WIP: Impact of Generative AI on Learning: Foci and Parameters for an Assessment Tool	The development of a structured assessment tool based on GAI to help educators measure outcomes.

continued on following page

Table 4. Continued

Author-year	Title	Relevant findings
Krugmann et al. (2024)	Sentiment analysis in the age of generative AI. Customer Needs and Solutions	GAI is revolutionising sentiment analysis by offering superior performance, new capabilities and new methodologies.
Papathanasiou et al. (2024)	Utilization of Generative AI for enabling knowledge contextualization among stakeholders for enhancing circularity in the construction industry	GAI is a key enabler for breaking down information silos.
Paramesha et al. (2024)	Enhancing resilience through generative artificial intelligence such as ChatGPT	GAI can bolster resilience by scenario planning, communication and knowledge management.
Thangaraj et al. (2024)	Cardiovascular care with digital twin technology in the era of generative artificial intelligence	GAI can help create highly personalised "digital twins" of a patient's heart by integrating various data.
Vallverdú (2024)	Generative AI and Causality. In Causality for Artificial Intelligence: From a Philosophical Perspective	GAI as a useful supplementary tool for generating plausible counterfactual hypotheses based on pattern recognition, but it is not a tool for causal reasoning This support requires human validation and the integration with formal causal methods.
van Breugel et al. (2024)	Synthetic data in biomedicine via generative artificial intelligence. Nature Reviews Bioengineering	GAI can generate synthetic data for biomedical research, without compromising patient privacy.
Wang (2024)	Prompts and large language models: a new tool for drafting, reviewing and interpreting contracts?	LLMs can facilitate drafting standard clauses, reviewing contracts, summarising lengthy documents, and interpret legal language.
Wolff (2024)	Preparing future lawyers to draft contracts and communicate with clients in the era of generative AI	Supports the use of GAI in legal practice in terms of legal contract drafting and analysis, regulatory compliance, due diligence, litigation, validation of interpretation; This support calls for human oversight.
Borowy (2025)	Generative AI as a Driver of Trust in Innovation	GAI build trust from an intangible feeling to a quantifiable and justifiable asset, thereby securing the investment necessary to drive innovation forward.
Cavadi (2025)	Strengthening resilience in healthcare organizations through an AI-enhanced performance management framework	GAI can help foresee potential crises and recommend actions; Use GAI to build more resilient healthcare organizations.
Cummins et al. (2025)	Beyond the Table: Insights on Negotiated Terms, Synthetic Scenario Simulations, and Future Competencies in Contract Management	Using GAI to analyse contract terms to identify trends, standards, and potential risks; Using GAI to create simulated negotiation scenarios and "what-if" analyses.
Demirel et al. (2025)	From optimism to concern: Unveiling sentiments and perceptions surrounding ChatGPT on Twitter	A social sentiment analysis of public perception using GAI.

continued on following page

Table 4. Continued

Author-year	Title	Relevant findings
Eapen & Finkenstadt, (2025)	Managing difficult conversations on new technology integration: the case of generative AI	GAI can support negotiation among complex stakeholders.
Li et al. (2025)	Generative AI empowered network digital twins: Architecture, technologies, and applications	GAI creates realistic simulations and scenarios, and optimise network behavior and configuration.
Taeihagh (2025)	Governance of generative AI	Governance of generative AI: Risks identification, concentration of power, etc.
te Marvelde (2025)	Designing LLM driven tools to support collaboration in complex multi-stakeholder systems	LLMs as mediation and facilitation tools to enhance mutual understanding and productive collaboration in complex environments.
Ulnicane (2025)	Governance fix? Power and politics in controversies about governing generative AI	A critical analysis of the power dynamics and political struggles inherent in the era of Generative AI.

PPPs in global health remain fragmented, unco-ordinated and donor-driven (Ruger, 2007). The conflicting goals and power-asymmetries made the global health partnerships (GHPs) significantly driven by private industries, narrowly targeting a specific issue or disease silos, rather than the wider global healthcare system (Stuckler et al., 2011). Moreover, the voice of weak partners is fully or partly ignored, which is against the value of globally equitable access (Buse & Walt, 2000b). The value of GHPs is thus diverted from the core ethical value of WHO and public sectors.

GHPs are characterised by long-term goals, very high institutional complexity and contextual shifts, which make a "one-size-fits-all" solution impossible to adopt. GHPs need to address not only health determinants, but also the social determinants based on the Gramscian conceptualisations of public/private (Ruckert & Labonté, 2014) and are also in line with One Health determinants of health (Wildlife Conservation Society, 2004). Unfortunately, GHP is still lacking necessary standards and norms to connect the whole PPP process in global health based on a coherent framework. In the context of Buse & Walt (2000b), such standardised guidelines that align the core ethical values promoted by the public sector with the private industry, are still under construction. The above issues call for the establishment of a connected digital ecosystem in global health, which can help the United Nations regain a central role in the international policy-making to achieve a universal, equitable health coverage. The details of the key aspects are presented below into 4 sub-sections.

3.1 Contextual Factors and Partnership Prerequisites Analysis

GHP progress is commonly delayed due to a lack of harmonised procedures (Paris Declaration, 2005) and poor alignment among different partners (Casper,

2004), leading to plenty of repetitive work and inefficiencies. The interagency competition also significantly undermines the effectiveness of the GHP (Buse & Walt, 2000a), while the serious competition among industry partners increases the opportunity costs (Olliario, 1997; Tarabusi & Vickery, 1998a; Tarabusi & Vickery, 1998b). Moreover, information asymmetries between the public and private sectors cause market failure in the GHPs. For example, public sectors perceive the market demand, while private industries might be unaware of the opportunity and hesitate to invest (Buse & Walt, 2000b). It calls for a transparent platform to equally share information among partners, in line with the ethical principles of World Health Organization (1999).

From a macroeconomic perspective, public sectors seek private investment to relieve the enormous financial pressure on the government (Dailami & Klein, 1998). It is still challenging to find suitable donors to guarantee a continued funding. Many healthcare projects implementations are constrained by short of funds, which is attributed to insufficient trusts among partners and the absence of data-sharing policies (Muinga et al., 2020). Attracting investment therefore requires a thorough investigation, analysis and prediction of the projects (Conway et al., 2006; World Bank, 2023). Additionally, many GHP projects initiated by private donors usually create plenty of siloed data and siloed implementations, which are not interoperable, further fragmenting the global health system.

GAI offers solutions to these challenges. It is capable to provide efficient environmental scanning and synthesise vast amounts of unstructured data from diverse sources (de Haan et al., 2024; Kar et al., 2023). In scenarios with insufficient data, GAI can generate synthetic data based on the existing data, without compromising privacy (Akkem et al., 2024; van Breugel et al., 2024). By mapping the stakeholder landscape, GAI can mediate conflicts, identify collaboration opportunities, and align divergent goals among various stakeholders (Papathanasiou, 2024; te Marvelde, 2025). The automatically generated synthetic data provide a comprehensive foundation for partnership prerequisites analysis, reducing information insufficiency. Beyond analysis, GAI provides a de-risk environment through scenario generation and creation of "digital twins", which can simulate partnership outcomes and foster collaborations (Li et al., 2025; Thangaraj et al., 2024). Besides, it can also help prevent overvalued capital and corruption schemes, which are considered as critical risks in GHPs (Glukhikh et al., 2021). By building a shared, comprehensive understanding of potential challenges and benefits, GAI can foster trust in investment (Borowy, 2025).

3.2 Structuring PPP Projects

Structuring PPP projects generally involves the outline of the whole project, including the technology intended to be used, the specification of output requirements, partner selection and the target customers, etc. (World Bank Group, 2023). Effective governance of the whole PPP project calls for the advance analysis of the three key aspects, containing legitimate representation, accountability and competence (Buse & Walt, 2000b). Representation in GHP should be selected carefully, since experts chosen from a certain profession may lack of neutral standpoint due to their funding source (Frost & Reich, 1998). Moreover, global health partners usually have different objectives, some of which are conflicted. It is still a challenge to align their goals under the core value of WHO and prevent the value from being eroded by any partner. The for-profit private corporates and large global health foundations sometimes make a strong voice in the committee (Caines et al., 2004), while the voice of recipient countries, particular the poor countries with inadequate infrastructure sometimes is neglected (Buse & Walt, 2000b). This can divert the limited domestic resources from national priorities, resulting in the national macroeconomic instability (Conway et al., 2006).

GAI can assist in structuring PPPs by drafting and analysing contracts, generating optimised project structures, and facilitating multi-stakeholder negotiation (Cummins et al., 2025; Papathanasiou, 2024; te Marvelde, 2025). These models have already been used for legal contract drafting and analysis, regulatory compliance, due diligence, litigation, validation of interpretation, etc. (Dwivedi et al., 2023; Wang, 2024; Wolff, 2024). It can also support the objective alignment and negotiation among complex stakeholders (Eapen & Finkenstadt, 2025). Building on the partnership prerequisites analysis outlined in Section 3.1, GAI can further create comprehensive partner profiles to facilitate partner selection and identify potential conflicts, thereby helping to avoid goal misalignment among partners (Glukhikh et al., 2021). By integrating each party's priorities, GAI can generate potential compromise frameworks and propose governance models that balance representation, thereby mitigating power imbalances and inequality among stakeholders (Taeihagh, 2025; Ulnicane, 2025).

3.3 Partnership Process & Performance Monitoring

According to a report from the *Bulletin of the World Health Organization*, the elements enable an effective PPP in global health remains unclear, highlighting an imperative to establish standards and norms by a systematic understanding of the whole PPP process (Buse & Walt, 2000b). Continuous setting standards and monitoring the whole partnership process are critical in the implementation of the

PPP (Jamali, 2004). Furthermore, PPP in global health requires highly complicated long-term contracts and multi-stage collaboration based in various institutionalised backgrounds (Bloomfield, 2006), making them distinct from the traditional areas with less change and uncertainty (Ross & Yan, 2020). Consequently, the goals and the context of GHP are highly dynamic, and partner roles may shift over time, necessitating frequent communication throughout the whole PPP lifecycle (Wang et al., 2018). Building an efficient network management and monitoring system thus exerts a significant impact on the PPP performance (Steijn et al., 2011).

A GAI platform can act as a central "knowledge pool," bridging information gaps across different types of data (Shefchek et al., 2020; Vasilevsky et al., 2020). The establishment of a connected and transparent digital system can promote the communications among different stakeholders and further solve the problems noted above (Glukhikh et al., 2021). Lack of accessibility to the relevant information is regarded as a significant drawback in the healthcare PPP based on a case study in Spain (Boardman et al., 2015). A further advantage that GAI can provide is analysing the content and tone of communications to perform sentiment and network analysis (Demirel et al., 2025; Krugmann & Hartmann, 2024). By continuously monitoring the project process and performance, and stakeholder communications, GAI can facilitate the project monitoring and management by automatically generating progress reports and highlighting potential risks (Bainey, 2024; Kanabar, 2023).

3.4 Measurement of Partnership Outcome and Value for Stakeholders

The measurement of GHP performance is highly complicated, partly due to the diversity of partnership types, which can be classified as goal-oriented, product-based, product development-based and issue/system-based (Buse & Walt, 2000b). GHPs need to ensure that private industries gain profit to incentivise continued innovation, while the outcome of the intervention should be measured systematically considering the wider global healthcare system. In addition, the globally equitable access is essential and cannot be diluted by any partners, and feedback from the recipient country should also be included in the measuring system.

Value for Money is a crucial assessment factor, encompassing costs, funds, risk sharing, timeframes, etc. (Santandrea et al., 2016). Efficiency and effectiveness are also significant metrics to evaluate PPP projects. Beyond these technical indicators, governance including engagement and accountability is equally important (Wang et al., 2018). The factors affecting the success of PPP performance are highly complicated and context related, making it impossible to directly transfer findings from one country to another (Kumar & Prasad, 2004).

A thorough evaluation containing both technical and governance parts is therefore necessary to identify context-specific factors exerting a significant impact on the PPP performance (Wang et al., 2018). Building a connected digital framework can facilitate the evaluation and measurement of the PPP outcomes. GAI can assess outcome and impact of the project based on the comprehensive database (Hao et al., 2024; Khan et al., 2024), improving the efficiency and effectiveness of healthcare project implementation (World Bank, 2023; Glukhikh et al., 2021). In addition, GAI model can generate counterfactual scenarios to answer the "What If?" questions (Vallverdú, 2024). It can continuously generate and compare multiple virtual scenarios incorporating not just the financial performance, determinants of health, but also broader social determinants of health, equity, and long-term systemic resilience, which are normally excluded from traditional evaluation methods (Cavadi, 2025; Paramesha et al., 2024). By comparing the real-world healthcare outcome with the simulated scenarios without this partnership, GAI provides a much richer and more comprehensive understanding of the value of the partnership.

4. DISCUSSION AND RECOMMENDATIONS

4.1 Discussion

The PPP in global health can neither be explained as the privatisation in neoliberal governance, nor as a new type of public health. The GHP should be understood as the rearrangement between private and public sector (Ruckert & Labonté, 2014). Public sector can utilise the expertise, resource and experience from private sector in some areas, such as product development, manufacturing, technology, marketing, etc. Whereas, it is not appropriate for the for-profit private sector to affect or decide the policy-making and regulatory approval for global health system based on the cautionary comment on PPPs from the WHO (Muula, 2006). Some governments or public sectors declared that they had no right to oversee the decisions made by the GHPs (Ruckert & Labonté, 2014). In this way, some countries even claimed that their government revenue was significantly reduced and the current global regulations are not in their favour (Bond, 1999; Ruckert & Labonté, 2014).

GHP involves multilateral stakeholders with different goals, and the voice from all the partners including the weak partners or the poor-country governments need to be considered. PPP in global health requires highly complicated long-term contracts and multi-stage collaboration based in various institutionalised backgrounds (Bloomfield, 2006), and the context and roles of partners may keep changing over time (Wang et al., 2018). In addition, process monitoring and evaluation are considered as overburdensome (Caines et al., 2004). The weak human resources system

(Caines et al., 2004) and large amounts of duty work for medical officers (Carlson et al., 2004) significantly reduced the efficiency of the GHP.

GAI models can potentially solve the above issues in GHPs. GAI models can facilitate GHP with structured communication, cooperation and engagement. It can support PPP project management by creating a structure of data and knowledge used for automating health informatics, routine tasks, generating progress reports, and facilitating collaboration among different stakeholders (Dwivedi et al., 2023). In addition, it can assist in planning, simulations, visualisations and forecasting, which improves overall efficiency, reduces the costs and wastes and enhances the success rate of partnerships (Alshuwaikhat & Abussaud, 2023). Besides, building a coherent digital platform can not only help in partners selection and resource allocation (Andres et al., 2017; Choy & Lee, 2002), but also assist in goal alignments (Glukhikh et al., 2021) and risk predictions (Tan et al., 2023). In this way, it is imperative to build a coherent, comprehensive, integrated and results-oriented system for the global health governance utilising the GAI models, which covers both health determinants and social determinants of health (Ruckert & Labonté, 2014).

4.2 Recommendations

4.2.1 Establish a Coherent Ontology

The findings support that the global health system need a coherent ontology aligning various ontologies including both health determinants and social health determinants. For example, Mondo ontology provides a structure of unifying various diseases together, which offers the possibility to extend relational query and inference across different ontologies (Shefchek et al., 2020; Vasilevsky et al., 2020). This is the foundation for the establishment of a coherent, integrated digital platform in global health system, exploiting the GAI models, Generative Adversarial Network models or large language models.

4.2.2 Standardisation in PPPs in Global Health

The findings indicate that the global health system still requires the necessary standards and norms to connect the whole GHP process based on a coherent ontological framework. The standardisation calls for the technological supports containing indicator identifications, monitoring and documentation systems, etc. This indicates that the GHP can benefit from the digital platform promoted by the GHDIF for connected innovation.

4.2.3 Cooperate With the United Nations

UN should take a central role in the standardisation process in global health. Cooperation with the UN can help UN regain a central role in the standardisation and legislation process. On the other hand, it can enhance the authority and legitimacy of the GHDIF digital platform. UN can also facilitate GHDIF to deploy its digital platform in the global health system, particularly in the private sectors and the healthcare providers based on the stakeholder analysis matrix (Table 1).

5. LIMITATIONS

This literature review aims to find evidence to identify the key aspects of the PPPs in global health that can benefit from GAI. Unfortunately, to the best of my knowledge there is few papers reported the association between GAI and PPPs in global health, as it is considered as a newly emerging area. I gathered the scientific evidence on the challenges of PPPs in global health and what benefits the GAI can bring. The limited number of data source is a limitation in this review.

This review is generated based on the publications reported full text in English. However, some studies published in other languages are not included in this report. Particularly, many studies in global health may publish in their local languages. This is considered as anther limitation.

Finally, this report does not systematically discuss the public panic about the widespread use of GAI models, including issues such as data privacy, bias, inequity in access, etc. It also does not include how to avoid negative side effects of GAI models from happening. This is considered as an important limitation.

6. CONCLUSION

This literature review aims to identify the key aspects in GHPs that benefit from GAI models, and generate recommendations to address them with the aim to promote the PPPs in global health. It generally contains 4 aspects, namely contextual factors and partnership prerequisites analysis, structuring PPP projects, partnership process & performance monitoring and measurement of partnership outcome and value for stakeholders. The findings support that the global health setting can benefit from the connected digital system proposed by GHDIF. This report offers 3 recommendations.

Firstly, establish a coherent ontology aligning various ontologies including both health determinants and social health determinants. Another key point is to build the necessary standards and norms to connect the whole GHP process based on a coherent ontological framework. Finally, cooperation with the United Nations can enhance the authority and legitimacy of the GHDIF digital platform. UN can also facilitate GHDIF to deploy its digital platform in the global health system, particularly in the private sectors and the healthcare providers.

The limited number of data source and restricted language source of the paper are regarded as the limitations of this study. Additionally, the literature review does not mention the ways to avoid negative side effects of GAI models from happening. Future studies should address these limitations.

6.1 Originality

To the best of my knowledge, there is few papers reported the association between GAI and PPPs in global health. This is the first paper reporting how PPPs in global health can benefit from the establishment of a connected digital system by the utilisation of GAI models or LLMs.

6.2 Significance

This report provides the scientific evidence on how global health system can benefit from building a connected digital system. It demonstrates how the fragmented, unco-ordinated and donor-driven GHPs can be converted into coherent, comprehensive and results-oriented patterns. The paper also bridges the gap among PPPs, global health and GAI models.

6.3 Rigour

This literature review is conducted based on a rigorous structure. The findings are supported by the sufficient scientific evidence and analysis, using an appropriate methodological framework. The Partnership Analysis Framework applied here is properly designed for the evaluation of the partnership relationships and outcomes on a holistic view.

REFERENCES

Ahmed, F., & Nisar, N. (2010). Public-private partnership scenario in the health care system of Pakistan, *EMHJ-. Eastern Mediterranean Health Journal, 16*(8), 910–912. DOI: 10.26719/2010.16.8.910

Akkem, Y., Biswas, S. K., & Varanasi, A. (2024). A comprehensive review of synthetic data generation in smart farming by using variational autoencoder and generative adversarial network. *Engineering Applications of Artificial Intelligence, 131*, 107881. DOI: 10.1016/j.engappai.2024.107881

Alshuwaikhat, H. M., & Abussaud, L. Z. (2023). *Generative urban design for smart, sustainable resilience cities, IAIA conference. Malaysia, 9-11 May*. International Association for Impact Assessment.

Andres, B., Poler, R., Camarinha-Matos, L., & Afsarmanesh, H. (2017). A simulation approach to assess partners selected for a collaborative network. *International Journal of Simulation Modelling, 16*(3), 399–411. DOI: 10.2507/IJSIMM16(3)3.382

Arksey, H., & O'Malley, L. (2005). Scoping studies: Towards a methodological framework. *International Journal of Social Research Methodology, 8*(1), 19–32. DOI: 10.1080/1364557032000119616

Babacan, H. (2020). Public-private partnerships for global health. In Haring, R., Kickbusch, I., Ganten, D., & Moeti, M. (Eds.), *Handbook of Global Health*. Springer International Publishing., DOI: 10.1007/978-3-030-05325-3_117-1

Bainey, K. (2024). *AI-driven project management: Harnessing the power of artificial intelligence and ChatGPT to achieve peak productivity and success*. John Wiley & Sons.

Bloomfield, P. (2006). The challenging business of long-term public-private partnerships: Reflections on local experience. *Public Administration Review, 66*(3), 400–411. DOI: 10.1111/j.1540-6210.2006.00597.x

Boardman, A. E., Greve, C., & Hodge, G. A. (2015). Comparative analyses of infrastructure public-private partnerships. *Journal of Comparative Policy Analysis, 17*(5), 441–447. DOI: 10.1080/13876988.2015.1052611

Bond, P. (1999). Globalization, pharmaceutical pricing, and South African health policy: Managing confrontation with US firms and politicians. *International Journal of Health Services, 29*(4), 765–792. DOI: 10.2190/4MA6-53E3-LE1X-C1YY

Borowy, M. (2025). Generative AI as a driver of trust in innovation. *Building Trust in the Generative Artificial Intelligence Era*, 53-66.

Bourgeois, D. M., Phantumvanit, P., Llodra, J. C., Horn, V., Carlile, M., & Eiselé, J. L. (2014). Rationale for the prevention of oral diseases in primary health care: An international collaborative study in oral health education. *International Dental Journal, 64*, 1–11. DOI: 10.1111/idj.12126

Breuer, J., Bishop, L., & Kinder-Kurlanda, K. (2020). The practical and ethical challenges in acquiring and sharing digital trace data: Negotiating public-private partnerships. *New Media & Society, 22*(11), 2058–2080. DOI: 10.1177/1461444820924622

Brinkerhoff, J. M. (2002). Assessing and improving partnership relationships and outcomes: A proposed framework. *Evaluation and Program Planning, 25*(3), 215–231. DOI: 10.1016/S0149-7189(02)00017-4

Buse, K., & Walt, G. (2000a). Global public-private partnerships: Part I-a new development in health? *Bulletin of the World Health Organization, 78*, 549–561.

Buse, K., & Walt, G. (2000b). Global public-private partnerships: Part II-what are the health issues for global governance? *Bulletin of the World Health Organization, 78*(5), 699–709.

Caines, K., Buse, K., Carlson, C., De Loor, R., Druce, N., Grace, C., Pearson, M., Sancho, J., & Sadanandan, R. (2004). *Assessing the impact of global health partnerships*. DFID Health Resource Centre.

Carlson, C., Druce, N., & Sadanandan, R. (2004). *Assessing the impact of global health partnerships. country case study report*. DFID Health Resource Centre.

Casper, T. (2004). Updated discussion paper on the core business model of a mature global fund, *Ninth board meeting of the Global Fund*. Arusha, 18-19 November. Geneva: The Global Fund.

Cavadi, G. (2025). Strengthening resilience in healthcare organizations through an AI-enhanced performance management framework. https://tesidottorato.depositolegale.it/handle/20.500.14242/187860

Charles, C., & McNulty, S. (1999). Partnering for results: assessing the impact of inter-sectoral partnering. Academy for Educational Development and United States Agency for International Development., https://pdf.usaid.gov/pdf_docs/Pnacd344.pdf, Retrieved October 15, 1999, from.

Choy, K., & Lee, W. B. (2002). A generic tool for the selection and management of supplier relationships in an outsourced manufacturing environment: The application of case based reasoning. *Logistics Information Management, 15*(4), 235–253. DOI: 10.1108/09576050210436093

Conway, M. D., Gupta, S., & Prakash, S. (2006). Building better partnerships for global health. *The McKinsey Quarterly*, •••, 1–8.

Cummins, T., Conrad, K., & Finkenstadt, D. (2025). *Beyond the table: Insights on negotiated terms, synthetic scenario simulations, and future competencies in contract management.*

Dailami, M., & Klein, M. (1998). *Government support to private infrastructure projects in emerging markets.* World Bank Publications.

de Haan, E., Padigar, M., El Kihal, S., Kübler, R., & Wieringa, J. E. (2024). Unstructured data research in business: Toward a structured approach. *Journal of Business Research, 177*, 114655. DOI: 10.1016/j.jbusres.2024.114655

Demirel, S., Kahraman-Gokalp, E., & Gündüz, U. (2025). From optimism to concern: Unveiling sentiments and perceptions surrounding ChatGPT on Twitter. *International Journal of Human-Computer Interaction, 41*(12), 7292–7314. DOI: 10.1080/10447318.2024.2392964

Dwivedi, Y. K., Kshetri, N., Hughes, L., Slade, E. L., Jeyaraj, A., Kar, A. K., Baabdullah, A. M., Koohang, A., Raghavan, V., Ahuja, M., Albanna, H., Albashrawi, M. A., Al-Busaidi, A. S., Balakrishnan, J., Barlette, Y., Basu, S., Bose, I., Brooks, L., Buhalis, D., & Wright, R. (2023). "So what if ChatGPT wrote it?" Multidisciplinary perspectives on opportunities, challenges and implications of generative conversational AI for research, practice and policy. *International Journal of Information Management, 71*, 102642. DOI: 10.1016/j.ijinfomgt.2023.102642

Eapen, T. T., & Finkenstadt, D. J. (2025). Managing difficult conversations on new technology integration: The case of generative AI. *Strategy and Leadership, 53*(2), 174–187. DOI: 10.1108/SL-07-2024-0062

Engel, N., & van Lente, H. (2014). Organisational innovation and control practices: The case of public-private mix in tuberculosis control in India. *Sociology of Health & Illness, 36*(6), 917–931. DOI: 10.1111/1467-9566.12125

Federspiel, F., Mitchell, R., Asokan, A., Umana, C., & McCoy, D. (2023). Threats by artificial intelligence to human health and human existence. *BMJ Global Health, 8*(5), e010435. DOI: 10.1136/bmjgh-2022-010435

Freedhoff, Y., & Hébert, P. C. (2011). Partnerships between health organizations and the food industry risk derailing public health nutrition. *Canadian Medical Association Journal, 183*(3), 291–292. DOI: 10.1503/cmaj.110085

Frost, L., & Reich, M. (1998). *Mectizan donation program: origins, experiences, and relationships with co-ordinating bodies for onchocerciasis control.* Harvard School of Public Health.

Ganguly, P., Jehan, K., de Costa, A., Mavalankar, D., & Smith, H. (2014). Considerations of private sector obstetricians on participation in the state led "Chiranjeevi Yojana" scheme to promote institutional delivery in Gujarat, India: A qualitative study. *BMC Pregnancy and Childbirth, 14*(1), 1–13. DOI: 10.1186/1471-2393-14-352

Gidado, M., & Ejembi, C. (2009). Tuberculosis case management and treatment outcome: Assessment of the effectiveness of Public-Private Mix of tuberculosis programme in Kaduna State, Nigeria. *Annals of African Medicine*, *8*(1), 25–31. DOI: 10.4103/1596-3519.55760

Glukhikh, I. N., Tolstolesova, L. A., & Arzikulov, O. A. U. (2021). Systems engineering methodology for designing digital public-private partnership platforms. *Applied System Innovation*, *4*(1), 1–13. DOI: 10.3390/asi4010004

Goth Itoi, N. (2022). Could stable diffusion solve a gap in medical imaging data? Stanford University., https://hai.stanford.edu/news/could-stable-diffusion-solve-gap-medical-imaging-data, Retrieved November 29, 2022, from.

Hao, J., von Davier, A. A., Yaneva, V., Lottridge, S., von Davier, M., & Harris, D. J. (2024). Transforming assessment: The impacts and implications of large language models and generative AI. *Educational Measurement: Issues and Practice*, *43*(2), 16–29. DOI: 10.1111/emip.12602

Imtiaz, A., Farooq, G., Haq, Z. U., Ahmed, A., & Anwer, S. (2017). Public private partnership and utilization of maternal and child health services in district Abbottabad, Pakistan. *Journal of Ayub Medical College, Abbottabad*, *29*(2), 275–279.

Jamali, D. (2004). Success and failure mechanisms of public private partnerships (PPPs) in developing countries: Insights from the Lebanese context. *International Journal of Public Sector Management*, *17*(5), 414–430. DOI: 10.1108/09513550410546598

Joudyian, N., Doshmangir, L., Mahdavi, M., Tabrizi, J. S., & Gordeev, V. S. (2021). Public-private partnerships in primary health care: A scoping review. *BMC Health Services Research*, *21*(1), 1–18. DOI: 10.1186/s12913-020-05979-9

Kamya, C., Shearer, J., Asiimwe, G., Carnahan, E., Salisbury, N., Waiswa, P., Brinkerhoff, J., & Hozumi, D. (2017). Evaluating global health partnerships: A case study of a Gavi HPV vaccine application process in Uganda. *International Journal of Health Policy and Management*, *6*(6), 327–338. DOI: 10.15171/ijhpm.2016.137

Kanabar, V. (2023). *The AI revolution in project management: Elevating productivity with generative AI.* Sams Publishing.

Kar, A. K., Varsha, P., & Rajan, S. (2023). Unravelling the impact of generative artificial intelligence (GAI) in industrial applications: A review of scientific and grey literature. *Global Journal of Flexible Systems Managment*, *24*(4), 659–689. DOI: 10.1007/s40171-023-00356-x

Khan, M. M., Ford, C., Dong, Y., & Afsarimanesh, N. (2024). *WIP: Impact of generative AI on learning: Foci and parameters for an assessment tool.* 2024 IEEE Frontiers in Education Conference (FIE), DOI: 10.1109/FIE61694.2024.10893560

Krugmann, J. O., & Hartmann, J. (2024). Sentiment analysis in the age of generative AI. *Customer Needs and Solutions*, *11*(1), 3. DOI: 10.1007/s40547-024-00143-4

Kumar, S., & Prasad, C. J. (2004). Public-private partnerships in urban infrastructure, *Kerala Calling*, 36-37.

Levac, D., Colquhoun, H., & O'Brien, K. K. (2010). Scoping studies: Advancing the methodology. *Implementation Science : IS*, *5*(1), 1–9. DOI: 10.1186/1748-5908-5-69

Li, B., & Akintoye, A. (2003). An overview of public-private partnership. In Akintoye, A., Beck, M., & Hardcastle, C. (Eds.), *Public-private partnerships: managing risks and opportunities*. Blackwell Publishing Ltd., DOI: 10.1002/9780470690703.ch1

Li, T., Long, Q., Chai, H., Zhang, S., Jiang, F., Liu, H., Huang, W., Jin, D., & Li, Y. (2025). Generative ai empowered network digital twins: Architecture, technologies, and applications. *ACM Computing Surveys*, *57*(6), 1–43. DOI: 10.1145/3711682

Lönnroth, K., Uplekar, M., Arora, V. K., Juvekar, S., Lan, N. T., Mwaniki, D., & Pathania, V. (2004). Public-private mix for DOTS implementation: What makes it work? *Bulletin of the World Health Organization*, *82*(8), 580–586.

Morley, J., DeVito, N. J., & Zhang, J. (2023). Generative AI for medical research. *BMJ (Clinical Research Ed.)*, *382*, 1551. DOI: 10.1136/bmj.p1551

Mudyarabikwa, O., & Regmi, K. (2016). Public-private partnerships and efficiency in public procurement of primary healthcare infrastructure: A qualitative research in the NHS UK. *Journal of Public Health (Berlin)*, *24*(2), 91–100. DOI: 10.1007/s10389-015-0701-8

Muinga, N., Magare, S., Monda, J., English, M., Fraser, H., Powell, J., & Paton, C. (2020). Digital health systems in Kenyan Public Hospitals: A mixed-methods survey. *BMC Medical Informatics and Decision Making*, *20*(1), 1–14. DOI: 10.1186/s12911-019-1005-7

Muula, A. S. (2006). Will Africa achieve the millennium development goals? *Croatian Medical Journal*, *47*(1), 194–196.

Newell, J. N., Pande, S., Baral, S., Bam, D., & Malla, P. (2005). Leadership, management and technical lessons learnt from a successful public-private partnership for TB control in Nepal. *The International Journal of Tuberculosis and Lung Disease : The Official Journal of the International Union against Tuberculosis and Lung Disease*, *9*(9), 1013–1017.

Olliario, P. (1997). Will the fight against tropical diseases benefit from orphan drug status? *Tropical Medicine & International Health : TM & IH*, *2*(2), 113–115. DOI: 10.1046/j.1365-3156.1997.d01-234.x

Papathanasiou, D. (2024). Utilization of generative AI for enabling knowledge contextualization among stakeholders for enhancing circularity in the construction industry.

Paramesha, M., Rane, N., & Rane, J. (2024). Enhancing resilience through generative artificial intelligence such as ChatGPT. DOI: 10.2139/ssrn.4832533

Paris Declaration. (2005). Paris declaration on aid effectiveness: ownership, harmonisation, alignment, results and mutual accountability, *High level forum on joint progress toward enhanced aid effectiveness: harmonization, alignment and results. 2nd high level forum on aid effectiveness*. Paris, 28 February-2 March. Paris: OECD Publishing.

Ramiah, I., & Reich, M. R. (2006). Building effective public-private partnerships: Experiences and lessons from the African Comprehensive HIV/AIDS Partnerships (ACHAP). *Social Science & Medicine*, *63*(2), 397–408. DOI: 10.1016/j.socscimed.2006.01.007

Rangan, S., Juvekar, S., Rasalpurkar, S., Morankar, S., Joshi, A., & Porter, J. (2004). Tuberculosis control in rural India: Lessons from public-private collaboration. *The International Journal of Tuberculosis and Lung Disease : The Official Journal of the International Union against Tuberculosis and Lung Disease*, *8*(5), 552–559.

Ross, T. W., & Yan, J. (2020). Comparing public-private partnerships and traditional public procurement: efficiency vs. flexibility. In Geva-May, I., Guy Peters, B., & Muhleisen, J. (Eds.), *Institutions and Governance in Comparative Policy Analysis Studies*. Routledge., DOI: 10.4324/9780429441622-9

Ruckert, A., & Labonté, R. (2014). Public-private partnerships (PPPs) in global health: The good, the bad and the ugly. *Third World Quarterly*, *35*(9), 1598–1614. DOI: 10.1080/01436597.2014.970870

Ruger, J. P. (2007). Global health governance and the World Bank. *Lancet*, *370*(9597), 1471–1474. DOI: 10.1016/S0140-6736(07)61619-5

Santandrea, M., Bailey, S., & Giorgino, M. (2016). Value for money in UK healthcare public-private partnerships: A fragility perspective. *Public Policy and Administration*, *31*(3), 260–279. DOI: 10.1177/0952076715618003

Shefchek, K. A., Harris, N. L., Gargano, M., Matentzoglu, N., Unni, D., Brush, M., Keith, D., Conlin, T., Vasilevsky, N., Zhang, X. A., Balhoff, J. P., Babb, L., Bello, S. M., Blau, H., Bradford, Y., Carbon, S., Carmody, L., Chan, L. E., Cipriani, V., & Osumi-Sutherland, D. (2020). The Monarch Initiative in 2019: An integrative data and analytic platform connecting phenotypes to genotypes across species. *Nucleic Acids Research*, *48*(D1), D704–D715. DOI: 10.1093/nar/gkz997

Sheikh, K., Porter, J., Kielmann, K., & Rangan, S. (2006). Public-private partnerships for equity of access to care for tuberculosis and HIV/AIDS: Lessons from Pune, India. *Transactions of the Royal Society of Tropical Medicine and Hygiene*, *100*(4), 312–320. DOI: 10.1016/j.trstmh.2005.04.023

Silow-Carroll, S. (2008). *Iowa's 1st five initiative: Improving early childhood developmental services through public-private partnerships*. Commonwealth Fund.

Simcik Arese, N. (2018). Seeing like a city-state: Behavioural planning and governance in Egypt's first affordable gated community. *International Journal of Urban and Regional Research*, *42*(3), 461–482. DOI: 10.1111/1468-2427.12601

Steijn, B., Klijn, E. H., & Edelenbos, J. (2011). Public private partnerships: Added value by organizational form or management? *Public Administration*, *89*(4), 1235–1252. DOI: 10.1111/j.1467-9299.2010.01877.x

Stuckler, D., Basu, S., & McKee, M. (2011). Global health philanthropy and institutional relationships: How should conflicts of interest be addressed? *PLoS Medicine*, *8*(4), e1001020. DOI: 10.1371/journal.pmed.1001020

Taeihagh, A. (2025). Governance of generative AI. *Policy and Society*, *44*(1), 1–22. DOI: 10.1093/polsoc/puaf001

Tan, T. F., Thirunavukarasu, A. J., Jin, L., Lim, J., Poh, S., Teo, Z. L., Ang, M., Chan, R. P., Ong, J., Turner, A., Karlström, J., Wong, T. Y., Stern, J., & Ting, D. S.-W. (2023). Artificial intelligence and digital health in global eye health: Opportunities and challenges. *The Lancet. Global Health*, *11*(9), e1432–e1443. DOI: 10.1016/S2214-109X(23)00323-6

Tarabusi, C. C., & Vickery, G. (1998a). Globalization in the pharmaceutical industry, part I. *International Journal of Health Services*, *28*(1), 67–105. DOI: 10.2190/7JDR-2TFN-2B3X-TYF5

Tarabusi, C. C., & Vickery, G. (1998b). Globalization in the pharmaceutical industry, part II. *International Journal of Health Services*, *28*(2), 281–303. DOI: 10.2190/B6VR-NND7-46BL-PY5G

te Marvelde, K. (2025). Designing LLM driven tools to support collaboration in complex multi-stakeholder systems, MS Thesis, Delft University of Technology, Delft, Netherlands, 2025.

Thangaraj, P. M., Benson, S. H., Oikonomou, E. K., Asselbergs, F. W., & Khera, R. (2024). Cardiovascular care with digital twin technology in the era of generative artificial intelligence. *European Heart Journal*, *45*(45), 4808–4821. DOI: 10.1093/eurheartj/ehae619

Tredinnick, L., & Laybats, C. (2023). The dangers of generative artificial intelligence. *Business Information Review*, *40*(2), 46–48. DOI: 10.1177/02663821231183756

Ullah, A. N. Z., Huque, R., Husain, A., Akter, S., Islam, A., & Newell, J. N. (2012). Effectiveness of involving the private medical sector in the National TB Control Programme in Bangladesh: Evidence from mixed methods. *BMJ Open*, *2*(6), e001534. DOI: 10.1136/bmjopen-2012-001534

Ulnicane, I. (2025). Governance fix? Power and politics in controversies about governing generative AI. *Policy and Society*, *44*(1), 70–84. DOI: 10.1093/polsoc/puae022

Uplekar, M. (2016). Public-private mix for tuberculosis care and prevention. What progress? What prospects? *The International Journal of Tuberculosis and Lung Disease : The Official Journal of the International Union against Tuberculosis and Lung Disease*, *20*(11), 1424–1429. DOI: 10.5588/ijtld.15.0536

Vallverdú, J. (2024). Generative AI and causality. In *Causality for Artificial Intelligence: From a Philosophical Perspective* (pp. 55–61). Springer., DOI: 10.1007/978-981-97-3187-9_6 van Breugel, B., Liu, T., Oglic, D., & van der Schaar, M. (2024). Synthetic data in biomedicine via generative artificial intelligence. *Nature Reviews Bioengineering, 2*(12), 991–1004. DOI: 10.1038/s44222-024-00245-7

van Heerden, A. C., Pozuelo, J. R., & Kohrt, B. A. (2023). Global mental health services and the impact of artificial intelligence-powered large language models. *JAMA Psychiatry, 80*(7), 662–664. DOI: 10.1001/jamapsychiatry.2023.1253

Vasilevsky, N., Essaid, S., Matentzoglu, N., Harris, N. L., Haendel, M., Robinson, P., & Mungall, C. J. (2020). Mondo Disease Ontology: Harmonizing disease concepts across the world. *CEUR Workshop Proceedings, 2807*, 1–2.

Wang, B. T. (2024). Prompts and large language models: A new tool for drafting, reviewing and interpreting contracts? *Law. Technology and Humans, 6*(2), 88–106. DOI: 10.5204/lthj.3483

Wang, H., Xiong, W., Wu, G., & Zhu, D. (2018). Public-private partnership in public administration discipline: A literature review. *Public Management Review, 20*(2), 293–316. DOI: 10.1080/14719037.2017.1313445

Wildlife Conservation Society. (2004). *One World, One Health: building inter-disciplinary bridges to health in a globalized world, One World One Health. The Rockefeller University, 29 September*. Wildlife Conservation Society.

Wolff, K. (2024). Preparing future lawyers to draft contracts and communicate with clients in the era of generative AI. *Transactions: The Tennessee Journal of Business Law, 25*(3), 8.

World Bank. (2023). *Digital-in-health: unlocking the value for everyone*. Washington, DC: World Bank Publications. https://openknowledge.worldbank.org/handle/10986/40212 (Accessed 18 August 2023).

World Bank Group. (2023). *Structuring PPP projects*. Public-Private Partnership Legal Resource Center. https://ppp.worldbank.org/public-private-partnership/structuring-ppp-projects (Accessed 23 May 2023).

World Economic Forum. (2023). *Scaling smart solutions with AI in health: unlocking impact on high potential use cases*. Geneva: World Economic Forum. https://www.weforum.org/reports/scaling-smart-solutions-with-ai-in-health-unlocking-impact-on-high-potential-use-cases/#:~:text=26%20June%202023-,Scaling%20Smart%20Solutions%20with%20AI%20in%20Health%3A%20Unlocking,on%20High%20potential%20use%20cases&text=The%20healthcare%20sector%20is%20grappling,potential%20to%20tackle%20these%20issues (Accessed 26 June 2023).

World Health Organization. (1978). Declaration of Alma-Ata, *primary health care: report of the International Conference on Primary Health Care*. Alma-Ata, 6-12 September. Geneva: WHO Press.

World Health Organization. (1999). *WHO guidelines on collaboration and partnerships with commercial enterprises*. WHO Press.

Zafar Ullah, A., Newell, J. N., Ahmed, J. U., Hyder, M., & Islam, A. (2006). Government-NGO collaboration: The case of tuberculosis control in Bangladesh. *Health Policy and Planning*, *21*(2), 143–155. DOI: 10.1093/heapol/czj014

Chapter 3
Overview of Telemedicine in Central Africa, Specifically in Democratic Republic of Congo

Samuel Kajama Tshikuta
http://orcid.org/0009-0004-6949-0623
Coppin State University, USA

A. K. Sharadhi
http://orcid.org/0000-0002-9412-1449
University of Arizona, USA

ABSTRACT

Technology through telemedicine makes it possible to conduct efficient interventions that contribute to narrowing health inequalities conditioned by various geopolitical aspects. Most central African countries, including the Democratic Republic (DR) of Congo, experience a shortage of healthcare professionals, especially in rural regions. This is caused by the non-advancement of technology, poor infrastructure, electricity outages, and the limited number of graduate students enrolling in medical institutions. To minimize this impact, telemedicine is used and implemented in some areas to facilitate easy access to healthcare. Even though telemedicine was booming during COVID-19, there are still areas of imbalance, especially in central African countries. The purpose of this research is to bring more insight into the complete adoption of telemedicine in DR Congo healthcare systems.

DOI: 10.4018/979-8-2600-2238-2.ch003

INTRODUCTION

The importance of healthcare services, promoting well-being, preventing illnesses, caring for the sick, reducing pain, and looking after people with disabilities is globally accepted. Yet, for decades, the healthcare system has been facing problems such as inequity, cost, and quality. Indeed, these are some of the reasons for telemedicine. DR Congo is constantly growing and evolving. Telemedicine represents the hope for the healthcare system. With the implementation of telemedicine, the DR of Congo will be able to foster immediate care for under-representative patients, facilitate ongoing medical monitoring for patients, reduce the cost of labor, and break the waiting time in hospitals and medical centers (Blandford et al., 2020). Despite the promises of telemedicine, its implementation remains slow due to the electricity outages, lack of financial support, and internet problems. These are the major challenges to telemedicine. Moreover, only rich and average people have access to good healthcare services, which exposes a substantial proportion of the population to diseases and premature death. This is one of the reasons that pushes adults in rural regions to trust more traditional medicine than the modern medical system.

Telemedicine helps healthcare professionals provide care to patients while being in their residences, and this was proven to be effective in reducing the cost of labor, reducing the time of consultations (Omboni et al., 2022), Other attributes of telemedicine have been seen in balancing work life and increasing the number of patients being consulted with simple interfaces. Some studies certified the utility of telemedicine as timesaving, and the cost of travel has been significantly reduced (The American Telemedicine Association, ATA 2017 Telehealth 2.0 Conference Abstracts, 2017b). Half of the patients who were consulted using video-consultation were satisfied with the timing; 5 to 10 minutes was enough to complete a medical consultation, and because of this, they were ready to reuse telemedicine for the long term. There are many advantages to telemedicine, such as: saving, cost-effectiveness, and reduced time to travel.

This research seeks to provide evidence of the resistance to telemedicine adoption in DR Congo and how socioeconomic, cultural, and technological aspects influence patients' acceptance of telemedicine.

Review of Telemedicine

Telemedicine, which is the practice of providing healthcare remotely, might feel like a new concept, fueled by the internet and sophisticated communication technologies. However, the concept of delivering care at a long distance has deep roots, going far before the initiation of smartphones and high-speed internet. So, tracing the historical perspective of telemedicine reveals an interesting evolution, driven by innovation, necessity, and an ultimate desire to overcome geographical barriers to access (Jagarapu & Savani, 2021). This establishes a parallel between implementation and adoption of telemedicine. As of now, DR Congo is in the process of implementing this tool in the medical system, so understanding what was done decades ago can serve as a template and therefore help save time and reduce cost.

Pre-Digital Era

Telemedicine was born out of sheer practicality. In the late 19th century, telephone lines were rapidly adopted, and medical professionals recognized the potential of telemedicine. Rural communities, struggling with limited access to healthcare, started using telephones to get treatment from specialists residing in Urban areas. This was true, particularly in remote regions of Australia, where the royal family flew in a doctor to provide specific services. These initiatives were slow to be implemented, but invaluable. They displayed the fundamental principle of telemedicine: emphasizing technology to bridge between patients and providers, especially in situations where physical consultation was impossible (Abouzid et al., 2022).

The mid-20th century produced advancements in television technology, opening new opportunities for remote healthcare. Universities and hospitals started experimenting with closed-circuit television to facilitate medical consultations, education, and remote monitoring within their reach. The University of Nebraska Medical Center pioneered the use of interactive television to establish a connection with patients in rural health centers (Abouzid et al., 2022).

The Digital Era

The internet and digital technologies have changed telemedicine in the late 21st century. The advent of the internet and digital technologies revolutionized telemedicine. A platform to secure real-time communication was provided by the World Wide Web to enable the development of sophisticated telemedicine platforms. Video conferencing, Email, and remote monitoring devices became accessible at an affordable price, which facilitated rapid, widespread integration into remote health systems (Abouzid et al., 2022).

METHODOLOGY

A literature review method was utilized for this research to assess the implementation, barriers, and potential of telemedicine, specifically in DR Congo. This research consists of reviewing the comprehensive synthesis of existing data on telemedicine. The selection of sources of information was based on the year of publication, peer-reviewed articles of the past two decades, journals from local and international institutions, and book chapters were the main sources of information. A comprehensive search strategy was developed using databases such as Web of Science, Google Scholar, ResearchGate, and Parlet Moore Library.

Inclusion and Exclusion Criteria

Inclusion

- Studies on telemedicine implemented in Central Africa.
- Research on hurdles and constraints to telemedicine adoption in regions.
- Research published in peer-reviewed journals, conference proceedings.

Exclusion

- Studies focused on regions other than African countries.
- Studies that failed to address the impediments to telemedicine implementation.
- Research published in Spanish.

Telemedicine is categorized into three types: Remote monitoring, Real-time interactive, and Store and Forward. They are categorized based on when the information is being forwarded (WHO, Regional Office for Africa, 2025).

1. Store and Forward

This is a strong and powerful means to deliver healthcare services, especially in the underserved areas with limited access to medical professionals. It allows healthcare providers to obtain data such as lab reports, screening results, and images and transfer it to another region for evaluation. Store and forward does not require both side of providers to be present at the same time. What exactly is Store-and-Forward? It is a data transmission method where an intermediate device (router, switch, server) receives a complete data packet, stores it temporarily, and then forwards it to the next destination (Kontaxakis et al., 2006). For instance, in rural territories, a general physician or specialist can obtain a biopsy and send it to another provider operating in an urban region for evaluation. When the process of evaluating the sample is completed, the results are sent back to the sender (Kruse et al., 2018). This telemedicine consists of storing data like bio-signals and clinical imagery after receiving them from patients being forwarded. The medical record of patients is an essential element to make this process complete, and it is worthy noting that the sender and the receiver are communicating at the same time, except when the sample is sent for evaluation. Certain departments in the hospital, such as Pathology, Radiology, and Dermatology, utilize this sort of telemedicine most of the time (World Health Organization, 2016). In Democratic Republic of Congo where many providers are serving in urban regions, Store and forward can bridge the gap, maintaining the connection between physicians and patients. It is also a way to prioritize health equity to make healthcare services efficient for everyone

2. Real-time interactive services

This is a vital feature of telemedicine, allowing healthcare professionals and patients to have a live chat or talk using audio calls, video conference. It is a replica of face-to-face consultation through which healthcare services are provided, decisions are taken, immediate interaction between two parties, and clinical evaluations are interpreted (Kruse et al., 2018). In territories with not enough access to medical infrastructure, such in DR Congo, these features can be of a huge importance in the nation. The Real-time interactive services involve instant interaction between physicians and clients, obtaining medical history, consultation, follow-up, and discussion of the management plan. Meaning, patients' satisfactions are enhanced because of the immediacy that provide this method of telemedicine, and this lead to quick interventions especially for acute conditions. For patients with chronic illnesses, regular checkups minimize the need to travel for hours, helping in saving time and money while promoting wellness through consistent monitoring. Real-time telemedicine minimizes the risks that come with physical touch for both patients and healthcare workers. Maintaining low latency is essential for practical user experience (Aljohani, 2023). Real-time telemedicine requires robust infrastructure, optimized network connections, and careful consideration of geographical factors. Moreover, security is of huge importance, especially when dealing with sensitive data.

3. Remote Monitoring

This method is also called remote patient monitoring (RPM), this branch of telemedicine is swiftly evolving to allow medical professionals to track clients' health information outside the traditional health centers or clinics. This is particularly effective for patients with chronic diseases such as diabetes, hypertension, asthma, COPD, and heart diseases can be managed using this sort of telemedicine. Wearable devices, mobile apps enable physicians to monitor blood glucose, heart rate, and oxygen levels. The key power of remote monitoring emphasizes improving patient convenience and clinical outcomes. Rather than waiting for the long queue of in-person appointments, feedback is provided to client spontaneously and tailored care recommendations are suggested based on the ongoing data (Krick et al., 2019). In countries like the Democratic Republic of Congo, where challenges to infrastructure and geography often limit access to medical professionals, this sort of telemedicine offers a reliable solution. This connects the urban medical systems to residents in villages in order to maintain continuous monitoring for the wellbeing of everyone. Combining existing local telemedicine platforms with RPM can truly facilitate the detection of complications to patients using wearable devices. It is worth noting that individuals can monitor themselves and notify physicians of any sudden change. The chances of getting false clinical results are so high (Kontaxakis et al., 2006).

CATEGORIES OF TELEMEDICINE AND BENEFITS

Teleradiology

Teleradiology is one of the most transformative fields of telemedicine. This type of telemedicine refers to sending or transferring radiology images that include CT, MRI, X-rays, and PET scans from one hand to the other. Tele radiology application represents half of the proportion of all sorts of telemedicine in both synchronous and asynchronous (Kontaxakis et al., 2006). With the advancement of technology, those who review clinical images can remotely access them. In Lualaba, which is a mineral province in DR Congo, clinics and hospitals lack specialists who can play a leading role in the evaluation process of patients' clinical results (Adambounou et al., 2024). Such a situation might mislead professionals in diagnosing patients and worsening their conditions. Clinics and hospitals that lack radiology department or radiologists can still maintain the workflow efficiently by sending out diagnostic images to specialists elsewhere for a possible diagnosis. This not only minimizes waiting time but also ameliorate the clinical outcomes by facilitating rapid diagnose and treatment (Thrall et al., 2020). And thus, this telemedicine plays an essential role in these types of situations to maintain the well-being of patients. Moreover, teleradiology works best in collaboration with other teams, allowing radiologists of different institutions to review a clinical case and come up with a solid possible diagnosis, not forget that in case of emergency, teleradiology is needed provide rapid interpretation of clinical images in order to save lives.

Despite the challenges that teleradiology faces, such as the data privacy, licensure procedures, cost-effectiveness and efficacy of telemedicine, some other features are needed to transmit the radiological images, including video conference tools, software, and hardware. The cost of teleradiology poses a huge problem as the government is not funding the establishment of this type of telemedicine (Ryu, 2012). Apart from this, recent research by Fuentes (2003) showed that the issues of patient information, security, and confidentiality, and qualitative training must be tackled to facilitate a successful integration of tele radiology in Central Africa.

Teledermatology

This is a growing field of telemedicine that helps dermatologists to provide remote medical services to clients through telecommunications tools. It plays an essential role in addressing the needs of clients living in areas with limited access to medical services. Chanussot-Deprez and Contreras-Ruiz (2013) demonstrated that various skin issues are being evaluated and treated with the help of telecommunication technology; this has been demonstrated with enough benefits. In countries such as DR Congo and other low- resource regions, tele dermatology is utilized to link patients to their specialists. This can lead to Patients' satisfaction in terms of waiting time in the hospital or medical centers, and transportation. Moreover, the usage of real-time interaction and store-and-forward has satisfied dermatologists with their effectiveness and accurate diagnosis. However, there is still doubt about how to remotely manage cancer. A recent study stated that diagnosing cancer remotely (teledermatology) comes with less accuracy as compared to clinical diagnosis.

Telecardiology

This is another branch of telemedicine that particularly emphasizes the diagnosis and management of cardiovascular diseases using digital technology. This type of telemedicine includes three areas: Pre-admission, during the hospital stay, and after (Molinari et al., 2017). The first phase has shown efficacy in providing treatment to remote patients, especially those suffering from heart problems, or supporting healthcare providers in making decisions. In comparison, teleconsultation that involves ECG imageries requires a brief time to be completed, and a patient with ST elevation (Myocardial infarction) will be identified at a higher speed, which in turn reduces sudden death rates (Terkelsen et al., 2002). When patients' data are transmitted from real-time or store forward department, telecardiology closes the gap between a specialist and a primary healthcare provider. For instance, a doctor working in a village can upload an ECG on a secure platform, and on the other hand, a cardiology specialist will review the case and provide suggestions and treatment plans (Scalvini et al., 2020). This prevents unnecessary referral of patients and speed up the diagnosis process, thus reducing the healthcare cost and ameliorates patients' satisfaction.

In-hospital applications used telecardiology, referring to the real-time echocardiogram transmissions in tertiary care centers and rural minor hospitals, especially for diagnosis purposes. In addition, a few studies have shown the effectiveness of post-hospital telecardiology in improving outcomes and decreasing visits of patients, especially those with arrhythmia, heart failure, or implanted devices.

Telepathology

This branch of telemedicine allows healthcare providers to examine cell and tissue samples through digital telecommunication technologies. Africa suffers from a shortage of pathologists; it has been proven that an African specialist in the field of pathology covers up to 500,000 individuals or even more. In developing countries, the number exceeds five hundred thousand people per pathologist (Adesina et al., 2013). This form of telemedicine will reduce the strain on pathologists and make virtual meetings an asset, as this telecommunication requires less time to meet needs. In the U.S, telepathology is defined as the interaction between clients and their physician, and this enables the transfer of clinical data and images of different procedures, including but not limited to diagnosis, histology interpretation, and opinion from a second consultant (Evans et al., 2015). Congo needs this.

Telepsychiatry

This is also called telemental health. It is noteworthy to mention that mental health is still a big challenge worldwide since the knowledge or education on mental illnesses is growing. The usage of telemedicine can be of huge importance in mental science in helping with therapies (individual, group, and family), medication management, educating patients, and follow-ups for individuals living in rural areas (Malhotra et al., 2013). Many of the psychiatry applications are using synchronous (real-time interaction). In a country such as the USA, telepsychiatry is considered one of the most utilized forms of telemedicine because the rate of mental illness is significant (Yellowlees et al., 2010). Telepsychiatry has been effective in the assessment and treatment of mental diseases. One of the greatest benefits of this branch of telemedicine is its easy way to minimize barriers that relate to mobility, stigma and regions. Patients who are not comfortable travelling long distances are now served by this means. Telepsychiatry was a key solution in maintaining the ongoing monitoring of patients with anxiety, depression, and other form mental disorders during the Covid-19 pandemic (Shore et al., 2020).

APPLICATIONS IN DR CONGO

The democratic Republic of Congo, a rich nation in Central Africa is facing barriers in meeting the needs of its population and in delivering the required health-care services.

Hospitals and medical centers in the country have incorporated Telemedicine applications, and here is a concise list of some of the available telemedicine applications (International Telehealth Projects | UVA Health, n.d.).

CongoRx

This platform offers online medical consultations, allowing patients to access quality care without leaving their homes. This is not just another telemedicine application; it is a complete healthcare system made to meet the unique needs of the Democratic Republic of the Congo and its population. Here is the impact that CongoRx is making in the country (Congo Medika RDC, n.d.):

Vision

The platform envisions providing and making accessible quality healthcare to everybody, in the urban and rural areas. Strategies are implemented to overcome geographical barriers and resource constraints. The CongoRx team is committed to bridge the gap between clients and physicians or specialists, ensuring timely, dependable, and effective medical services.

Modes of consultation

Video consultations: this connects patients to the physicians and specialists
Clinic visits: patients schedule in person appointments at medical center or hospital
Home visits: Doctors visit patients in their homes

Available Specialties

Neurology, Cardiology, Psychiatry, Geriatrics, Family medicine, Endocrinology, Pain management

Consultation Fee and Payment Options

Physicians and consultants at CongoRx set their own rate which depends on the type of consultation and services provided. Doctors are also paid based on years of experience. As of now, the easy means of payment on the platform is M-Pesa, which enables clients to make an online payment or transfer money . However, the organization has a plan to incorporate Airtel Money and Debit/Credit cards to facilitate payments.

Why is CongoRX different?

CongoRx is not just another telemedicine app; it is a comprehensive healthcare ecosystem designed to meet the unique needs of the DRC and its people. Here is what sets them apart:

This platform is not just like any other telemedicine application. It has an ecosystem that is comprehensive and specifically made to meet the needs of the country and its communities. A backup system is available to ensure that personal information is well-secured and protected; there are strong security and privacy measures in place to prevent breaches from happening (CongoRX I Consultation Vidéo Médecins Locaux Internationaux, n.d.).

1. Global Research: This platform connects healthcare professionals with their patients not only in the country but all over the world. This can be useful for patients seeking opinions from international specialists.
2. Pharmaceutical Partnership: The platform works in collaboration with local and international pharmacies that enable patients to place an online order and receive the package at their doorstep.
3. User-friendly interface: This application is well-designed to keep, store, and secure patient information. It has an easy and friendly interface to navigate, which enables people to access it with limited clicks. Easy navigation and clear interfaces reduce the odds of medical errors, misinterpretation of data, or invalid data entry.
4. Insurance integration: The platform works closely with the main insurance companies in the country to make healthcare more accessible and affordable to all. The platform has a plan to incorporate the insurance service into the application to simplify the complexities of health coverage. This will help reduce overspending and make healthcare more accessible, especially in underserved locations. Moreover, patients and healthcare professionals will easily track the utilization of insurance and make the reimbursement process less complex.
5. ISO-certified data center: The ISO-certified Data Center is utilized to host patients' data; this is to ensure that the information is well-secured and stored in a good environment. Possessing the ISO certification means this application meets rigorous universal standards in terms of data security and management.

6. HIPAA compliance: CongoRx understands the crucial importance of health data privacy, which is why CongoRx is compliant with HIPAA. HIPAA sets strict standards for the protection of patients' data in the United States, and the commitment to these standards ensures that the health information is treated with the utmost care and integrity.

Practitioners at CongoRX believe that a successful therapeutic relationship requires trust, which is true. The platform is committed to ensuring that patients' information is lawfully accessed, and only a limited number of professionals deal with the governmental and sensitive data. Therefore, people should be at peace knowing that security and privacy are maintained (Congo Medika RDC, n.d.).

Congo Medika

The population in DR Congo benefits from this platform, and the lower price of home healthcare services enables individuals to meet with their physicians. Kinshasa is the first place where these services are available. The futuristic goal of this App is to provide services to nearby cities and countries (Congo Medika RDC, n.d.).

The Congo Medika application is available on the Apple-Store and Google Play. Receiving requests for medical care at home is one of its functionalities from multidisciplinary medical providers. The team consists of twenty nurses, six lab technicians, four physiotherapists, and one hundred and ten doctors from different towns. The main goal of this platform is to establish a physician per family.

There are policies to follow while using this App before initiating home medical care. The medical team must evaluate the condition of the patient to ensure there's no evidence of an existing life-threatening condition that requires close attention. Now that a life-threatening condition has been dismissed, home care is recommended for the patient. This care does not present a considerable risk; it is always important to check on the infection/contamination risk levels that are present in the environment and people around the patient (Congo Medika RDC, n.d.).

As stated, the platform is functional in Kinshasa, it provides affordable services with a multidisciplinary team. Congo Medika is one of the first Apps to offer remote services to Congolese residents. In 2019, a conference was held by the scientific research institution. The ministries of Industry, Innovation, and Invention. The Congo Medika was selected among the best; it is compliant and follows ethical regulations to ensure efficient clinical development of patients.

Every drug purchased is traceable on the App before placing the order; the client must upload an identity and justify the reason for the purchase. There are some exceptions where the bill is found on the prescription slip; all patients are advised to upload a photo of the prescription with the physician's stamp.

Available Services

Homes Healthcare visits
Health Education
Medication delivery
Direct communication
Pricing

Congo Medika focuses on the quality of services provided to patients. A video consultation with physicians, price varies based on the condition and services provided to patients. The price for a general consultation varies between $10 and $50.

Targeted Medical Issues

Primary healthcare, malaria, infectious diseases, maternal/child health, cardiovascular diseases, cancer, mental health, emergencies, and access to quality medicine/pharmacy.

Synwell

This platform enables people to have online consultations and schedule appointments with their medical providers.

Sophia (2023) stated that the limited number of trained medical professionals, improper infrastructure, and poor access to decent medical services are the serious issues that residents are facing; because of these reasons, the rate of infection and mortality is extremely high in the country.

DR Congo is among countries with high infant mortality and morbidity rates worldwide, and life expectancy is short (Vakaniaki et al., 2024). In addition to malnutrition, which remains one of the leading causes of death, there are numerous diseases, epidemics, and infections. Illnesses, if left untreated, kill thousands of people every day. It is noteworthy that there are high rates of low digital literacy, lack of trust, lack of information, and lack of resources that lead people to consult unqualified local professionals for a possible medical solution. Traditional medicine is well-respected and widely used, which has led rural residents to self-medication and therefore increased the mortality rate (Sophia, 2023).

On the other hand, healthcare providers have few solutions to meet the needs of patients. Doctors, nurses, radiologists, pathologists, and all other healthcare professionals lack the knowledge to operate modern technologies. The infrastructure to support telemedicine is poor, electricity is not dependable. These are preventing the country from experiencing the full potential of novel tech.

This platform was launched to fight major medical killers in the country. The main objective of Synwell is to make available an easily accessible, secure, and equitable system in the DR Congo, where every individual can be consulted at a low cost (Sophia 2023).

How Does This Work?

To start with, a few clicks to register for a consultation. First, get the app from the Google Play Store or the Apple store. Once this step is completed, create an account. Patients have access to a range of services on the platform, to locate a specialist, an advanced search is to be done, and Synwell is well-equipped with healthcare professionals ready to serve (Sophia 2023).

H J Hospital

This Hospital is one of a kind. It is a well-known hospital in DR Congo that offers services to diagnose diseases. This setting has digital equipment for two purposes (VFMatch, n.d.):

- Adding various departments to the medical center
- Making telemedicine consultation possible

This hospital is one of the first to provide an EMR (electronic medical record), a telemedicine application that enables individuals to go through virtual consultations with healthcare providers. Additionally, medicine can be ordered on this platform, and all reports are found on the patient portals (HOPS Healthcare, 2021)

CHALLENGES

In underserved region where a nearest clinic is at hundreds of kilometers, pregnant women travel this long distance to receive prenatal care, along this long journey, accidents are inevitable causing the rate of maternal mortality and morbidity to increase. To bridge the gap between patients and their healthcare professionals, telemedicine is an option.

The pandemics have posed multifaceted challenges for hospitals. Healthcare systems and medical practitioners were overburdened to tackle the outbreak. Amidst the challenging times, the hospital wanted to upgrade to an EMR system that could integrate all departments and deal with the crisis at hand. It faced a two-pronged challenge (VFMatch, n.d.):

- To integrate telemedicine into the existing healthcare system
- To provide patients with access to doctors through telemedicine consultation.

To reduce the strain on healthcare professionals and prevent the staff and patients from catching the infection, telemedicine ought to be implemented, especially in rural areas where having access to quality healthcare is a big challenge (HOPS Healthcare, 2021). It is important to mention that the strain on doctors is due to the insufficient number of professionals to treat patients.

IMPACT

More than 20.000 patients have access to their electronic records. With an easily accessible application, after clients are screened, the clinical imagery results are discussed through video consultation. This hospital has incorporated all the required departments, hardware, and software that make the exchange of information from one system to the other via Health Level 7 (HL7) and a HIPAA-compliant system. This was useful, especially during the pandemic; patients' needs were met (HOPS Healthcare, 2021).

Why Should People Use Telemedicine in DR Congo?

Telemedicine comes with numerous benefits in a Congolese context, especially in improving access to healthcare in underserved regions and building a framework of trained healthcare professionals. Telemedicine in the DR Congo could represent a major asset, as far as the population is concerned. In Africa, and particularly in the Democratic Republic of Congo, access to health care remains a significant challenge. Adults in rural areas face barriers such as limited time to meet a physician, and they lack financial resources to afford a consultation (Sophia 2023).

Several Individuals share a brief time of consultation, making this difficult for the patient to completely express their concerns. There is a need for longer, more personalized conversations between healthcare providers and patients to ensure that client needs are sufficiently met. Telemedicine would also be beneficial for DR Congo, in the sense that individuals will be able to remotely access it on time and have regular follow-ups without constantly travelling.

Sophia (2023) also mentioned that to be seen by a doctor is not cheap, and not every individual in the country can afford a consultation. This is one of the reasons that leads people to solely rely on traditional medicine rather than seeking advice from educated and well-trained doctors.

Pregnant women in underserved regions must travel for miles to reach a nearby hospital, this is just for a follow-up. While travelling, many accidents have been registered, and this has increased the proportion of premature birth, maternal death, and infant mortality rate in the whole country (VFMatch, n.d.).

CHALLENGES OF TELEMEDICINE IN DR CONGO

A quick reminder, Democratic Republic of Congo is the second largest countries in Africa, one of the richest countries in the world with natural resources such Copper, Diamont, Coltan, Uranium, and many more. Still the country has limited infrastructure, and an ongoing shortage of medical professionals exposing average and poor individuals to either traditional medicine or self-treatment.

The reasons that prevent people from welcoming telemedicine are many:

Culturally, many people in the Democratic Republic of Congo are reticent to adopt digital healthcare. Digital breaches have become a trend; individuals are increasingly cautious about sending their confidential health information on an online platform, so sharing individual health information with a person using the internet is not reassuring (Mehta et al., 2024).

Psychological features also play a key role. Some people think meeting and facing a doctor in the face or being examined by physical touch contributes to a placebo effect in healing. As a result, consulting an online doctor who cannot examine by physical touch is a problem to many individuals. This is a major problem because many residents are still comfortable using traditional medicine; with that being said, physical touch is crucial (Kumari et al., 2022).

The fear of running into untrained and unqualified practitioners who can prescribe medicine that can be harmful. Due to a lack of training, some healthcare professionals have been misdiagnosing people and prescribing medicines that, instead of improving the state of people's condition, made them worse (Ayat et al. 2024). The Socioeconomic challenges delay the adoption of telemedicine. To be consulted, patients must already have a phone with access to the internet, but also the means to afford a stable connection. The country itself does not have stable and reliable internet, and the cost is exorbitant; therefore, it poses a barrier to telemedicine (Ayat et al. 2024).

Finally, the proportion of illiteracy is significantly vast. Only educated people master the term telemedicine and its potential. To address this problem, welfare programs should be implemented to make sure the leaders of clans receive specific tailored training, involving them in the process will boost residents' trust, therefore facilitating the process of implementation (Adong et al., 2024).

IMPACT OF TELEMEDICINE APPLICATION ON HEALTH SYSTEMS IN AFRICAN COUNTRIES

The table provides the outcomes on written scientific papers that emphasized the impact and the capacity that telemedicine has built to strengthen healthcare systems across African countries.

Table 1. Impact of Telemedicine in African Countries

Author(s) and Year of Publication	**Title**	**Research Method**	**Outcome of healthcare systems**
Abouzid et al. (2022) West Africa / north Africa	Telemedicine applications in North/West Africa areas: advantages and barriers encountered.	A literature review of medical related papers was conducted; the main databases consisted of Google scholar, PubMed	- Despite the inability of Telemedicine to replace the in-person consultations, its implementation can still meet the needs of underserved individuals in rural regions. - It is also noteworthy that telemedicine still is a tool that healthcare providers can utilize for ongoing medical consultation and scientific research.
Alboraie et al. (2021) Northeast Africa	Egypt: barriers of Telemedicine, and the application of knowledge a local survey	Among the Egyptian men and women, a cross-sectional method was conducted: list of questions	- The population is well educated on the use of Telemedicine. Additionally, many Egyptians attribute positive outcomes to Telemedicine and are fully willing to use it for a long term.
Alphol et al. (2019) West Africa	Senegalese doctors provide their opinion on the implementation of Telemedicine.	In 2014, from January to June, Men and Women participated in interviews conducted by doctors: Descriptive Method. This study consisted of thirty-seven doctors serving in the health centers sector, thirty-two doctors serving in public medicals, and most importantly the outcome of the interviews was recorded and securely stored and coded for future use.	- The conducted research provide clarity on how Senegalese doctors think about the use of Telemedicine and its benefits in the underserved regions, such a facility is useful in improving access to quality healthcare services and minimize the cost of labor.

continued on following page

Table 1. Continued

Author(s) and Year of Publication	Title	Research Method	Outcome of healthcare systems
Maia et al. (2019) Portugal and African countries (Portuguese language)	How to establish a strong and sustainable telemedicine program? Operations of Telecardiology for children: exploratory study	An assessment was conducted in public environment to evaluate to track the effectiveness of telemedicine, this brought clarity on the crucial elements to successfully implement and sustain telemedicine in the regions to meet individual needs.	- This study affirms that a solid and reliable telemedicine program depends on the motivation of workers, the commitment and support from local and international bodies. - Future research prospects should focus on keeping an eye on the development of technology, most importantly the modern ones such as the usage of apps.
M.M et al. (2022) South Africa	South Africa: a survey was conducted on the use and impact of Telemedicine by physicians in the neighbor region: KwaZulu.	A survey by 143 healthcare providers was done while serving in twenty-two medical centers. Cross sectional	- The advantages of instantly responding to messages must maintain the balance in keeping the security and confidentiality of patients' information, this should comply with privacy regulations to maintain clients' records.
Todd et al. (2018)	Addiction case: the implementation and impact of telemedicine to patients with addiction.	Cross sectional: A survey on telemedicine, benefits of technology, utilization, and adoption in institutions.	- There is a need for the result to be improved, reducing the number of sudden deaths. Telemedicine could be one of the keys to responding to and addressing these issues or at least provide another means to deliver remote services and maintain health equity.
Ncube et al. (2023) Southern Africa	Opinions and behaviors of healthcare providers and patients regarding the implementation and use of telemedicine in southern Africa Botswana Exploratory study	Multiple surveys (questions, interviews) were conducted using an exploratory method on clients and doctors, nurses, clinicians, and therapists. the questions were both open and closed-ended	- These outcomes fit well for implementing telemedicine. Well-tailored strategies to initiate the digital Health in Botswana, this will help the rapid adoption of telemedicine and the use of apps in the country.

continued on following page

Table 1. Continued

Author(s) and Year of Publication	Title	Research Method	Outcome of healthcare systems
Odhiambo & Mars (2018) East Africa	Patients' understanding of telemedicine terms required for filling and signing documents when translated into Kiswahili	An approximate of forty computerized terms and terminologies were utilized while providing explanation on telemedicine when patients were signing documents for approval. Translation was required to make the process simple for residents, the language of choice was Kiswahili.	- Language is the main barrier that prevents the adoption of telemedicine. Innovative ideas and solutions are required to tackle these issues, if not addressed this process will fail to meet patients' needs, and filling and signing the consent documents requires understanding. - Specific program should be implemented to help reduce the proportion of illiteracy. Moreover, simplifying the process of signing and filling documents will benefit both healthcare providers and clients.
Onsongo et al. (2023) Eastern Africa	Kenya: the outcome on the usages and challenges of telemedicine in healthcare system	Cross sectional: this study was done using a self-web with questions to individuals in different regions. The web was shared through email	- This study demonstrates that Kenyan physicians and other healthcare workers are well informed about the utility and benefits of telemedicine. As of now the main goal of telemedicine in Kenya is to support medical consultations and make sure the needs of patients are met. Although this has been of huge significance, there are still areas of improvement.
Tchao et al. (2019) Western Africa	On Telemedicine Implementations in Ghana	Peer review papers, articles and journals were collected to analyze the data on the implementation on telemedicine in the healthcare system of Ghana. The objective of collecting literature was to have enough information on how well telemedicine added to the current healthcare system.	- This paper presented the number of telemedicine applications being used in Ghana. All the applications being active in Ghana are being discussed in this paper. Nevertheless, some of the papers lack elements in how these telemedicine applications were implemented.

continued on following page

Table 1. Continued

Author(s) and Year of Publication	Title	Research Method	Outcome of healthcare systems
Scott et al. (2005) West Central Africa	Cameroon: There is a need of an assessment on the digital health on men and women	A real-life situation series of questions were developed to collect relevant data. Exiting datas were reviewed using a simple survey method	- A telemedicine solution was introduced based on low cost to improve and maximize the effectiveness of mobile phone use, authorizing easy access to medical records and allowing the transfer of clinical images to respond to the needs of residents, and this should firstly be implemented. - in the underserved regions of Cameroon
Vincent et al. (2019) Southeast Africa	Uganda: An assessment was conducted on medical professionals on how ready they are with telemedicine services	Facilities of a public healthcare: a descriptive and cross-sectional study was done in Uganda. A random sampling was taken on both northern and western localities of Uganda.	- The readiness on the adoption of telemedicine was displayed differently by each healthcare provider, this is because of their role, specialty, and number of years of experience. Adoption of telemedicine was easily completed in the administration facility and the referral centers. Although physicians that serve in the administration are shown to be ready with telemedicine, they lack knowledge on the use and benefits, and no service was initiated. These factors need attention. Moreover, Nurses, clinicians, radiologists, physiotherapists, and other allied healthcare workers should be evaluated for readiness.

RECOMMENDATIONS

I worked as a student nurse at Prakriya Hospital in the city of Bengaluru (India). Telemedicine was the perfect key solution that facilitated ongoing healthcare services as well as reduced infection risk. The average men and women in India are well educated on telemedicine, which has helped the rapid adoption of telemedicine throughout the country. The price for a remote consultation is affordable to all, and English was not the only language that was utilized; Kannada, Hindi, Urdu, and Malayalam were among the best languages in meeting patient needs. Individuals with Chronic illnesses such as cardiovascular diseases, diabetes, psychiatric disorders, respiratory disease, and even pregnant women obtain excellent quality of healthcare services through Telemedicine. Lukas et al. (2020) demonstrated that during the pandemic, telemedicine was a key success in maintaining the cycle of medical follow-ups. Some countries, such as Ghana and Kenya, have implemented this technique in monitoring and providing remote treatment, which reduces the load on hospitals and healthcare professionals. Learning from these countries can help DR Congo gain time and make sound decisions.

Partnerships and Training

Governments should collaborate with NGOs and private sector players to foster an environment that will encourage telemedicine to grow. By using available resources and expertise, stakeholders will address infrastructure gaps and, therefore, promote awareness about the proper usage and efficacy of Telemedicine. Intelligent investment in training programs for healthcare professionals on digital health technologies can equip them with the knowledge and skills to utilize Telemedicine effectively and confidently. Training on telemedicine should be incorporated into medical student curricula to make them familiar with the operation of technology, and for this to be realistic, international collaborations with developed nations such USA and Australia are required to enforce these trainings in central African countries, especially in the Democratic Republic of Congo. Some studies from countries such as Ghana, Nigeria, South Africa, and even Kenya suggested regular and supervised training. Additionally, the number of specialists in the field has negatively affected the practice of telemedicine. Thus, regular training is of high significance to equip healthcare professionals and patients with skills and awareness by increasing the efficacy of technology usage.

Regulatory Body

The government should be involved in the process of integrating telemedicine into healthcare systems, which will remove the strain on individuals (private investors) and healthcare providers. The absence of a clear regulatory body slows the integration of telemedicine into the existing medical system. The government should establish comprehensive legislation to address fundamental issues. Moreover, healthcare professionals of different specialties should be able to follow a clear scope to ensure quality of care and prevent medical errors. Developing a strong policy and framework for virtual consultations and incorporating telemedicine into the curriculum of medical students to make them familiar with the system.

Mobile Applications Initiative

The rapid adoption of mobile phones provides a pathway for innovative mobile health ideas that facilitate the transfer of healthcare information, teleconsultation, and monitoring of health statuses in real time. Schoolap, a mobile app that was developed and launched in DR Congo (internet free) to bridge the gap in the education system, can be considered for healthcare services to help both patients and health workers to easily navigate healthcare systems easily. CongoRx and H J Hospital have implemented these techniques despite facing challenges due to a lack of trust among patients and healthcare professionals.

Technology and Infrastructure

In Western Africa, countries such as Nigeria and Ghana, the designs of telehealth applications are simple and user-friendly, and support both patients and healthcare providers. Implementing this feature in the medical system of DR Congo will enable even uneducated patients to easily navigate the system and maintain contact with their healthcare providers. Reliable internet is the solid foundation of telemedicine. Providing appropriate and adequate infrastructure is essential for health technology. For instance, Providers should incorporate real-time monitoring in underrepresented regions to boost patients' trust, as this connects them to both healthcare providers and specialists. Furthermore, it will reduce doubt among individuals on telemedicine, thus facilitating rapid adoption. The government must also invest in extending partnerships with some existing telecom companies, such as Airtel, Vodacom, Orange, and Africell, to help provide stable, ongoing internet at low cost. Another aspect of the infrastructure is the power supply and equipment that must be powerful and consistent in supplying energy, not limited to urban regions, but also rural areas. The government can also invest in solar systems that provide stable electricity to hospitals and medical centers that utilize telemedicine. Moreover, equipment such as incubators, computers, printers, and diagnostic machines is needed for a successful telemedicine consultation.

CONCLUSION

Telemedicine represents a beacon of hope for healthcare delivery in the Democratic Republic of Congo. With a considerable number of factors delaying its implementation, the ongoing advancement of technology provides a compelling opportunity for healthcare reform. By working on these barriers head-on through collaborative efforts and strategic investment, Central African countries, specifically the DR Congo, can harness Telemedicine's potential to produce a more equitable and effective healthcare delivery system for all. Resilience, innovation, and commitment will be the cornerstones on which a brighter healthcare future can be built. The literature review played a key role in displaying to what extent telemedicine has been useful in Central Africa, to be precise in DR Congo, and exposing the areas that require improvement.

The services provided by telemedicine, including teleconsultation, teledermatology, telepsychiatry, and telecardiology, have been efficient in improving the delivery of healthcare services, precisely during the pandemic when physical consultation was a big challenge. Moreover, the overall integration of telemedicine is not complete due to the challenges mentioned. Telemedicine has indeed seen light in nearby countries; therefore, making this easy to access will facilitate rapid change and maximize treatment in underserved areas.

REFERENCES

Abouzid, M. R., Elshafei, S. M., Elkhawas, I., & Elbana, M. K. (2022). Applications for telemedicine in the Middle East and North Africa region: Benefits gained and challenges faced. *Cureus, 14*(7), e26611. Advance online publication. DOI: 10.7759/cureus.26611 PMID: 35936169

Adambounou, K., Farin, F., Boucher, A., Adjenou, K. V., Gbeassor, M., N'dakena, K., Vincent, N., Adesina, A., Chumba, D., Nelson, A. M., Orem, J., Roberts, D. J., Wabinga, H., Wilson, M., Adong, G., Odoyo, C., & Ondulo, J. (2024). Factors influencing the successful implementation of eHealth in healthcare facilities in developing countries: A scoping review. Journal of Science. *Innovation and Creativity, 3*(2), 8–17.

Alboraie, M., Allam, M. A., Youssef, N., Abdalgaber, M., El-Raey, F., Abdeen, N., Mahdy, R. E., Elshaarawy, O., Elgebaly, A., Haydara, T., Abd-Elsalam, S., Nassar, Y. A., Shabana, H., & Zaky, S. (2021). Knowledge, applicability, and barriers of telemedicine in Egypt: A national survey. *International Journal of Telemedicine and Applications, 2021*, 5565652. Advance online publication. DOI: 10.1155/2021/5565652 PMID: 34211550

Aljohani, A. M. (2023). Barriers and challenges to adopting telemedicine in Saudi Arabia.

Bhaskar, S., Bradley, S., Chattu, V. K., Adisesh, A., Nurtazina, A., Kyrykbayeva, S., Sakhamuri, S., Yaya, S., Sunil, T., Thomas, P., Mucci, V., Moguilner, S., Israel-Korn, S., Alacapa, J., Mishra, A., Pandya, S., Schroeder, S., Atreja, A., Banach, M., & Ray, D. (2020). Telemedicine across the globe—Position paper from the COVID-19 Pandemic Health System Resilience PROGRAM (REPROGRAM) International Consortium (Part 1). *Frontiers in Public Health, 8*, 556720. Advance online publication. DOI: 10.3389/fpubh.2020.556720 PMID: 33178656

Blandford, A., Wesson, J., Amalberti, R., AlHazme, R., & Allwihan, R. (2020). Opportunities and challenges for telehealth within, and beyond, a pandemic. *The Lancet. Global Health, 8*(11), e1364–e1365. DOI: 10.1016/S2214-109X(20)30362-4 PMID: 32791119

Chanussot-Deprez, C., & Contreras-Ruiz, J. (2013). Telemedicine in wound care. *Advances in Skin & Wound Care, 26*(2), 78–82. DOI: 10.1097/01.ASW.0000426717.59326.5f PMID: 23337648

Congo, R. X. | Consultation vidéo Médecins locaux internationaux. (n.d.). https://www.congorx.com/

Congo Medika, R. D. C. (n.d.). https://congomedika.com/

Dodoo, J. E., Al-Samarraie, H., & Alsswey, A. (2022). The development of telemedicine programs in Sub-Saharan Africa: Progress and associated challenges. *Health Technology (Hong Kong)*, *12*(1), 33–46. DOI: 10.1007/s12553-021-00626-7 PMID: 34849325

Evans, A. J., Krupinski, E. A., Weinstein, R. S., & Pantanowitz, L. (2015). 2014 American Telemedicine Association clinical guidelines for telepathology: Another important step in support of increased adoption of telepathology for patient care. *Journal of Pathology Informatics*, *6*(1), 13. Advance online publication. DOI: 10.4103/2153-3539.153906 PMID: 25838965

Fuentes, A. (2003). Remote interpretation of ultrasound images. *Clinical Obstetrics and Gynecology*, *46*(4), 878–881. DOI: 10.1097/00003081-200312000-00019 PMID: 14595230

Health, U. V. A. (n.d.). International telehealth projects. https://uvahealth.com/services/telemedicine/international-health

HOPS Healthcare. (2021, June 3). Introducing one of its kind EMR platform integrated with telemedicine patient app in Congo. https://hops.healthcare/blogs/introducing-one-of-its-kind-emr-platform-integrated-with-telemedicine-patient-app-in-kinshasa-d-r-congo

Jagarapu, J., & Savani, R. C. (2021). A brief history of telemedicine and the evolution of teleneonatology. *Seminars in Perinatology*, *45*(5), 151416. Advance online publication. DOI: 10.1016/j.semperi.2021.151416 PMID: 34006382

Kontaxakis, G., Visvikis, D., Ohl, R., Sachpazidis, I., Suarez, J., Selby, P., Rest, C. C., Santos, A., Ortega, F., Diaz, J., & Pan, L. (2006). Integrated telemedicine applications and services for oncological positron emission tomography. *Oncology Reports*, *15*(4), 1091. DOI: 10.3892/or.15.4.1091 PMID: 16525707

Krick, T., Huter, K., Domhoff, D., Schmidt, A., Rothgang, H., & Wolf-Ostermann, K. (2019). Digital technology and nursing care: A scoping review on acceptance, effectiveness and efficiency studies of informal and formal care technologies. *BMC Health Services Research*, *19*(1), 400. Advance online publication. DOI: 10.1186/s12913-019-4238-3 PMID: 31221133

Kruse, C. S., Krowski, N., Rodriguez, B., Tran, L., Vela, J., & Brooks, M. (2018). Telehealth and patient satisfaction: A systematic review and narrative analysis. *BMJ Open*, *7*(8), e016242. Advance online publication. DOI: 10.1136/bmjopen-2017-016242 PMID: 28775188

Kumari, R., Singh, A. K., Verma, R., & Fetais, A. H. M. (2022). Enablers and challenges for e-health services: A systematic literature review. *International Journal of Electronic Government Research, 18*(1), 1–17. DOI: 10.4018/IJEGR.298626

Lukas, H., Xu, C., Yu, Y., & Gao, W. (2020). Emerging telemedicine tools for remote COVID-19 diagnosis, monitoring, and management. *ACS Nano, 14*(12), 16180–16193. DOI: 10.1021/acsnano.0c08494 PMID: 33314910

Maia, M. R., Castela, E., Pires, A., & Lapão, L. V. (2019). How to develop a sustainable telemedicine service? A pediatric telecardiology service 20 years on—An exploratory study. *BMC Health Services Research, 19*(1), 681. Advance online publication. DOI: 10.1186/s12913-019-4511-5 PMID: 31547824

Malhotra, S., Chakrabarti, S., & Shah, R. (2013). Telepsychiatry: Promise, potential, and challenges. *Indian Journal of Psychiatry, 55*(1), 3. DOI: 10.4103/0019-5545.105499 PMID: 23441027

Mehta, A., da Silva Dias, L., Espinal, M., Jillellamudi, R., Mathew, R., Chauhan, A., Dhingra, K., & Verma, S. (2024). E-health implementation challenges: A comprehensive review of digital healthcare in the United States. *Journal of Knowledge Learning and Science Technology, 3*(4), 233–246. DOI: 10.60087/jklst.v2.n3.p233

Molinari, G., Molinari, M., Di Biase, M., & Brunetti, N. D. (2017). Telecardiology and its settings of application: An update. *Journal of Telemedicine and Telecare, 24*(5), 373–381. DOI: 10.1177/1357633X16689432 PMID: 28084886

Ncube, B., Mars, M., & Scott, R. E. (2023). Perceptions and attitudes of patients and healthcare workers towards the use of telemedicine in Botswana: An exploratory study. *PLoS One, 18*(2), e0281754. Advance online publication. DOI: 10.1371/journal.pone.0281754 PMID: 36795740

Ncube, B., Mars, M., & Scott, R. E. (2023). Recommendations for developing a telemedicine strategy for Botswana: A meta-synthesis. *International Journal of Environmental Research and Public Health, 20*(18), 6718. Advance online publication. DOI: 10.3390/ijerph20186718 PMID: 37754578

Odhiambo, R., & Mars, M. (2018). Patients' understanding of telemedicine terms required for informed consent when translated into Kiswahili. *BMC Public Health, 18*(1), 588. Advance online publication. DOI: 10.1186/s12889-018-5499-1 PMID: 29720139

Omboni, S., Padwal, R. S., Alessa, T., Benczúr, B., Green, B. B., Hubbard, I., Kario, K., Khan, N. A., Konradi, A., Logan, A. G., Lu, Y., Mars, M., McManus, R. J., Melville, S., Neumann, C. L., Parati, G., Renna, N. F., Ryvlin, P., Saner, H., & Wang, J. (2022). The worldwide impact of telemedicine during COVID-19: Current evidence and recommendations for the future. *Connected Health.* Advance online publication. DOI: 10.20517/ch.2021.03 PMID: 35233563

Onsongo, S., Kamotho, C., Rinke de Wit, T. F., & Lowrie, K. (2023). Experiences on the utility and barriers of telemedicine in healthcare delivery in Kenya. *International Journal of Telemedicine and Applications, 2023*, 1487245. Advance online publication. DOI: 10.1155/2023/1487245 PMID: 37180825

Ryu, S. (2012). Telemedicine: Opportunities and developments in member States: Report on the second Global Survey on eHealth 2009 (Global Observatory for eHealth Series, Volume 2). *Healthcare Informatics Research, 18*(2), 153. DOI: 10.4258/hir.2012.18.2.153

Scott, R. E., Ndumbe, P., & Wootton, R. (2005). An e-health needs assessment of medical residents in Cameroon. *Journal of Telemedicine and Telecare, 11*(2_suppl, Suppl 2), S78–S80. DOI: 10.1258/135763305775124911 PMID: 16375807

Shore, J. H., Schneck, C. D., & Mishkind, M. C. (2020). Telepsychiatry and the coronavirus disease 2019 pandemic—Current and future outcomes of the rapid virtualization of psychiatric care. *JAMA Psychiatry, 77*(12), 1211–1212. DOI: 10.1001/jamapsychiatry.2020.1643 PMID: 32391861

Sophia. (2023, August 28). The future of healthcare in Congo: The era of telemedicine. SYNWELL. https://www.synwell-sante.com/en/post/the-future-of-healthcare-in-congo-the-era-of-telemedicine

Tchao, E. T., Acquah, I., Kotey, S. D., Aggor, C. S., & Kponyo, J. J. (2019). On telemedicine implementations in Ghana. *International Journal of Advanced Computer Science and Applications, 10*(3). Advance online publication. DOI: 10.14569/IJACSA.2019.0100325

Terkelsen, C. J., Nørgaard, B. L., Lassen, J. F., Gerdes, J. C., Ankersen, J. P., Rømer, F., Nielsen, T. T., & Andersen, H. R. (2002). Telemedicine is used for remote pre-hospital diagnosing in patients suspected of acute myocardial infarction. *Journal of Internal Medicine, 252*(5), 412–420. DOI: 10.1046/j.1365-2796.2002.01051.x PMID: 12528759

The American Telemedicine Association. (2017). ATA 2017 Telehealth 2.0 Conference abstracts. *Telemedicine Journal and e-Health : The Official Journal of the American Telemedicine Association*, *23*(4), A-78. DOI: 10.1089/tmj.2017.29005-A.abstracts PMID: 28410061

Thrall, J. H., Boland, G., & Larson, D. B. (2020). Teleradiology: Expanding the reach of radiology. *Radiology*, *295*(3), 636–641. DOI: 10.1148/radiol.2020192652

Vakaniaki, E. H., Kacita, C., Kinganda-Lusamaki, E., O'Toole, Á., Wawina-Bokalanga, T., Mukadi-Bamuleka, D., Amuri-Aziza, A., Malyamungu-Bubala, N., Mweshi-Kumbana, F., Mutimbwa-Mambo, L., Belesi-Siangoli, F., Mujula, Y., Parker, E., Muswamba-Kayembe, P.-C., Nundu, S. S., Lushima, R. S., Makangara-Cigolo, J.-C., Mulopo-Mukanya, N., Pukuta-Simbu, E., & Mbala-Kingebeni, P. (2024). Sustained human outbreak of a new MPXV clade I lineage in eastern Democratic Republic of Congo. *Nature Medicine*, *30*(10), 2791–2795. DOI: 10.1038/s41591-024-03130-3 PMID: 38871006

VFMatch. (n.d.). VFMatch. https://vfmatch.org/explore/facilities/5e5d6ecfaf007f0082810279

World Health Organization. (2016). Global diffusion of eHealth: Making universal health coverage achievable. https://apps.who.int/iris/handle/10665/252529

World Health Organization. (2025, March 13). Telemedicine: Opportunities and developments in Member State. WHO Regional Office for Africa. https://www.afro.who.int/publications/telemedicine-opportunities-and-developments-member-state

Yellowlees, P., Shore, J., & Roberts, L. (2010). Practice guidelines for videoconferencing-based telemental health—October 2009. *Telemedicine Journal and e-Health : The Official Journal of the American Telemedicine Association*, *16*(10), 1074–1089. DOI: 10.1089/tmj.2010.0148 PMID: 21186991

Chapter 4
Strengthening Telemedicine and Remote Patient Monitoring in Nigeria With Artificial Intelligence

Basil Osayin Daudu
http://orcid.org/0009-0000-9162-9426
Kogi State Univerisity, Nigeria

Esther Besty Anaiye
National Open University of Nigeria, Nigeria

ABSTRACT

The advancement of telemedicine empowers healthcare providers to treat patients remotely via telecommunication technology, thus bridging the healthcare gap for patients in remote regions of Nigeria. As such, the objectives of the chapter are to: (i) assess the compliance of Nigerian healthcare providers with telemedicine and remote patient monitoring practices, (ii) evaluate the proficiency of Nigerian healthcare providers in utilizing telemedicine practices, and (iii) retrieve patient opinions on telemedicine and remote monitoring services that Nigerian healthcare providers offer. The methodology used in this chapter primarily involves quantitative analysis. The collected data were analyzed critically and descriptively using tools such as chi-square. Based on the research findings, there is a need for the government to intensify telemedicine practices and invest more in artificial intelligence as a facilitator of telemedicine and a solution to the challenges hindering its implementation in Nigeria.

DOI: 10.4018/979-8-2600-2238-2.ch004

INTRODUCTION

Health informatics plays a key role in transforming healthcare globally, enabling seamless systems and health professionals to offer solutions to problems and improve customer services. This technology allows professionals to manage various functions more effectively and efficiently (Daudu et al., 2025). The significance of health to human life and well-being cannot be overstated. Ensuring access to healthcare facilities regardless of location is a hallmark of a responsible and responsive government. This is why a substantial portion of the national budget is allocated to improving the health sector, as good health enables one to be effective in their work, while poor health incapacitates.

In Nigeria, the provision of health assistance in remote areas proves difficult due to some limiting factors like insecurity, poor road conditions, and environmental hazards (floods and erosion). Despite advancements in technological adoption, especially in the 21st century, these concerns still persist, especially the location of health centers being far away. For example, the distance of Etsu Gudu community from Minna, the capital of Niger State, is a two-hour drive with rough roads, obstructed by small rivers. Another hour of travel along narrow dirt roads (pitch black) is needed to reach the community (Malaria Consortium, 2019).

Telemedicine, however, has greatly enhanced the Nigerian health system, enabling in-person communication between healthcare providers and patients, between patients and health technologies or tools, which allows users to receive medical attention from the comfort of their homes. Notably, machine learning advances healthcare systems in Nigeria and Africa at large (Daudu, Osimen & Anaiye, 2024). Healthcare is delivered by people for people. Sometimes, healthcare is intensive, such as for individuals with severe acute diseases hospitalized as inpatients. Other times, it is less intensive, such as for individuals with chronic diseases requiring regular medication or therapeutic measures (Winter et al., 2023).

Ukaoha and Egbokhare (2012) noted that, despite the wide range of ICT applications in Nigeria, with approximately 45,000 medical doctors serving a population exceeding 150 million, this technology has had a minimal impact on the health sector. In addition to a shortage of doctors, the country also lacks other health workers and medical facilities, with the few available being unevenly distributed, primarily in urban areas. Consequently, rural communities, where many Nigerians live, struggle to access quality healthcare. Telemedicine, as a means of delivering health services to remote locations, has the potential to improve Nigeria's health services and prospects if harnessed through existing mobile telephony services.

The medical profession is highly specialized and is suited only for trained medical personnel, operating in accordance with the Hippocratic Oath that certified medical practitioners and healthcare providers are required to comply with, extending to the adoption of telemedicine and remote patient monitoring practices. Interestingly, Nigeria has a large number of medical practitioners and healthcare facilities like clinics, hospitals, and pharmaceutical companies. In 2007, telemedicine practice was adopted in Nigeria when the National Space Research and Development Agency (NASRDA) and the Federal Ministry of Health launched a pilot project in two teaching hospitals (University College Hospital, Ibadan, and University Teaching Hospital, Maiduguri) and six federal medical centers (Owo, Gombe, Makurdi, Yenagoa, Birnin Kebbi, and Owerri) across the country's six geopolitical zones. Private establishments like Lagoon Hospital, Lagos, and Igbinedion University Teaching Hospital, Benin, also adopted telemedicine.

Thus, this chapter centers on three key issues (noncompliance, lack of technological proficiency, and patient dissatisfaction), which serve as the objectives of the chapter:

i. To examine the level of compliance among Nigerian healthcare providers with telemedicine and remote patient monitoring practices.
ii. To evaluate the proficiency of Nigerian healthcare providers in using telemedicine technology.
iii. To gather patients' opinions on telemedicine and remote monitoring services that Nigerian healthcare providers provide.

BACKGROUND

Innovative healthcare solutions like telemedicine and remote patient monitoring are designed to close the gap between patients and medical personnel, especially in areas of limited access to quality healthcare services (Chauhan, 2023).

Telemedicine

Telemedicine practice is rapidly gaining recognition in developed countries, but resource-limited countries like Nigeria are yet to integrate it fully (Ezeani et al., 2022). In 1879, telemedicine began with the use of telephones to minimize unnecessary doctor visits and evolved via innovations like radio consultations and early remote diagnosis. Major milestones included the use of radios for ship-based care, World War II image transmissions, and 1950s developments in teleradiology and teleconsultation by institutions like the University of Nebraska. NASA's initiatives in the 1970s and 1980s expanded telemedicine for rural and space healthcare.

The emergence of ICT in the 1990s greatly accelerated its growth, leading to wider global adoption and investment. Historically, telemedicine adopted wired communication technologies like plain old telephone systems (POTS) and integrated services digital networks (ISDN), but recent applications have expanded to include diverse wireless systems like ZigBee, Bluetooth, VSAT, WLAN, WiMAX, GPRS, and UMTS. In this sense, telemedicine depicts a developing technology merging telecommunications and information technologies to increase healthcare delivery, mostly benefiting patients in remote areas (Pandian, 2016).

The term "telemedicine" is derived from the Greek prefix 'tele,' meaning at a distance; thus, telemedicine refers to medicine conducted at a distance. It encompasses a wide range of medical activities, including diagnosis, treatment, disease prevention, continuing education for healthcare providers and consumers, and research and evaluation. Telemedicine facilitates the delivery of healthcare and the exchange of healthcare information across distances. Similar terms include telecare and telehealth. Telecare provides nursing and community support from a distance, and telehealth refers to public health services delivered remotely to people who wish to remain well and independent. Essentially, telemedicine involves transferring health-related information between locations via telecommunications networks, rather than moving the providers or recipients of healthcare (Craig & Patterson, 2005).

Telemedicine consists of delivering healthcare and exchanging healthcare information over distance. It is not a distinct technology or a separate branch of medicine. It can be grouped based on client and expert engagement (real-time or prerecorded), and the type of information transmitted via text, audio, and video (Craig & Patterson, 2005). Telemedicine has proven to reduce patient wait times, leading to more cost-effective healthcare (Akintosin, 2015). Telemedicine-based devices include (i) store-and-forward/asynchronous devices like x-ray images, cardiology results, and laboratory test results; (ii) remote monitoring devices like electronic sphygmomanometers and digital glucometers; and (iii) interactive/synchronous or live service devices like enabling virtual consultations, live phone, video, and online communication.

Currently, most telemedicine is practiced in industrialized countries like the USA, but its use is growing in developing countries. Telemedicine should be considered in two main situations: (i) when no alternative exists (e.g., emergencies in remote areas), and (ii) when it is superior to conventional services (e.g., teleradiology for rural hospitals). Telemedicine can enhance equity of access to healthcare, the quality of care, and the efficiency of its delivery. It allows doctors in remote areas to consult with specialists without extensive travel (Miller & Derse, 2002).

Telehealth aims not to create new healthcare services but rather to enhance the delivery of existing ones using technology. On the clinical side, telehealth facilitates patient access to healthcare providers remotely, enabling patients to receive care without traveling far from their communities (Exner-Pirot, 2022). Remote monitoring through telehealth offers benefits such as enhanced patient surveillance, cost-effectiveness, and improved patient satisfaction. However, drawbacks include potential inaccuracies in self-conducted tests, the risk of incorrect diagnoses when symptoms overlap across different conditions, among other concerns.

Notably, telemedicine increases medical services by allowing patients to consult healthcare providers remotely through video, phone, or online platforms. Before COVID-19, its utilization was limited to specific cases, but the pandemic accelerated adoption as countries removed regulatory and financial barriers to support remote care (Keelara, Sutherland & Almyranti, 2025). Teleconsultations across OECD nations more than doubled between 2019 and 2021 and continued to rise even after in-person services resumed. The bone of contention is integrating telemedicine sustainably into routine healthcare and developing evidence-based policies for equitable delivery (Organization for Economic Cooperation and Development, 2023).

Remote Patient Monitoring

A recent advancement in healthcare is remote patient monitoring, which is particularly beneficial in an aging global population with increasing health complexities. This technology involves sensors that monitor vital signs such as electrocardiogram readings, heart rate, respiration rate, blood pressure, temperature, blood glucose levels, and neural activity. The essential components of a remote monitoring system include a data acquisition system with sensors capable of wireless data transmission, a data processing system, and end-terminals at healthcare facilities, all connected via a communication network (Lakmini, Naeem & Keshav, 2019).

Remote patient monitoring is a vital advancement in modern healthcare, using information technologies for early disease detection and continuous health tracking. It helps prevent complications, reduces hospitalizations and costs, and improves healthcare efficiency through real-time communication. The system is especially beneficial for patients with chronic conditions, mobility issues, or those needing constant supervision, such as post-surgical, newborn, and elderly patients, allowing them to live more comfortably and independently (Gouveia et al., 2025).

In West Africa, remote patient/physiologic monitoring (RPM) enhances healthcare quality and helps manage healthcare costs, thereby significantly advancing telemedicine (Idris-Umarfarouq et al., 2022). Today in Nigeria, telemedicine advancements enable RPM from patients' homes, supporting the expansion of RPM in managing non-life-threatening illnesses. RPM targets various patient groups requiring continuous monitoring, including those with chronic diseases, mobility limitations, post-surgical patients, newborns, and elderly individuals (Molefi, 2015).

Figure 1. Key Components, Limitations, and Benefits of Remote Patient Monitoring (RPM)

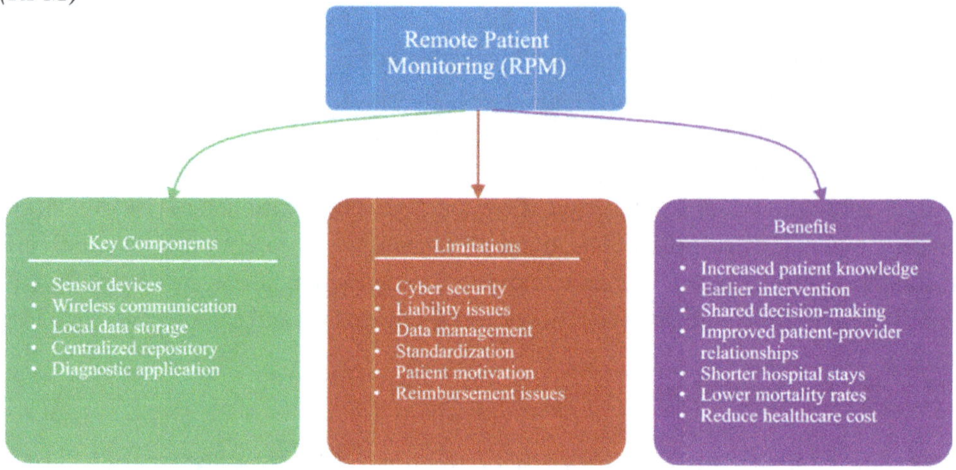

Source: Authors' creation

Figure 1 displays key components, limitations, and benefits of RPM. Remote patient monitoring involves several key components, like devices with sensors that measure physiological parameters; wireless communication to transmit data from sensors to a central database; local data storage at the patient's location; a centralized repository for data storage; and diagnostic application software for data analysis and recommendations. RPM is utilized for managing conditions such as cancer, COVID-19, chronic obstructive pulmonary disease (COPD), dementia and falls, diabetes, congestive heart failure, infertility, and post-surgery care. The benefits of RPM include increased patient knowledge, earlier interventions, shared decision-making, improved patient-provider relationships, shorter hospital stays, lower mortality rates, and reduced healthcare costs. However, RPM also faces limitations such as patient motivation, liability issues, data management, standardization, cybersecurity, and reimbursement challenges.

Further, in the Remote Patient Monitoring (RPM) ecosystem, the patient is the central focus around which all activities revolve. A patient-centered approach is essential not only for improving health outcomes but also for ensuring program success and provider performance. The ecosystem involves several key players: patients who generate health data and whose engagement is vital; providers who analyze this data in real-time to guide care; distributors who supply software, devices, and monitoring services; and data and device manufacturers who design and produce technologies that collect and transmit patient information. Ultimately, the RPM model begins and ends with the patient; without their active participation and ease of device use, the system cannot function effectively.

Brief History of Telemedicine and Remote Patient Monitoring Practices in Nigeria

Between 2009 and 2010, Lagos University Teaching Hospital in Idiaraba, Lagos, initiated Nigeria's first public telemedicine project in collaboration with universities in India. Akin Osibogun, who served as the hospital's Chief Medical Director at the time, highlighted the potential of telemedicine in Nigeria, which was demonstrated during the program. Osibogun noted that the telemedicine project allowed Lagos University Teaching Hospital to engage in seminars with leading hospitals in India. Subsequently, the National Hospital in Abuja partnered with the Sickle Cell Foundation to conduct a live interactive diagnostic session for a 13-year-old sickle cell patient in Lagos, using teleconferencing technology linking medical experts from the National Hospital in Abuja and the National Sickle Cell Foundation in Lagos. The teleconferencing setup was facilitated by Suburban West Africa, an Indian communications provider.

By 2015, Hudibia, a Nigerian telemedicine organization founded by Dr. Ahjoku Amadi-Obi, developed the first telemedicine digital application for accessing healthcare services digitally. During the peak of the COVID-19 pandemic in 2020, the Hudibia application saw a reported 400% increase in downloads (Adegbite, 2021). Notably, the Nigerian Federal Government partnered with Canadian firm Ethnomet to launch NigComHealth, a digital healthcare platform aimed at providing millions of Nigerians with access to quality healthcare digitally. NigComHealth is expected to revolutionize patient-provider connections by offering convenient and accessible medical consultations by licensed healthcare professionals via a mobile app, anytime and anywhere. Presently, several business entities in Nigeria offer telehealth services, including Sesame Care, MeMD, Amwell, MDLive, Health Tap, Telehealth Ambassadors, Medisr, MyMedicalBank, 1Dokita Healthcare Ltd, and Medtech Africa (Ahanwa & Okoloma, 2023).

Nigeria's telemedicine practice faces major challenges, primarily due to poor technological infrastructure, including weak internet connectivity, a lack of telemedicine devices, and high setup and maintenance costs. The absence of specific telemedicine laws further complicates issues related to clinical liability, practitioner credentialing, and provider indemnity. Additionally, there is no comprehensive policy integrating telemedicine into the national health framework. Data security risks, such as hacking and privacy breaches, remain significant concerns. Limited physical examination and reliance on patient self-reporting can hinder accurate diagnosis, while doctors also fear potential malpractice issues during virtual consultations.

Legal Regulatory Bodies

There is a myriad of legal monitoring bodies of telemedicine practices in Nigeria, such as the National Information Technology Development Agency Act (2007), Code of Medical Ethics (2008), Evidence Act (2011), and Data Protection Act (2023).

National Information Technology Development Agency Act 2007

The National Information Technology Development Agency (NITDA) Act of 2007 significantly impacts the regulation and advancement of telemedicine services in Nigeria. Section 1 of this Act established the NITDA, which is primarily responsible for creating regulations concerning electronic governance and overseeing the use of information technology and electronic data within the country. Telehealth, which involves the provision of healthcare services through digital systems, naturally falls under the purview of the NITDA Act.

Specifically, Section 6 details the functions of the NITDA, highlighting its authority to formulate regulations governing telehealth practices in Nigeria: (i) Planning, developing, and regulating IT practices and systems nationwide, with emphasis on universal access, including underserved areas. (ii) Providing guidelines for IT development and application across the public and private sectors. (iii) Promoting electronic governance and data exchange to replace paper-based systems. (iv) Facilitating the networking of institutions and standardizing IT systems, including software escrow and certification. (v) Offering advisory services and creating incentives to boost IT use and investment. (vi) Supporting the establishment of IT and knowledge parks. (vii) Encouraging private sector involvement through regulatory policies. (viii) Collaborating with stakeholders to achieve IT development goals. (ix) Identifying critical research areas and advising on relevant legislation to enhance national security and industry growth. (x) Promoting internet penetration and sound internet governance. (xi) Carrying out additional necessary functions to fulfill the agency's mandate (NITDA, 2007).

Code of Medical Ethics 2008

The Code of Medical Ethics (2008) endorses the relevance of telemedicine in transforming healthcare delivery across the country. As such, guideline 22 of the Code specifically addresses telemedicine and offers guidance for its application as follows: Telemedicine, an emerging professional opportunity stemming from modern advancements in computer and telecommunication technology, is gradually becoming integrated into professional practice in Nigeria. It involves the practice of medicine at a distance and is especially beneficial for patient care and management by general practitioners and specialists. Through tele-support, they can access specialist consultations in various fields of medicine and dentistry as needed in their daily practices.

Evidence Act 2011

In Nigeria, Section 84 of the Evidence Act outlines the requirements for admitting electronically generated evidence in judicial proceedings. Section 84 (1) establishes the general admissibility of electronic evidence. Section 84 (2) (a) – (d) specifies the conditions under which such evidence is admissible. Section 84 (3) addresses the treatment of electronic evidence originating from multiple computers as if from a single source. Section 84 (4) requires a certificate of authentication to verify the source of the electronically generated evidence. Consequently, if telehealth practices are involved in litigation, Section 84 of the Evidence Act governs the submission of relevant electronic evidence (NLB, 2011).

Data Protection Act 2023

The Data Protection Act of 2023 establishes the legal framework for safeguarding the personal data of Nigerian citizens. As the primary data protection law in Nigeria, it outlines the guidelines and standards for collecting, processing, storing, and transferring personal data within the country. This Act applies to all data controllers and processors handling personal data in Nigeria, including healthcare providers involved in telehealth. Section 1 of the Act outlines its objectives, which include ensuring that data controllers and processors meet their obligations to data subjects. Generally, Section 2 of the Data Protection Act applies to the processing of personal data, whether automated or not. Section 2 (2) specifies that the Act is applicable when: (a) the data controller or processor is based, ordinarily resident, or operating in Nigeria; (b) the processing of personal data takes place within Nigeria; or (c) the data controller or processor is not based, ordinarily resident, or operating in Nigeria but processes the personal data of a data subject in Nigeria. Notably, Section 2 (1) (e) extends the Act's provisions to data controllers or processors not based, ordinarily resident, or operating in Nigeria if they process personal data of data subjects in Nigeria. This provision addresses the involvement of health personnel located outside Nigeria who conduct telehealth sessions with patients in Nigeria.

Legal and Moral Concerns Arising

Informed consent, confidentiality, the relationship between parties, and data privacy are some of the legal and ethical concerns arising from telemedicine practices.

Informed Consent

Informed consent is the procedure by which a healthcare provider informs a patient about the risks, benefits, and alternatives of a particular treatment or intervention (Shah, Thornton, Kopitnik & Hipskind, 2023). Typically, medical professionals are required to obtain the patient's consent before initiating any treatment to avoid potential legal issues such as assault or battery claims. Telehealth, which involves virtual consultations between healthcare providers and patients, also necessitates obtaining consent before beginning the consultation to protect the interests of both parties. It is recognized that the importance and benefits of informed consent apply to telehealth just as they do to traditional, in-person medical care (Cascella, 2023).

Furthermore, the informed consent process in telehealth should address risks specific to the use of telecommunication technologies for care delivery. The World Medical Association, in its 1999 Statement on Accountability, Responsibilities, and Ethical Practice of Telemedicine, emphasized that patient consent is required when a physician needs to seek the expertise of a distant specialist during a telemedicine session. In summary, obtaining informed consent in telehealth is crucial to prevent legal issues and other complications that may arise without it.

Confidentiality

During routine medical consultations, healthcare professionals collect patients' details, including their medical history. As part of their professional ethics, medical personnel are required to maintain the confidentiality of patients' information. For doctors, this obligation is reinforced by the Hippocratic Oath, taken upon entering the medical profession. The Code of Medical Ethics in Nigeria, as well as other international jurisdictions, also mandates this duty of confidentiality. Specifically, Rule 44 of the Nigerian Code of Medical Ethics stipulates this obligation. Essentially, healthcare providers must keep a patient's personal health information private unless the patient consents to its release (Bord, Burke & Dudzinski, 2023). The primary reason for this duty is to encourage patients to provide honest and complete information during medical consultations.

However, the duty of confidentiality is not absolute. In Nigeria, Rule 44 of the Code of Medical Ethics and Section 26 (2) of the National Health Act outline situations where disclosure without patient consent is permitted. These situations include a. when a court order mandates disclosure. b. At the request of a parent or guardian for a minor or someone unable to give consent. c. When non-disclosure poses a threat to public health. Similar to physical consultations, confidentiality must also be maintained in digital health interactions. Telehealth poses additional risks because it is typically internet-based, and the digital platforms used for communication are not entirely controlled by healthcare providers. The risk of information interception by internet fraudsters is significant, potentially compromising the confidentiality of telehealth sessions. Therefore, telehealth service providers must implement robust measures to protect the channels through which patients share their information.

Relationship between the Parties Involved

According to Rules I-IV of the American Code of Medical Ethics, a patient-doctor relationship is established when a physician attends to a patient's medical needs. During traditional medical consultations, this relationship brings with it specific duties and obligations. For example, once a legal relationship is established, several duties are imposed on medical personnel, including the duty of care and the duty of confidentiality. These duties also arise when a relationship is established between a healthcare provider and a patient.

Ordinarily, the lack of a physical meeting during telehealth sessions should not negate the duties and rights inherent in a doctor-patient relationship during in-person consultations. However, many medical personnel believe that a doctor-patient relationship is only fully formed during physical consultations. One perspective is that since a doctor cannot thoroughly examine a patient or effectively prescribe treatment during a telehealth session, a full doctor-patient relationship does not exist. This view holds that physical medical examination is essential to the doctor-patient relationship, and its absence renders the relationship incomplete (Menage, 2020). Consequently, there is uncertainty about whether a doctor-patient relationship, with its associated rights and duties, fully arises in telehealth settings.

Data Privacy

During medical consultations, patients share a significant amount of personal information. In telehealth sessions, healthcare providers also obtain personal details from patients over the internet, where complete security cannot be assured. Consequently, information exchanged online is vulnerable to interception by unauthorized third parties. This raises the risk of unauthorized access and illegal disclosure of health data. Therefore, telehealth providers must implement measures to secure the data exchanged during these sessions (van Daalen, 2023).

Theoretical Framework

This chapter anchors its foundation on Rogers' diffusion of innovations theory, which explains how innovations spread and are adopted within society. El Malouf and Bahemia (2025) assert that diffusion of innovation research seeks to identify the factors that drive the adoption of new ideas or products and to examine how these adoption decisions influence social structures and contexts.

The diffusion of innovations theory (IDT) originated from American sociologist Everett M. Rogers, who first observed how agricultural innovations were gradually accepted by farmers in his hometown of Carroll, Iowa. While studying the adoption of hybrid maize, Rogers interviewed 148 farmers about their use of new agricultural products like herbicides. By examining innovation diffusion across various fields such as education, driving schools, and healthcare, he found that, despite industry differences, the diffusion process followed similar patterns. These included variations in information sources at different adoption stages, an "S-shaped" adoption curve, and the tendency for early adopters to be knowledgeable and experienced individuals.

Drawing from extensive studies on technology adoption, social communication, and interdisciplinary insights from sociology, communication, economics, and education, Rogers developed the diffusion of innovations theory in the early 1950s and presented it comprehensively in his 1962 book *The Diffusion of Innovations*, introducing a general model of how innovations spread over time and within social systems. Thus, the diffusion of innovation should include four core elements: innovation, communication channel, time, and social system. The diffusion of innovations theory provides a structured framework to explain how individuals and organizations adopt new ideas or technologies through five stages: knowledge, persuasion, decision, implementation, and confirmation.

A study carried out by Peter et al. (2025) revealed that telemedicine remains underused in Nigeria despite high rates of childhood mortality. Using a mixed-methods design with surveys and interviews in urban and rural Abuja, the study revealed that telemedicine awareness was significantly higher among urban mothers. However, many participants viewed it as inferior to in-person consultations, with barriers including limited awareness, high costs, and resource shortages. Therefore, increasing public awareness and improving resource access are key to expanding telemedicine use in pediatric care.

Dodoo, Al-Samarraie and Alzahrani (2021)'s research revealed that while telemedicine proved valuable during the COVID-19 pandemic, its overall use and effectiveness in Sub-Saharan Africa (SSA) remain limited. An analysis of 66 studies showed broad adoption of telemedicine technologies but little evidence of their impact on COVID-19 control. Aanuoluwapo et al. (2024) reported that telemedicine enhances nursing practice through teletriage, remote monitoring, virtual consultations, and telepsychiatry, which improve care efficiency and accessibility, particularly in rural areas. Tele-education supports nurses' ongoing learning, while ethical concerns such as privacy, consent, and data security remain key challenges.

Fostina, Okon and Chikaodili (2024) assert that telemedicine is vital for addressing the shortage of skilled medical professionals and improving healthcare access in developing countries. In their cross-sectional study of 150 clinicians at the Federal Medical Centre, Yenagoa, most respondents were female nurses with 6-10 years of experience. Findings revealed that 23.3% had high awareness of telemedicine, 69.3% had moderate awareness, and 7.3% had low awareness. Overall, participants showed a positive attitude toward telemedicine, though most were not actively providing telemedicine services. A study on Health Professionals in LAUTECH Teaching Hospital, Osogbo, Nigeria, by Abodunrin and Makanjuola (2009) revealed that although many healthcare professionals supported the use of telemedicine and e-health, they lacked adequate knowledge to implement these technologies effectively. Therefore, improving healthcare workers' access to a reliable power supply and modern communication tools is essential.

Noel et al. (2024) discovered that while telemedicine has strong potential to enhance equitable healthcare in developing nations, its use is limited by low awareness and understanding. Among 305 medical students studied at the University of Jos, only about one-third demonstrated good knowledge, perceived benefits, or ease of use. Those with better knowledge were more likely to hold positive views. Their study underscores a gap in medical education and calls for improved training and curriculum development to strengthen telemedicine awareness and adoption. Obotu (2019) found that telemedicine availability significantly improves medical service delivery in Federal Medical Centers across North Central Nigeria.

Lawani-Luwaji and Okafor (2025) conducted a descriptive cross-sectional study involving 42 fourth-year Medical Laboratory Science students. Participants completed a structured questionnaire evaluating their awareness, familiarity, perceived benefits, and challenges of telemedicine, as well as its potential use in rural Bayelsa. Results showed that although 60.5% of respondents were aware of telemedicine, their knowledge of specific forms, such as asynchronous and synchronous telehealth, was limited. The most recognized benefits included improved healthcare access (48.8%) and cost reduction (18.6%). Overall acceptance was mixed, with 47.6% supporting telemedicine, while others remained uncertain or sceptical.

Agbeyani and Lukose (2025) identify telemedicine as a transformative approach to improving healthcare access in Sub-Saharan Africa's underserved regions. Their critical appraisal shows that South Africa leads in adoption, emphasizing specialist consultations, chronic disease management, and mental health services. Kenya excels in mobile health (mHealth) integration, particularly for maternal health, HIV care, and reproductive health, supported by mobile technology and systems like M-Pesa. Nigeria, despite infrastructural and regulatory challenges, is progressing in remote diagnosis and teleconsultation innovations. Together, South Africa, Kenya, and Nigeria represent the region's leading examples of telemedicine development, each reflecting unique strengths and barriers within the broader African context.

The myriad of studies revealed the use of telemedicine and remote patient monitoring within the Nigerian healthcare system and beyond, alongside its noticeable challenges. Not much emphasis is placed on the remarkable impact of artificial intelligence at work in the process. This gap is what this chapter tends to close by promoting artificial intelligence as an enhancer or strengthener of telemedicine and remote patient monitoring in Nigeria.

PROBLEM STATEMENT

In the 21st century, lack of quality healthcare is a key challenge facing humanity (WHO, 1997). Other hindrances in the developing countries include a shortage of health workers, demand for quality healthcare, and geographical barriers in favour of remote areas in accessing medical services (Khemapech, Sansrimahachai & Toahchoodee, 2019; Moahi, 1999). Many governments, especially in developing economies, are seeking better and more affordable alternatives for delivering health services. The advent of Information and Communications Technology (ICT) has introduced innovative ways to provide healthcare at lower costs and with a greater reach, particularly in remote areas (Adewale, 2004).

Across Africa and Asia, the use of digital health solutions such as mobile health and virtual consultations has grown, particularly after COVID-19 (Iyengar, Jain & Vaishya, 2020). Although nations like Rwanda, Ghana, and India have implemented national digital health strategies, challenges such as weak internet connectivity, insufficient funding, and low technical literacy hinder widespread adoption. In Nigeria, where rural healthcare access remains limited, telemedicine offers significant potential for improvement (WHO, 2021).

A significant percentage of Nigerians live in remote rural areas with limited or no access to modern healthcare facilities. Geographic isolation, a scarcity of physicians and hospitals, and difficulties traveling to larger cities where care is available are among the factors limiting access. Federal, state, and local governments have focused on improving healthcare in these remote rural areas to ensure equal access for citizens in both rural and urban areas (Anaiye & Daudu, 2025). However, these efforts have only been partially successful.

Currently, telemedicine is gaining attention in Nigeria, with private healthcare providers increasingly incorporating it into their services. Over 20 telemedicine startups are now operational in Nigeria, some locally focused and others with international reach. While these advancements aim to bridge the healthcare gap between professionals and remote areas, a significant portion of the population remains disconnected due to a lack of access to the necessary virtual devices (Rasid & Woodward, 2005). Therefore, this chapter centers on the formulated research questions:

1. What is the level of compliance among Nigerian healthcare providers with telemedicine and remote patient monitoring practices?
2. What is the proficiency of Nigerian healthcare providers in using telemedicine technology?
3. What are patients' opinions on telemedicine and remote patient services that Nigerian healthcare providers provide?

HYPOTHESES

Ho: The level of compliance among Nigerian healthcare providers with telemedicine and remote patient monitoring practices is significantly low.

Hi: The level of compliance among Nigerian healthcare providers with telemedicine and remote patient monitoring practices is significantly high.

Ho: The level of proficiency in the use of telemedicine technology among Nigerian healthcare providers is significantly low.

Hi: The level of proficiency in the use of telemedicine technology among Nigerian healthcare providers is significantly high.

RESULTS AND DISCUSSION

Results

Objective 1

To determine the level of compliance among Nigerian healthcare providers to telemedicine and remote patient monitoring practices, questionnaires were distributed via online platforms to 200 respondents from the six geopolitical zones of Nigeria: North Central, North East, North West, South West, South East, and South South, using the rating scale of "very often", and "Not often."

Table 1. The level of compliance of Nigerian healthcare providers with telemedicine and remote patient monitoring practices

S/N	Items	Very often	Not often	Total (%)
1	How often do you prescribe drugs to your patients?	160 80%	40 20%	200 100
2	How often do you do follow-up calls?	90 45%	110 55%	200 100
3	How often do you engage in emergency care?	95 47.5%	105 52.5%	200 100
4	How often do you counsel your patients?	70 35%	130 65%	200 100
5	How often do you diagnose your patients?	170 85%	30 15%	200 100

Source: (Survey, 2025)

Based on the data in Table 1, it can be seen that 160 individuals, comprising 80% of the surveyed Nigerian healthcare providers, often prescribe drugs to their patients, while 40 individuals, or 20%, expressed uncertainty. 90(45%) of healthcare providers frequently conduct follow-up calls while 110(55%) do not. 95(47.5%) often engage in emergency care while 105(52.5%) do not. 70(35%) often counsel patients while 130(65%) do not. 170(85%) often diagnose their patients while 30(15%) do not.

Objective 2

To determine the level of proficiency in the use of telemedicine technology among Nigerian healthcare providers, questionnaires were distributed through e-platforms to 200 respondents from the six geopolitical zones of Nigeria: North-Central, North East, North West, South West, South East, and South-South using the rating scale of "very often", "Not often", and "Not at all."

Table 2. The level of proficiency in the use of telemedicine technology among Nigerian healthcare providers

S/N	Items	Very often	Not often	Not at all	Total (%)
1	How often do you participate in video conferencing via Zoom, Microsoft Teams, Skype, Google Meet, free conference calls, and the like?	80 40%	90 45%	30 15%	200 100
2	How often do you make telephone calls and send messages via WhatsApp, WeChat, BBM, and the like?	110 55%	70 35%	20 10%	200 100
3	How often do you use wearable devices and sensors such as heart rate monitors, blood pressure cuffs, scales, glucose meters, pulse oximeters, thermometers, and the like?	100 50%	70 35%	30 15%	200 100
4	How often do you use mobile health apps like MyChat, Health Tap, and the like?	15 7.5%	100 50%	85 42.5%	200 100
5	How often do you rely on electronic health records EHRs like Eyecare Live, Teladoc, and the like?	15 7.5%	95 47.5%	90 45%	200 100

Source: (Survey, 2025)

Based on the provided data in Table 2, 80 individuals, making up 40% of the surveyed Nigerian healthcare providers, frequently use video conferencing tools such as Zoom, Microsoft Teams, Skype, Google Meet, and Free Conference Call. Conversely, 90 respondents, or 45%, do not frequently use these tools, and 30 respondents, or 15%, do not use them at all. Regarding telephone calls and messaging via WhatsApp, WeChat, BBM, and similar platforms, 110 respondents, representing 55%, often use these methods, while 70 respondents, or 35%, do not often use them, and 20 respondents, or 10%, do not use them at all. When it comes to wearable devices and sensors like heart rate monitors, blood pressure cuffs, scales, glucose meters, pulse oximeters, and thermometers, 100 respondents, or 50%, use them frequently, 70 respondents, or 35%, do not use them often, and 30 respondents, or 15%, do not use them at all. Only 15 respondents, or 7.5%, frequently use mobile health apps like MyChat and HealthTap, while 100 respondents, or 50%, do not often use these apps, and 85 respondents, or 42.5%, do not use them at all. Lastly, 15 respondents, or 7.5%, often rely on electronic health records (EHRs) like Eye Care Live and Teladoc, while 95 respondents, or 47.5%, do not often rely on EHRs, and 90 respondents, or 45%, do not use them at all.

Objective 3

To sample patients' opinions about telemedicine and remote monitoring services, questionnaires were distributed via in-person and online platforms to 200 respondents from the six geopolitical zones of Nigeria: North Central, North East, North West, South West, South East, and South-South, using the rating scale of "Yes" and "No."

Table 3. Patients' opinions about telemedicine and remote monitoring services

S/N	Items	Yes	No	Total (%)
1	Telemedicine and remote monitoring services are very effective and result-oriented.	120 60%	80 40%	200 100
2	Nigerian telemedicine practitioners always follow up.	180 90%	20 10%	200 100
3	Most times, there is an internet connection during conversations with telemedicine practitioners.	95 47.5	105 52.5%	200 100
4	The cost of medical treatment via telemedicine is high.	120 60%	80 40%	200 100
5	Most Nigerian telemedicine practitioners are good at what they do.	150 75%	50 25%	200 100

Source: (Survey, 2025)

From the data in Table 3, 120(60%) of patients agreed that telemedicine and remote monitoring services are effective and result-oriented, while 80(40%) disagreed. 180(90%) agreed that Nigerian telemedicine practitioners consistently follow up, whereas 20(10%) disagreed. 95(47.5%) agreed that the internet is available during conversations most time, while 105(52.5%) disagreed. 120(60%) agreed that the cost of medical treatment via telemedicine is high, while 80(40%) disagreed. 150(75%) agreed that most Nigerian telemedicine practitioners are skilled, whereas 50(25%) disagreed.

Hypothesis Testing

To make a generalized conclusion, the hypotheses were reviewed and tested in the light of all available evidence for acceptance or rejection. The hypotheses were tested at 5% level of significance, and the statistical method used is the Chi-square.

Restatement of Hypothesis:

> Ho: The level of compliance among Nigerian healthcare providers with telemedicine and remote patient monitoring practices is significantly low.
> Hi: The level of compliance among Nigerian healthcare providers with telemedicine and remote patient monitoring practices is significantly high.

To test the hypothesis, Table 1 above is used.

Expected frequency is $0 = 1+2......$

Hypothesis One

Whether the level of compliance among Nigerian medical workers with telemedicine and remote patient monitoring practices is significantly high or low.

$$fe = \frac{(90 + 110)}{2}$$

$$fe = \frac{200}{2}$$

fe=100

x^2=

Table 4. Chi-square table value

Fo	Fe	Fo-Fe	$(Fo\text{-}Fe)^2$	$\frac{(Fo - Fe)^2}{Fe}$
70	100	-30	900	9
110	100	10	100	1
				$X^2 = 10$

X^2 tab n-1 at 5% significance
3-1 under 0.05
Therefore, x^2 tab = 5.99
Under 0.5
X^2 Cal = 10

Decision Rule

From the provided tested hypothesis, the compliance level among Nigerian healthcare providers with telemedicine and remote patient monitoring practices is significantly high. According to the decision rule, if the calculated value exceeds the table value, the null hypothesis (Ho) should be rejected, and the alternative hypothesis (Hi) should be affirmed, and vice versa. In this case, since the calculated (X2) chi-square value is greater than the table value, it indicates that the compliance level among Nigerian healthcare providers with telemedicine and remote patient monitoring practices is significantly high.

Hypothesis Two

Ho: The level of proficiency in the use of telemedicine technology among Nigerian healthcare providers is significantly low.

Hi: The level of proficiency in the use of telemedicine technology among Nigerian healthcare providers is significantly high.

$$fe = \frac{(110 + 70 + 20)}{3}$$

$$fe = \frac{200}{3}$$

fe=66.7

$$X^2 = \frac{(fo - fe)^2}{fe}$$

x^2=

Table 5. Chi-square table value

Fo	Fe	Fo-Fe	$(Fo-Fe)^2$	$\frac{(Fo - Fe)^2}{Fe}$
110	66.7	43.3	1874.89	28.10
70	66.7	3.3	10.89	0.16
20	66.7	-46.7	280.89	4.211
				$X^2 = 32.47$

X^2 tab n-1 at 5% significance
3-1 under 0.05
Therefore, x^2 tab = 5.99
$X^2 = 32.47$

Decision Rule

Based on the hypothesis tested using Table 2, it can be inferred that the level of proficiency significantly influences the use of telemedicine technology among Nigerian medical practitioners. The acceptance of the alternative hypothesis (Hi) over the null hypothesis (Ho), due to the calculated X2 value exceeding the table

X2 value, indicates that proficiency in telemedicine use among Nigerian healthcare providers is notably high.

Discussion of Findings

As shown in Table 3 titled "Opinions about Telemedicine and Remote Monitoring Services," the findings indicate that 120 patients (60%) find telemedicine and remote monitoring services to be very effective and result-oriented, 180 patients (90%) believe Nigerian telemedicine practitioners consistently follow up, and 150 patients (75%) think most Nigerian telemedicine practitioners are skilled at their work. These results strongly support the first and second objectives: (i) that the level of compliance among Nigerian healthcare providers with telemedicine and remote patient monitoring is significantly high, and (ii) that the level of proficiency in the use of telemedicine among Nigerian healthcare providers is also significantly high.

Digital technologies, particularly AI, have transformed remote healthcare through telemedicine, telehealth, and mobile health. AI-driven tools such as machine learning, natural language processing, and computer vision have enhanced diagnostic accuracy, real-time decision-making, and patient engagement, signifying a major shift in healthcare delivery and connectivity (Chaturvedi, Chauhan & Singh, 2025). Artificial intelligence is revolutionizing healthcare by improving research, training, prevention, diagnosis, and patient care. The growing adoption of innovative healthcare solutions, artificial intelligence (AI), has become a leading force among medical service providers. This is largely due to its ability to use multiple algorithms to address complex problems quickly and efficiently (Odunuga et al., 2024).

AI holds great potential (Daudu & Osimen, 2025) to transform Nigeria's healthcare system by addressing key challenges and enhancing the quality, accessibility, and efficiency of healthcare delivery. In Nigeria, various AI-based healthcare innovations are improving clinical decision-making and service delivery. Xolani Health provides cloud tools for medical imaging and diagnosis, while ARONE uses AI-powered drones to deliver medical supplies. Pronov offers a telehealth platform with diagnostic and prescription services, and 10mg applies AI to optimize pharmaceutical logistics and financing. Hub Care Health enables teleconsultations, lab tests, and home care through a digital platform that also supports remote patient monitoring (Baballe, Ayagi & Musa, 2023).

Additional examples of telemedicine and remote patient monitoring in rural Nigeria include Barau Dikko telemedicine in Kaduna State, which links tertiary hospitals to rural hospitals and PHCs via digital imaging and e-stethoscopes (Musa et al. 2023). In Ondo State, there is Abiye (safe motherhood project) that enables mobile communication between pregnant women and health workers via mobile phones and SMS (Oyeyemi & Wynn, 2014). Then Kwara Telehealth platform, an online consultation between rural patients and urban doctors through Teleconsult apps and smartphones (Oyinlola, 2024).

Therefore, the integration of IoT into healthcare is crucial for improving patient outcomes, enhancing efficiency, and addressing current challenges, serving as a key driver of innovation and progress in the field (Lawal, 2023). The Web-based Remote Patient Monitoring System (WB-RPMS) is an effective tool for enhancing access to affordable healthcare in Nigeria, especially for orthopaedic outpatients, by providing continuous care during and after pandemics (Onyeabor et al., 2024). The primary challenges facing telemedicine and remote patient monitoring practices in Nigeria are poor internet connectivity and high medical costs (Emmanuel et al., 2025). However, with strategic investments in technology, training, and community involvement, Nigeria can leverage telemedicine to create a stronger and more equitable healthcare system (Ukpe, 2025).

SOLUTIONS AND RECOMMENDATIONS

From the findings, this chapter recommends the following:

i. There should be a result-oriented collaboration between healthcare providers, AI developers, and policy makers to revolutionize telemedicine and remote patient monitoring practices in Nigeria.
ii. All stakeholders and the Federal government should intensify AI-assisted training programs for healthcare professionals to improve their skills.
iii. The need to perfect data security with AI-driven encryption and access control alongside better access to reliable internet facilities.
iv. Establishment of transparent ethical regulatory frameworks for the responsible adoption of telemedicine technology to address content and privacy issues.
v. All stakeholders, including the government, should alleviate patients' financial burden.

FUTURE RESEARCH DIRECTIONS

The need to optimize local needs in Nigeria's health sector via AI-driven technological advancement calls for urgent attention. As such, future studies should boil down to designing and validating AI algorithms centered on Nigeria-specific health data that would enhance diagnostic precision for diseases. Again, a study of a comprehensive national strategy for AI integration into healthcare with clear ethical guidelines for positive results will serve as a welcome idea.

CONCLUSION

Every individual has the right to quality health. Telemedicine and remote patient monitoring have benefited man's well-being. AI adoption in Nigeria has transformed telemedicine in diverse ways, like detecting hepatitis B in disadvantaged populations by using AI algorithms. AI enhances connected healthcare by integrating patient data and strengthening holistic healthcare. Additionally, AI assists proactive healthcare systems and enhances personalized care by facilitating human capacities.

REFERENCES

Aanuoluwapo, C. D.-O., Olawade, D. B., Yanuoluwa, O. O., Famujimi, M. E., Olawumi, T. T., & Esan, D. T. (2024). Nursing in the Digital Age: Harnessing telemedicine for enhanced patient care. *Informatics and Health, 1*(2), 100–110. DOI: 10.1016/j.infoh.2024.07.003

Abodunrin, L. O., & Makanjuola, T. A. (2009). Knowledge and Perception of E-Health and Telemedicine among Health Professionals in LAUTECH Teaching Hospital, Osogbo, Nigeria. *International Journal of Health Research, 2*(1), 51–58. DOI: 10.4314/ijhr.v2i1.55388

Adegbite, T. (2021). 'Telemedicine – A Panacea for Nigeria's Healthcare Ills?' https://www.thisdaylive.com/index.php/2021/03/21/telemedicine-a-panacea-for-nigeriashealthcare-ills

Adewale, O. S. (2004). An internet-based telemedicine system in Nigeria. *International Journal of Information Management, 24*(3), 221–234. DOI: 10.1016/j.ijinfomgt.2003.12.014

Ahanwa, E. S., & Okoloma, H. C. (2023). Telehealth in Nigeria: A Legal Perspective. [IJOLACLE]. *International Journal of Law and Clinical Legal Education, 4*, 136–143.

Akintosin, J. (2015). The status of telemedicine in Africa: The role of broadband. http://nuviun.com/content/ the-status-of-telemedicine-in-africa/

Anaiye, E. B., & Daudu, B. O. (2025). Medical Care and Patients' Health Correlation in Anyigba Community Health Sectors of Kogi East in Nigeria. *Tanzania Journal of Health Research, 26*(4), 2277–2288. https://www.ajol.info/index.php/thrb/article/view/269962. DOI: 10.4314/thrb.v26i4.15

Baballe, A. M., Ayagi, S. H., & Musa, U. F. (2023). Using artificial intelligence (AI) technology in the health sector has several goals. *Global Journal of Research in Engineering & Computer Sciences, 3*(5), 31–35. DOI: 10.5281/zenodo.10048487

Bord, J. D., Burke, W., & Dudzinski, D. M. D. M. (2023). Confidentiality. https://depts.washington.edu/bhdept/ethics-medicine/bioethicstopics/detail/58

Cascella, L. M. (2023). Risk Perspectives in Telehealth: Informed Consent. https://www.medpro.com/telemedicine-informedconsent

Chaturvedi, U., Chauhan, S. B., & Singh, I. (2025). The impact of artificial intelligence on remote healthcare: Enhancing patient engagement, connectivity, and overcoming challenges. *Intelligent Pharmacy, 3*(5), 323–329. DOI: 10.1016/j.ipha.2024.12.003

Chauhan, M. (2023). Emerging Trends in Telemedicine and Remote Patient Monitoring: Improving Access to Healthcare Services. *International Research Journal of Basic and Clinical Studies, 8*(3), 1–5.

Craig, J., & Patterson, V. (2005). Introduction to the practice of telemedicine. *Journal of Telemedicine and Telecare, 11*(1), 3–9. DOI: 10.1177/1357633X0501100102

Daudu, B. O., Amodu, S. A., Ojochenemi, P. Y., & Anaiye, E. B. (2025). Leveraging Data-Driven Approaches: A Case Study on Enhancing Water Governance in Africa. In Agarwal, S., & Garg, M. C. (Eds.), *The Handbook of AI for Clean Water: Innovations in Treatment and Monitoring* (pp. 293–306). CRC Press., DOI: 10.1201/9781003600718-24

Daudu, B. O., & Osimen, G. U. (2025). Combatting Cyberthreats in African Digital Space with Artificial Intelligence. In Vajjhala, N. R., & Strange, K. D. (Eds.), *Cybersecurity in Knowledge Management: Cyberthreats and Solutions* (pp. 115–130). CRC Press., DOI: 10.1201/9781003498094-8

Daudu, B. O., Osimen, G. U., & Anaiye, E. B. (2024). Sustainable Smart Cities in African Digital Space. In Whig, P., Sharma, P., Aneja, N., Elngar, A. A., & Silva, N. (Eds.), *Artificial Intelligence and Machine Learning for Sustainable Development: Innovations, Challenges, and Applications* (pp. 100–111). CRC Press., DOI: 10.1201/9781003497189-8

Dodoo, J. E., Al-Samarraie, H., & Alzahrani, A. I. (2021). Telemedicine use in Sub-Saharan Africa: Barriers and policy recommendations for Covid-19 and beyond. *International Journal of Medical Informatics, 151*, 104467. DOI: 10.1016/j.ijmedinf.2021.104467

El Malouf, N., & Bahemia, H. (2025). Diffusion of Innovations: A review. In S. Papagiannidis (Ed), *TheoryHub Book*. https://open.ncl.ac.uk

Emmanuel, A. K., Abdul, S. O., Obasi, D. E., Jokoh, P. E., Omoze, E. M., Usoh, A. E., Ashimi, A. A., & Adisa, A. A. (2025). Investigating the challenges and opportunities of telemedicine in enhancing health care access in Nigeria. *Int J Clin Med Case Stud., 2*(1), 1004. DOI: 10.52768/3067-3852/1004

Exner-Pirot, H. (2022). Challenges of Telehealth. https://openpress.usask.ca/northernhealthcare/chapter/chapter-25-challenges-totelehealth-implementation/

Ezeani, I. U., Okwuonu, G. C., Chukwuonye, I. I., & Nkpozi, M. O. (2022). The Impact of Telemedicine during the COVID-19 Pandemic in Nigeria: A Review. *Annals of Health Research*, *8*(4), 260–268. DOI: 10.30442/ahr.0804-02-177

Fostina, P., Okon, E. U., & Chikaodili, A. I. (2024). Knowledge, Attitude, and Use of Telemedicine among Health Care Professionals in Federal Medical Center, Bayelsa State, Nigeria. GPH -. *International Journal of Health Sciences and Nursing*, *7*(05), 62–140. DOI: 10.5281/10.5281/zenodo.14237894

Gouveia, A. J., Ribeiro, J., Sousa, G., Barbosa, D., & Machado, M. (2025). Advancing Healthcare through Remote Patient Monitoring: A brief literature review. *Procedia Computer Science*, *256*, 893–899. DOI: 10.1016/j.procs.2025.02.192

Idris-Umarfarouq, I., Afolabi, A. A., Olorunfemi, D. O., & Akinola, A. I. (2022). Systematic Overview of Remote Patient Monitoring in Nigeria (West Africa). *Telehealth and Medicine Today*, *7*(3), 359. DOI: 10.30953/tmt.v7.359

Iyengar, K., Jain, V. K., & Vaishya, R. (2020). Pitfalls in telemedicine consultations in the era of COVID-19 and how to avoid them. *Diabetes & Metabolic Syndrome*, *14*(5), 797–799. DOI: 10.1016/j.dsx.2020.06.007

Keelara, R., Sutherland, E., & Almyranti, M. (2025). Leading practices for the future of telemedicine: Implementing telemedicine post-pandemic. OECD Health Working Papers No. 173. DOI: 10.1787/18152015

Khemapech, I., Sansrimahachai, W., & Toahchoodee, M. (2019). Telemedicine – Meaning, Challenges, and Opportunities. *Siriraj Medical Journal*, *71*(3), 246–252. DOI: 10.33192/Smj.2019.38

Lakmini, P. M., Naeem, R., & Keshav, D. (2019). Remote patient monitoring: A comprehensive study. *Journal of Ambient Intelligence and Humanized Computing*, *10*(1), 57–76. DOI: 10.1007/s12652-017-0598-x

Lawal, R. (2023).Transformative Potential of IoT on Smart Healthcare and Remote Patient Monitoring in Nigeria: A Literature MSC Internet of Things with Data Analytics. DOI: DOI: 10.13140/RG.2.2.24453.52966

Lawani-Luwaji, E., & Okafor, C. F. (2025). Perceptions of Telemedicine and Rural Healthcare Access in a Developing Country: A Case Study of Bayelsa State, Nigeria. *Barw Medical Journal*, *3*(4), 21–25. DOI: 10.58742/bmj.vi.187

Malaria Consortium. (2019). How remote villages in Nigeria can beat malaria through community health. https://malariamustdie.com/nigeria-community-health

Menage, J. (2020). Why Telemedicine Diminishes the Doctor-Patient Relationship. *British Medical Journal*. https://www.bmj.com/content/371/bmj.m4348

Miller, T. E., & Derse, A. R. (2002). Between Strangers: The practice of medicine online. *Health Affairs (Project Hope)*, *21*(4), 168–179. DOI: 10.1377/hlthaff.21.4.168

Moahi, K. H. (1999). Health Information Networks for Telehealth in Africa-Challenges and Prospects: A Review of the Literature. *Libri*, *49*(1), 43–50. DOI: 10.1515/libr.1999.49.1.43

Molefi, D. M. (2015).The status of telemedicine in Africa. https://nuviun.com/content/the-status-of-telemedicine-in-africa

Musa, S., Ramatu, A., Haliru, L., Abigail, D., & Gumbi, S. (2023). Establishing a paediatric telemedicine centre in a low-resource setting: Experience and challenges from a teaching hospital in Kaduna, Nigeria. *Sri Lanka Journal of Child Health*, *52*(2), 155–160. DOI: 10.4038/sljch.v52i2.10548

National Information Technology Development Agency. (2007). ACT 2007 ACT NO. 28. Federal Republic of Nigeria Official Gazette No. 99, Vol. 94 Lagos. https://nitda.gov.ng/wp-content/uploads/2020/11/NITDA-ACT-2007-2019-Edition1.pdf

National Legislative Bodies. (2011). Nigeria: Evidence Act, 2011. https://www.refworld.org/legal/legislation/natlegbod/2011/en/104226

Nigeria Data Protection Act. (2023). Explanatory Memorandum. https://placng.org/i/wp-content/uploads/2023/06/Nigeria-Data-Protection-Act-2023.pdf

Noel, N. B., Maryam, N. B., Yila, E., Nkala, C. A., & Banwat, M. E. (2024). Knowledge and Perception of Telemedicine among Medical Students of the University of Jos, Plateau State, Nigeria. *Nigerian Medical Journal : Journal of the Nigeria Medical Association*, *64*(6), 816–824.

Obotu, A. S. (2019). Perceived Effect of Telemedicine on Medical Service Delivery by Federal Medical Centers in North Central Zone of Nigeria. *Library Philosophy and Practice* (e-journal). 3051. https://digitalcommons.unl.edu/libphilprac/3051

Odunuga, K. V., Owoicho, O. E., Oredipe, F. B., Oke, O. E., Okogu, S. I., Anipole, O., Sunmola, M. A., Bamgbose, O. A., & Adebanjo, A. O. (2024). Artificial Intelligence in Nigeria's Health Sector, *Scholar. Journal of Computational Science*, *1*(8), 15–19. DOI: 10.5281/zenodo.13226114

Onyeabor, U. S., Okenwa, W. S., Onwuasoigwe, O., Lasebikan, O. A., Schaaf, T., Pinkwart, N., & Balzer, F. (2024). Telemedicine in the age of the pandemics: The prospects of web-based remote patient monitoring systems for orthopaedic ambulatory care management in the developing economies. *Digital Health*, *10*, 1–16. DOI: 10.1177/20552076241226964

Organization for Economic Cooperation and Development. (2023). *Health at a Glance 2023: OECD Indicators*. OECD Publishing., DOI: 10.1787/7a7afb35-

Oyeyemi, S. O., & Wynn, R. (2014). Giving cell phones to pregnant women and improving services may increase primary health facility utilization: A case-control study of a Nigerian project. *Reproductive Health*, *11*(1), 8. DOI: 10.1186/1742-4755-11-8

Oyinlola, A. (2024). Redefining healthcare delivery in rural areas through telemedicine.https://www.africanchangestories.org/2024/03/23/redefining-healthcare-delivery-in-rural-areas-through-telrmedicine/

Pandian, P. S. (2016). An Overview of Telemedicine Technologies for Healthcare Applications. *International Journal of Biomedical and Clinical Engineering*, *5*(2), 29–52. DOI: 10.4018/IJBCE.2016070103

Peter, I. D., Danjuma-Karau, K. J., Omokhuale, E. M., & Yakubu, J. C. (2025). A Mixed Methods Study of the Challenges and Prospects of Utilizing Telemedicine in the Delivery of Healthcare to Nigerian Children. *International Journal of Public Health*, *70*, 1607790. DOI: 10.3389/ijph.2025.1607790

Rasid, M. F., & Woodward, B. (2005). Bluetooth telemedicine processor for multichannel biomedical signal transmission via mobile cellular networks. *IEEE Transactions on Information Technology in Biomedicine*, *9*(1), 35–43. DOI: 10.1109/TITB.2004.840070

Rogers, E. M. (2003). *Diffusion of Innovations* (5th ed.). Free Press.

Shah, P., Thornton, I., Kopitnik, N. L., & Hipskind, J. E. (2023). Informed Consent. National Library of Medicine. https://www.ncbi.nlm.nih.gov/books/NBK430827/

Ukaoha, K. C., & Egbokhare, F. A. (2012). Prospects and Challenges of Telemedicine in Nigeria. *Journal of Medical and Biomedical Sciences*, *3*(1), 65–70. DOI: 10.7813/jmbs.2012/3-1/10

Ukpe, E. (2025). Transforming Healthcare: Telemedicine's Role and Impact in Nigeria. *IOSR Journal of Humanities and Social Science*, *30*(2), 20–26. DOI: 10.9790/0837-3002072026

Van Daalen, O. L. (2023). The right to encryption: Privacy as preventing unlawful access. *Computer Law & Security Review, 49*, 105804. DOI: 10.1016/j.clsr.2023.105804

Winter, A., Ammenwerth, E., Haux, R., Marschollek, M., Steiner, B., & Jahn, F. (2023). *Health Informatics: Health Information Systems Technological and Management Perspectives* (3rd ed.). Springer., DOI: 10.1007/978-3-031-12310-8

World Health Organization. (1997). *Health-for-all Policy for the 21st Century, HQ (document EB101/8)*. WHO.

World Health Organization. (2021). Global strategy on digital health 2020–2025. Geneva. https://www.who.int/publications/i/item/9789240020924

World Medical Assembly. (1999). Statement on Accountability, Responsibilities and Ethical Practice of Telemedicine 1999. https://www.wma.net/e/press/1999_5

ADDITIONAL READING

Amedari, M. I., & Ejidike, I. C. (2021). Improving access, quality, and efficiency in health care delivery in Nigeria: A perspective. *PAMJ - One Health : Pan African Medical Journal, 5*(3). Advance online publication. DOI: 10.11604/pamj-oh.2021.5.3.28204

Emery, S. (2020). *Telemedicine in Hospitals: Issues in Implementation*. Routledge.

Gwama, G. T., Olaboye, J. A., Maha, C. C., Ajegbile, M. D., & Abdul, S. (2024). Integrating electronic health records systems across borders: Technical challenges and policy solutions. *International Medical Science Research Journal, 4*(7), 788–796. DOI: 10.51594/imsrj.v4i7.1357

Heston, T. F., & Doarn, S. (2024). A Comprehensive Overview of Telemedicine. In *Biomedical Engineering*. IntechOpen., DOI: 10.5772/intechopen.1002138

Kumar, S. N., Zafar, S., Babulak, E., Alam, M. A., & Siddiqui, F. (2025). *Artificial Intelligence in Telemedicine Processing of Biosignals and Medical Images*. CRC Press.

Okwukwu, M., Oluwafemi, O. D., & Akintayo, T. A. (2025). Artificial Intelligence in Nigerian Healthcare: A Review of State, Challenges, and Opportunities. *EthAIca, 4*, 210. DOI: 10.56294/ai2025210

Onsongo, S., & Kagotho, E. (2024). *Telemedicine in Africa: Applications, Opportunities, and Challenges*. IntechOpen., DOI: 10.5772/intechopen.1005094

Zeshan, F., & Ahmad, A. (2023). *Recent Advancements in Smart Remote Patient Monitoring, Wearable Devices, and Diagnostics Systems*. IGI Global., DOI: 10.4018/978-1-6684-6434-2

KEY TERMS AND DEFINITIONS

Artificial Intelligence: Cognitive system

Healthcare Provider: A system or person who delivers healthcare.

Informatics: Data analysis

Patient: A client of a health professional.

Remote Area: A place far from cities with limited access.

Remote Patient Monitoring: Monitoring patient health data afar through technology.

Telemedicine: Adoption of digital communication systems to deliver healthcare.

Chapter 5
Enablers and Barriers to Digital Transformation of Integrated Care Systems (ICS) Across NHS England

Han Liew
http://orcid.org/0009-0002-7013-5050
National University Hospital, Singapore

Abdul M. Seckam
http://orcid.org/0000-0002-4516-9366
Healthcare Business Solutions, UK

Marzena Nieroda
University College London, UK

ABSTRACT

NHS England is shifting toward digital health technologies (DHT) to enhance care delivery, supported by both intrapreneurs and entrepreneurs. However, digital health companies face a key challenge: "no evidence, no implementation vs. no implementation, no evidence." The Health and Care Bill introduced 42 Integrated Care Systems (ICSs) to lead digital transformation, though barriers such as financial constraints, fragmented infrastructure, and leadership gaps persist. This scoping review analyzed 23 studies to identify enablers and barriers from digital health companies' perspectives, using the Service-Dominant logic and DEDHI framework. Findings were categorized across micro (patients, clinicians), meso

DOI: 10.4018/979-8-2600-2238-2.ch005

(organisations, providers), and macro (policymakers) levels. The study highlights the need for stakeholder collaboration, investment, and regulatory clarity to scale DHT adoption within ICSs.

1. PROBLEM STATEMENT

The National Health Service (NHS) England's journey towards digital transformation has been instrumental in driving improvements in healthcare delivery, patient outcomes, and operational efficiency (NHS England, 2022). The Integrated Care Systems (ICSs) are central to this transformation, a collaborative approach that seeks to integrate health and care services to provide more coordinated and patient-centred care (NHS England, 2021a). While the adoption of digital technologies and the implementation of ICS hold immense promise, significant challenges need to be addressed to fully leverage their potential.

Integrated Care Systems (ICSs)

ICSs are local partnerships between NHS trust, local government, and other relevant groups, to take collaborative responsibility for the health and care of the populations (Briggs et al., 2020). With the new Health and Care bill, there are a total of 42 ICSs areas have emerged and the creation of ICSs consists of i) Integrated Care Board (ICB), as a statutory NHS commissioning body, and ii) Integrated Care Partnership (ICP), as a statutory committee that responsible for developing a health and care strategy for the area (Briggs et al., 2020). However, there are some challenges ICSs are facing, firstly, financial constraints. For example, a survey of NHS trusts in 2022 found 98% expressed current financial allocations for 2022-2023 were insufficient to address inflationary pressure and 86% stated they would not achieve financial balance (National Audit Office, 2022). As a result, this leading to investment in digital transformation had not been sufficient to support the long-term ambitions of NHS digital transformation. For example, a study showed there was a significant variation in organisational digital maturity (e.g., readiness, capability, infrastructure) across hospitals in England. These findings demonstrate the potential challenges for the implementation of Digital Health Technology (DHT) in relation to the context of ICSs (Martin et al., 2019).

The purpose of this review is to investigate and analyse the enablers and barriers of digital transformation within NHS England's Integrated Care Systems. By conducting an in-depth study on the enablers and barriers of digital transformation in NHS England's ICS, this study aims to provide actionable insights in the market. Understanding the specific needs and challenges faced by NHS England will enable health-tech companies to address these requirements, maximise its value proposition, and contribute to the ongoing enhancement of healthcare services within the ICS framework.

2. BACKGROUND

Digital transformation has increasingly become an important phenomenon in the healthcare sector. Digital health involves tools and services that use information and communication technologies to improve the prevention, diagnosis, treatment, monitoring, rehabilitation, and management of health-related issues and to monitor and manage lifestyle habits that impact health (Collin and Varmus, 2015). One of the key priorities of the NHS Long-Term Plan (Briggs et al., 2020; NHS, 2019) is to support digital transformation and provide a step change in the way the NHS cares for citizens. Today, healthcare is at least 10 years behind other industries (e.g., hospitality, transport, retail, and banking) in the adoption of technologies in transforming the ways services are provided (Taylor, Hall and Siegel, 2019).

"Digital health" is an umbrella term that refers to the use of digital technology to improve the operation and quality of healthcare systems and services, as well as individual and population health (Hutchings and Morris, 2022). According to the NHS (2022), digital transformation envisions the use of technology to improve health and care professionals' communication better and enable patients to access the care they need quickly and easily when needed, by focusing on 3 key areas: working in more efficient ways, improving diagnosis and treatment, and improving services. Despite a robust policy push, substantial obstacles persist in achieving the political goal of positioning the NHS as the most innovative health system globally (Asthana, Jones and Sheaff, 2019). For example, following the disastrous National Programme for Information Technology (NPfIT) launched in 2002 and terminated in 2011 after an investment of £7.3bn, the NHS England moved away from the idea of top-down mandated IT systems and instead encouraged a 'let many flowers bloom' approach, in another word, this has led to led to a largely localised approach to digitalization (Asthana et al, 2019; Justinia, 2017).

Digital innovation plays a crucial role in the digital health ecosystem, Spena and Cristina (2020) explored that this is increasingly emerging from health tech companies with a focus on tech-enabled services. In healthcare systems like the NHS, innovation is driven by intrapreneurship, where members within the organisation actively create innovative ideas, such as Clinical Entrepreneur Programme for clinical and non-clinical NHS staff (Arora et al., 2021). In the meantime, innovation is also largely driven by entrepreneurs who generate novel concepts and collaborate with healthcare partners (Arora et al., 2021). Service-Dominant (SD) Logic is derived from the form of exchange of knowledge and services, and goods are merely an indirect way of providing a service (Joiner and Lusch, 2016). In the perspective of SD logic, it serves as a theoretical framework for understanding value co-creation in service-oriented systems like healthcare, emphasising the active involvement of a broad range of actors in the healthcare ecosystem (Nyende, 2018). Incorporating SD logic into this arena, digital health results in a complex ecosystem involving multiple actors, where diverse elements and behaviours intertwine, leading to novel forms of collaboration and value creation. For example, a digital healthcare company digitalise consent-taking for patients undergoing surgery, which has improved the efficiency of the surgical patient pathway and reduction in time spent on file storage, creation, and retrieval (Digital Health London, 2023). One of the key successes is through the support from Digital Pioneer Fellowship, the introduction of electronic consent-taking has demonstrated the value of co-creation and interactions between different players of the digital health ecosystem (e.g., patients, families, clinicians, hospitals, policymakers and digital health companies) to transform the conventional way of delivering care (Digital Health London, 2023; Kraus et al., 2021; Sebastiani and Anzivino, 2022). This is consistent with a systematic review of the adoption of telemedicine on cardiovascular patients, highlighting that the fundamental element of co-creating value in healthcare services is information and communication technology (e.g., data sharing, interoperability, integration to an existing workflow, and any management and exchange of health-related information) (Farabi et al., 2020).

In addition, Sebastiani and Anzivino (2022) explored that at the micro level, 'actor-role empowerment' plays a key role in the evolutionary process of the digital health ecosystem. To further elaborate, the role of the clinician in promoting and coordinating the other actors (e.g., patients) becoming increasingly vital, as healthcare professionals are often the sponsor of the adoption of DHT (Sebastiani and Anzivino, 2022). Besides that, the authors also underlined the importance of collaborative relationships at the meso level among service providers, hospitals, and health tech start-ups. For example, a study conducted in Germany has demonstrated that collaboration from multiple actors in the health ecosystem has promoted the opportunity to exchange information and experiences (Mühlensiepen et al., 2021). As a result, the transition to digital health services have contributed to the adoption of DHT by specialist, improve accessibility and successfully incorporated into clinical routine (Mühlensiepen et al., 2021). Drawing from a sociological perspective, sociologists conceptualised the nature of social problems are situated dynamics in three interrelated cycles that operate at the micro-, meso- and macro-level (Wijk et al., 2019). For example, scholars argued that the probability of being exposed to personal behavioural, and psychosocial risk factors (micro level) are significantly associated with the contextual factors (meso-level: such as societal organisation or institutions) as well as related to social determinants (macro-level) (Richter and Dragano, 2018). This demonstrates the importance of exploring the various mechanism (e.g., enabler and barriers) at different levels in the NHS ICSs context.

As the largest unified healthcare system, NHS. ICSs can appear as a place to innovate (Kelly and Young, 2017). To promote the invention, development and implementation of cost-effective technologies that improve healthcare delivery, there are several existing innovative routes that accelerate market entry for health tech companies (Arora et al., 2021). For example, Applied Research Collaboration, National Institute for Health Research Funding Scheme, Innovate UK, etc. However, it also brings along a unique set of challenges. Conversely, academic literature has evaluated the development and adoption of innovation in the healthcare sector. It remains significant barriers may be hindering the progression of the innovation pathway in NHS ICSs, such as lack of funding, lack of accountability and variation in digital maturity across regions. In the United Kingdom (U.K.), reports have shown that across all four nations varying degrees of success, in the use of digital technologies to modernize services (Taylor et al., 2019). While all nations have experienced challenges in digital transformation, England has seen significant variation in terms of the extent, quality, and scope of the solutions that have been implemented and the outcomes achieved (Taylor et al., 2019). Kelly and Young (2017), identified that for the successful implementation of innovation for digital health companies or start-ups, there are three stages such as invention, development, and implementation. In the NHS Context, works of literature showed that there are significant challenges in each stage. For instance, i) lack of access to funding and support (invention phase), ii) lack of access of clinical data for prototyping and clinical testing (development phase) and iii) the bureaucracy associated with the ability to achieve interoperability within the NHS (implementation phase) (Arora et el., 2021). To further elaborate, small and medium-sized enterprises (SMEs) prioritise their budget for product development, but wider implementation needs robust evidence of benefits, facing challenges due to new ventures and long approval times for evaluation (Guo et al., 2020). Scholars stated digital health companies face significant paradoxes in digital health, 'no evidence, no implementation versus no implementation, no evidence' (Guo et al., 2020). In general, this presents obstacles for digital health companies or start-ups as they strive to integrate their innovative solutions into ICSs in NHS England.

Taking the COVID-19 pandemic as an example, this pandemic acted as a catalyst that accelerated the digital transformation in healthcare. The healthcare industry experienced a significant shift in its usual practices such as virtual care, teleconsultation, remote monitoring, advancement of technology and improvement in clinical practices. For example, before the pandemic, approximately 80% of General Practice (GP) appointments took place in person (Hutchings, 2022). However, by June 2020, this percentage had decreased to slightly below 50%, with a similar proportion of appointments occurring via telephone (Hutchings, 2022). Undoubtedly, the remarkable digital healthcare companies' achievement of transitioning NHS services and the rapid integration of DHT to combat the Covid-19 pandemic raise important questions about the lasting impact on healthcare delivery and clinical practices. It is essential to consider the potential risks and disadvantages, especially when such transformations occur at an accelerated pace.

As ICSs adopt and implement system-wide digital leadership and transformation, we ask the question: "What are the enabler and barriers of digital transformation to the implementation of ICSs in NHS England?" There is limited research into the successful implementation of the digital transformation amongst ICSs. To further understand the role of digital health adoption in NHS England and the implication of ICS in digital transformation on digital healthcare companies, this study performed a scoping review to gain insights and explore the enablers and barriers in the art of digital transformation in healthcare.

The article is structured as follows. The next sections outline the objectives and the theoretical approach adopted in this study. Followed by the methodology used in this paper. We then present the secondary findings from the three databases, such as its enablers and barriers across micro, meso- and macro-levels. Then, conclusions and the implications of our findings for digital healthcare companies.

3. OBJECTIVES

1. To understand the enablers and barriers from a digital health companies' perspective in relation to the digital transformation in ICSs.
2. To identify and map the relevant stakeholders involved in the digital transformation process across the micro-, meso-, and macro-levels within NHS England.
3. To categorize and classify the various enablers and barriers of digital transformation across the micro, meso, and macro levels within ICSs NHS England.

4. THEORETICAL APPROACH

Service-Dominant (SD) Logic

SD Logic is derived from the form of exchange of knowledge and services, and goods are merely an indirect way of providing a service (Joiner and Lusch, 2016). In the perspective of SD logic, it serves as a theoretical framework for understanding value co-creation in service-oriented systems like healthcare, emphasising the active involvement of a broad range of actors in the healthcare ecosystem (Nyende, 2018).

In recent decades, the health system has undergone significant changes due to the integration of digital technologies (Botti and Monda, 2020). This transformation has made the system more intricate, dynamic, and involves multiple facets and stakeholders (Botti and Monda, 2020). For example, the patient's role within this environment has become increasingly active and central, signifying a shift towards patient empowerment and engagement. For this reason, customer value co-creation and SD logic have gained attention in healthcare (Joiner and Lusch, 2016). Value co-creation in healthcare is a complex process and not necessarily linear due to the wide range of actors with different and unique roles, skills and competencies involved in (Hardyman, Daunt and Kitchener, 2015). Studies on the role of healthcare technologies (e.g., electronic health records, mobile apps, telemedicine, wearable devices, remote monitoring and etc.) have shown the role of digital transformation for the development of value cocreation in a healthcare context (Nyende, 2018). In line with the aim of this paper, using SD logic, the authors would explore the various actors to understand the interactions and engagement of digital health transformation at micro-, meso- and macro- levels. Specifically, the exploration will be conducted from the perspective of NHS ICSs to inform and provide insights digital health companies and their impact in the context of the transformation.

5. METHODOLOGY

Design and Evaluation of Digital Health Intervention (DEDHI) Framework

In this scoping review, The DEDHI framework was adopted as an ideal approach for conceptualising the research topic, owing to its comprehensive nature and focus on DHT (Kowatsch, et al., 2019).

This framework emphasises the importance of interdisciplinary collaborations, bringing together stakeholders from various sectors. In this scoping review, the study team will involve digital health organisations, health insurance providers, patient organisations, and pharmaceutical companies. This diverse group of stakeholders will provide valuable insights into the real-world implementation and impact of DHT. Moreover, the DEDHI framework was developed from a wide range of field knowledge such as behavioural medicine, medical informatics, and information systems. These interdisciplinary perspectives will enhance the depth and accuracy of our findings, enabling us to understand the complexities of DHT from multiple angles.

In conclusion, the DEDHI framework serves as an ideal guide to structuring our research on DHT from a digital healthcare companies' standpoint. By utilising this framework, we can gain a comprehensive understanding of the enablers and barriers of DHT through the SD logic lens, to understand the evolution of value cocreation and interdisciplinary collaborations to advance digital health innovation and improve patient outcomes through digital transformation.

Exploring Terminology

According to DEDHI's framework, Digital Health Intervention (DHI) is described as the action of intervening with "tools and services that use information and communication technologies (ICTs) to improve prevention, diagnosis, treatment, monitoring and management of health and lifestyle", which is closely related to the notion of mHealth, telemedicine, telecare and health IT (Kowatsch, et al., 2019). This definition is consistent with the World Health Organization's (WHO) explanation of the term 'digital health', which encompass electronic health records, virtual care, remote monitoring, artificial intelligence, smart wearables, and tools enabling data exchange and storage and tools enabling remote data capture and sharing of relevant information across the health ecosystem (WHO, 2021). By employing this framework, we can gain a comprehensive overview of the evaluation criteria and implementation barriers related to DHT. The framework allows us to identify the key factors that influence the success and efficacy of DHT across NHS England ICS.

Design

A scoping review in line with Munn et al. (2018) was carried out to compile knowledge from previous research on the enablers and barriers to scaling up digital transformation in the healthcare sector. This methodology was chosen because it allowed the study team to review evidence in these emerging fields and identification of research gaps. In contrast to a traditional literature review, this methodology involved summarising various articles and publications on a specific topic, which could be considered subjective due to its reliance on the author's existing knowledge of the subject matter (Munn et al., 2018). The following keywords were used to explore this topic: "digital health", "digital transformation", "Integrated Care System (ICS)", "United Kingdom", "NHS", "enabler" and "barrier". The authors also incorporated practical perspectives from experts from various sources e.g., NHS Confederation, independent reviews, etc. in the context of ICSs.

Search Strategy

The study team searched the above-mentioned words on three prominent digital databases- Scopus, PubMed and EBSCON. To ensure an in-depth analysis of this study, Cochrane databases were initially included as the fourth database. However, while it is a valuable source, it is important to acknowledge that its primary emphasis remains on systematic reviews, randomised trials, and study protocol (Science Direct, 2023). Therefore, the Cochrane database was not included in the final selection as the information was not directly related to this study topic.

This review's search was done using Boolean operators and a list of keywords: "enabler", "barrier", "NHS", "Digital Transformation", and "Digital Health". As emphasised by Gusenbauer and Haddaway (2020), performing Boolean searches can effectively and efficiently enhance the performance of search systems such as the precision and reproducibility of our research. Furthermore, to make sure that all potentially relevant studies were identified, we adopted 4 search IDs as outlined in Table 1. This would enable a wider range of papers to be considered for inclusion, broaden our initial search strategy and produce more reliable findings (Bramer et al., 2018). We limit the search to the last 5 years (2017 - 2023), as the digital landscape has evolved rapidly with new technologies and tools constantly emerging, this allows the study team to capture the latest trends and best practices in relevant to the study topic. Searches were supplemented by manually screening the references of relevant articles. Only papers published in the English language were reviewed.

On study type, there was no restriction on the type of articles for inclusion. However, study titles and abstracts were screened based on predetermined inclusion and exclusion criteria which are outlined in table 2 below. The final reference list was generated based on originality and relevance to this viewpoint.

Table 1. Search IDs

	Search IDs
1	Digital Health AND Barrier* AND NHS
2	Digital Health AND Enabler* AND NHS
3	Digital Transformation AND Barrier* AND NHS
4	Digital Transformation AND Enabler* AND NHS

Table 2. Inclusion and exclusion criteria

Search Parameters	Inclusion criteria	Exclusion criteria
Population	Healthcare setting related	Non-healthcare setting
Date	2017-2023	N.A..
Intervention	Range of digital health/transformation	N.A.
Geographical areas/ location	UK/NHS	Non-UK based studies

Data Analysis

A scoping review in line with Munn et al. (2018) will be carried out to compile knowledge from previous research on the enablers and barriers to scaling up digital transformation in the healthcare sector. Our analysis was oriented by the DEDHI framework that serves to provide an overview of implementation barriers for DHT. Included studies were initially coded independently by the lead author under close guidance by the co-authors, identified themes were then synthesised below as shown.

Quality Appraisal

In line with scoping review practice, included studies were not quality appraised (Munn et al., 2018).

Ethical Approval

In the context of this scoping review, there is no involvement of human participants or the use of sensitive data. In addition, researchers did not collect new data or interact with human subjects directly. Instead, the study was analysed and synthesised from existing sources, it is considered as secondary research and less likely to raise ethical concerns (Taquette and Borges da Matta Souza, 2022). Therefore, ethical approval was not required. Nevertheless, it is essential to follow ethical guidelines for conducting literature reviews, such as proper citation and acknowledgement of the original authors' work and ensuring that the research is conducted with integrity and objectivity.

6. RESULTS & FINDINGS

Study Characteristics

A total of 868 articles were retrieved from three databases. In total, 52 articles that met the criteria were included for further screening. After reviewing full-text articles for eligibility, only 23 articles were included in the final stage. The flowchart is shown in Figure 1.

Figure 1. Scoping review flowchart

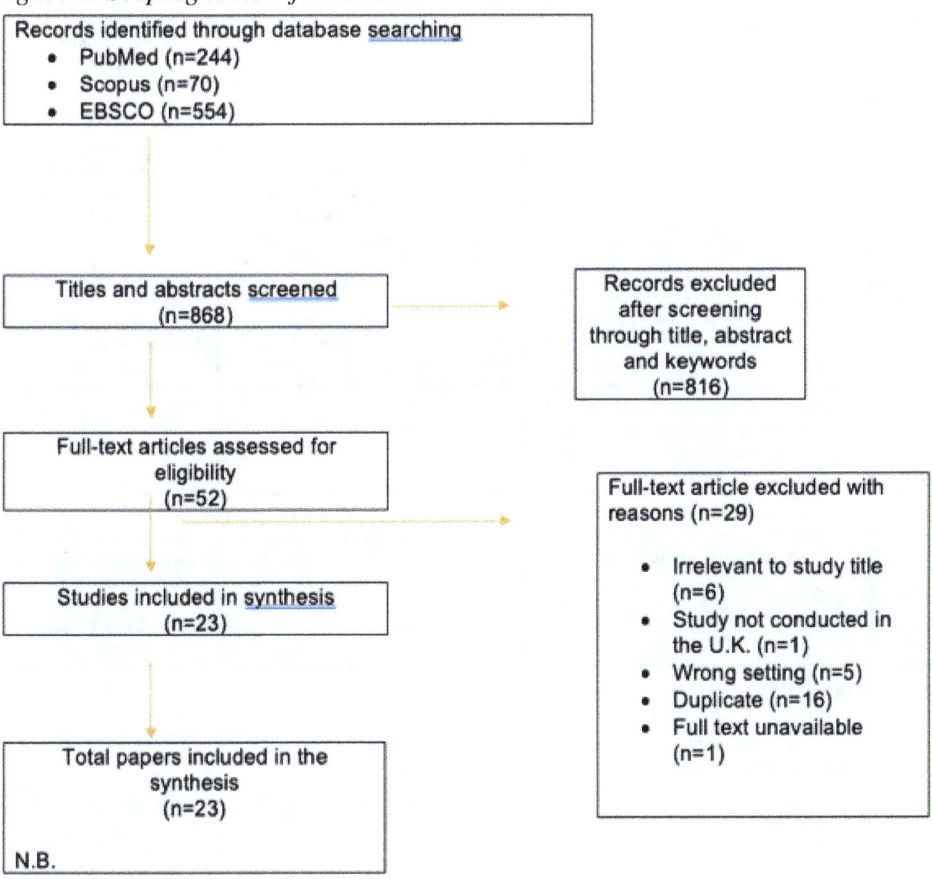

Overview Findings

A comprehensive analysis of 23 articles from three distinct databases has revealed a total of 26 barriers and 13 enablers. Upon further data analysis and synthesis, the identified categories encompassing barriers and enablers have been systematically allocated within three distinct societal contexts, namely micro, meso, and macro as shown in Table 3.

Table 3. Various groups of stakeholders were identified through this scoping review from 23 articles across micro, meso and maco societal contexts.

Societal levels	World Health Organization's definition*	Authors	Identified stakeholders/ actors
Micro	'...is the service users when they interact with service providers.'	(Pote et al., 2021; Twamley et al., 2022; O'Cathail et al., 2020; Sawyer et al., 2023; Turnbull et al., 2021; Leigh et al., 2020; Ibrahim et al., 2021; Buckingham et al., 2022; Nelson et al., 2023; Moody et al., 2022; Kanavos et al., 2022; Patel et al., 2022; Bucci et al., 2019; Joughin et al., 2021)	Clinician, patient, caregiver, family member, social worker, care coordinator, community worker, and social care worker.
Meso	'...the interaction between stakeholders is a critical determinant of the health system and its governance, such as public and private organizations, both for-profit and non-profit, offering clinical, para-medical, and non-clinical health services... unions, professional associations, and care or service networks.'	(Subbe et al., 2019; Leigh et al., 2020; Ibrahim et al., 2021; Buckingham et al., 2022; Dave et al., 2021; Tolley et al., 2023; Kanavos et al., 2022)	Local healthcare providers, commissioners, regulatory bodies, academic institutions, Information Technology experts
Macro	'...encompassing government organizations and agencies at both the central and sub-national levels.'	(Kanavos et al., 2022; Asthana et al., 2019)	NHS England, National commissioner, Clinical Commissioning Groups, Policy makers (e.g., National Institute for Health and Care Excellence)

Key: * WHO (2023)

Data Extraction

Table 4. Overview of micro-level of identified enablers and barriers

Categories *	Enablers	Authors	Barriers	Authors
Accessibility* The accessibility of technology, such as the ease of obtaining access (e.g., high accessibility (enabler), low accessibility (barrier).	#	(Bucci, et al., 2019)		(Dave et al., 2022)
Benefits* The presence or absence of benefits/incentives for healthcare providers to adopt digital health technology (e.g., presence (enabler), absence (barrier).)	#	(Bucci, et al., 2019; Joughin, et al., 2019)		N/A
Individual characteristics of end users* Characteristics of the patient (e.g., demographics, health status resistance to change and the healthcare provider (e.g., lack of willingness to cooperate, lack of trust in colleagues or politics (barriers); willing to cooperate, trust in healthcare providers or healthcare leaders (enablers).	#	(Bucci, et al., 2019)	#	(Sawyer et al., 2023; Harvey and Powell, 2020; William et al., 2020; Leigh et al., 2020; Buckingham et al., 2022; Dave et al., 2021; Watson et al., 2022; Bucci et al., 2020; Asthana et al., 2019)
Individual resources of users* Financial or temporal resources (e.g., low income, already high workload for rural healthcare providers (barriers); presence of digital literacy, able to afford electronic devices (enablers)	#	(Patel et al., 2022)	#	(Pote et al., 2021; Joughin, et al., 2021; Twamley et al., 2022; Sawyer et al., 2023; Turnbull et al., 2021; Buckingham et al., 2022; Nelson et al., 2023; Watson et al., 2023; Asthana et al., 2019; Bucci, et al., 2019)
Social interaction Interaction between patient and healthcare provider (e.g. limited personal connection, interaction, and relationship (barriers); positive experience or interaction among users (e.g., healthcare professionals, customers, patients and etc.) (enablers)	#	(Bucci et al., 2019)	#	(O'Cathail et al., 2020; Patel et al., 2022; Bucci et al., 2019; Joughin et al., 2021; Harvey & Powell, 2020)

continued on following page

Table 4. Continued

Categories *	Enablers	Authors	Barriers	Authors
Usability of technology Effort needed to use the technology according to its purpose (e.g., lack of user centred design, complex use, problems with technical supports (barriers); user-centred design approach, user-friendly DHT (enablers).	#	(Bucci et al., 2019; Bucking-ham et al., 2022)	#	(Joughin et al., 2021; Twamley et al., 2022; Nelson et al., 2023; Moody et al., 2023; Bucci et al., 2019)
Negative Association* Negative associations of healthcare providers, regarding the technology (barriers)	N/A	N/A	N/A	(Pote et al., 2021; Harvey & Powell, 2020; Bucci et al., 2021)

*: Kowatsch et al., 2019
#: identified categories
N/A- Not Applicable

Table 5. Overview of meso-level of identified enablers and barriers

Categories*	Enablers	Authors	Barriers	Authors
Cooperation Lack of cooperation between healthcare providers (e.g., lack of authority or conflict potential (barriers); collaboration, multidisciplinary team meetings, efficient resource utilisation (enablers)	#	(Pote et al., 2021; Subbe et al., 2019; Bucci et al., 2019; Ibrahim et al., 2021; Tolley et al., 2023; Kanavos et al., 2022; Patel et al., 2022; Cooper et al., 2022)	N/A	N/A
Social support Consideration of patient's Environment, presence of community support, social and support groups (enablers)	#	(Twamley et al., 2022; Turnbull et al., 2021)	N/A	N/A
Diseases Requirements due to patient's disease (e.g., special demands for group therapy)	#	(Bucci et al., 2019)	#	(Twamley et al., 2022; Bucci et al., 2019)

continued on following page

Table 5. Continued

Categories*	Enablers	Authors	Barriers	Authors
Human technical support Support for end user by humans (e.g., lack of skilled IT maintenance workforce) (barrier).	#	(Pote et al., 2021; Harvey & Powell, 2020)	#	(Kanavos et al., 2023)
Integration Integration of technology into healthcare system (e.g., technology isolated from care processes) (barriers); effectively integrate technology into existing workflow, enhance operational efficiency (enablers).	#	(Twamley et al., 2022)	#	(Pote et al., 2021; Tolley et al., 2023; Bucci et al., 2019)
Methodology: The availability or the process of proof of evidence (e.g., cost-effectiveness) (enablers); lack of clinical and cost-effectiveness evaluation of DHT (barriers).	#	(Leigh et al., 2020)	#	(Bucci, Schwannauer and Berry, 2019)
Planning: Administrative activities (e.g., lack of broad scope, technology isolated from care processes (barriers), proper planning of implementation of DHT, alignment with organisation vision, mission and goal, efficient time management (enablers).	#	(Patel et al., 2022)	#	(Kanvos et al., 2022; Bucci et al., 2019; Twamley et al., 2022)
Interoperability: The ability of technology to be used with existing infrastructure (lack of interoperability).	N/A	N/A	#	(Subbe et al., 2019; Tolley et al., 2023; Bucci et al., 2019)
Regional infrastructure: Infrastructure available for the end user (e.g., lack of technological infrastructure such as internet coverage).	N/A	N/A	#	(Pote et al., 2021; Tolley et al., 2023)
Accessibility: The accessibility of technology, such as the ease of obtaining access (e.g., low accessibility (barrier)).	N/A	N/A	#	(Patel et al., 2022; Buckingham et al., 2022; Bucci et al., 2019)
Usability of technology: Effort needed to use the technology according to its purpose (e.g., lack of user-centred design, complex use, problems with technical support (barriers); user-centred design approach, user-friendly DHT (enablers)).	#	(Tolley et al., 2023)	#	(Swayer et al., 2021)
Benefits: The absence of benefits/incentives for healthcare providers to adopt digital health technology (barrier).	N/A	N/A	#	(Dave et al., 2021; Kanvos et al., 2022)

continued on following page

Table 5. Continued

Categories*	Enablers	Authors	Barriers	Authors
Cost: Cost for start-up and maintenance, high cost of technology.	N/A	N/A	#	(Leigh et al., 2020)
Culture: Characteristics of the end user which are inherent in a group of users belonging together (e.g., language).	N/A	N/A	#	(Tolley et al., 2023; Harvey and Powell, 2020)
Funding: No funding, insufficient funding for equipment, lack of long-term funding.	N/A	N/A	#	(Pote et al., 2021; O'Cathail et al., 2020)
Guideline: Lack of consistency between clinicians and guidance, lack of policies, lack of training materials in adopting digital technologies (barriers).	N/A	N/A	#	(Pote et al., 2021; Patel et al., 2022)
Workforce: Professional people involved in the usage of the DHI (e.g., high turnover of medical staff).	N/A	N/A	#	(Tolley et al., 2023; Bucci et al., 2019)

*: Kowatsch et al., 2019
#: identified categories
N/A- Not Applicable

Table 6. Overview of macro-level of identified enablers and barriers

Categories*	Enablers	Authors	Barriers	Authors
Regulatory issues "Regulatory issues by governmental and non-governmental organisations which need to be followed (e.g., liability and jurisdiction) (enablers); Risk of cybersecurity issues, lack of credible, reliable in data privacy and data sharing (barriers)"	#	(Ibrahim et al., 2021)	#	(Moody et al., 2022; Kanavos, et al., 2022; Bucci, et al., 2019; Asthana et. al., 2019; Sawyer, et al., 2023; Subbe, et al., 2019; Bucci, Schwannauer, and Berry, 2019; Buckingham, et al., 2022; Ibrahim et al., 2021)
Funding "No funding insufficient funding for equipment, lack of long-term funding"	#	(Tolley et al., 2023)	#	(Harvey and Powell, 2020; Pote et al., 2021; O'Cathail et al., 2020; Asthana et. al., 2019)
Planning "Administrative activities (e.g., lack of broad scope, technology isolated from care processes (barriers), proper planning of implementation of DHT, alignment with organisation vision, mission and goal, efficient time management (enablers)"	#	(Asthana et al., 2019)	#	(Asthana et al., 2019)

continued on following page

Table 6. Continued

Categories*	Enablers	Authors	Barriers	Authors
Interoperability "Ability of technology to be used with existing infrastructure (lack of interoperability)"	N/A	N/A	#	(Asthana et al., 2019)
Regional infrastructure "Infrastructure available for the end user (e.g., lack of technological infrastructure)"	N/A	N/A	#	(Dave, et al., 2021)

*: Kowatsch et al., 2019
#: identified categories
N/A- Not Applicable

Overview Findings

A comprehensive analysis of 23 articles from three distinct databases has revealed a total of 26 barriers and 13 enablers. Upon further data analysis and synthesis, the identified categories encompassing barriers and enablers have been systematically allocated within three distinct societal contexts, namely micro, meso, and macro as shown in Table 3.

7. DISCUSSION

The categories of enablers and barriers have demonstrated that digital transformation across NHS England's ICS is influenced by different levels (micro, meso and macro) and actors (e.g., end-users, policymakers, regulatory bodies, software developers, commissioners, service managers, service providers and hospitals). Taking SD logic's perspective, provides broad applicability, extending to various stakeholders and encompassing the digital health ecosystem (Vargo and Lusch, 2017). From a digital health companies' perspective, SD logic can be described as a system comprising self-contained and adaptable actors who integrate resources, are connected by shared institutional arrangements, and are engaged in mutual value creation through service exchange (Vargo and Lusch, 2017). Scholars persuasively argued that the benefit (value) realised by a 'customer' (e.g., beneficiary) occurs through the integration of resources from many sources, thus resulting in a seamless holistic experience (Vargo and Lusch, 2017). From this concept, our study will further highlight the role and potential impact of DHT companies' role and its impact across the three different levels in this digital health ecosystem.

Micro-Level

As noted in Table 3. In this review, three groups of stakeholders were identified such as healthcare professionals, patients, and carers/ family members. This is consistent with Lennon et al. (2017) findings that under the micro-level, the stakeholder group was mainly health professionals, the public and patients

Bucci et al. (2019) examined clinicians' views about adopting and utilising DHT within mental health service delivery. Scholars identified that when staff valued the potential 'benefit' for DHT to be used as an adjunct therapy to traditional mental health service rather than a replacement would facilitate the adoption of DHT (Bucci et al., 2019). This study was conducted across three large NHS trusts, but the authors acknowledged that the majority of the study sample was amongst a White British cohort, which limits the generalisability of the findings across NHS England. From an end-user perspective, 'usability of technology' such as user-friendly and easy to use were perceived to be the key influence to achieving meaningful health goals at the community level (Buckingham et al., 2022). For example, wearable activity monitors (e.g., Fitbit ®) emerged as the top choice among users due to their perceived ease of use and usefulness in monitoring various aspects of health, including physical activity, sleep, and heart rate (Buckingham et al., 2022). Additionally, these devices were found to be motivating, providing individuals with the incentive to make behavioural changes (Buckingham et al., 2022). Moody et al. (2023) argued that the 'usability of technology' is seen as a barrier in the NHS context, especially the elderly for self-management of chronic diseases, such as diabetes and dementia. Besides that, Moody et al. (2023) reported that a lack of diversity in design such as English language-only apps would potentially be excluding ethnic minorities, people from low socio-economic backgrounds and those with low digital or literacy skills. Another study supported this argument that although 77% of elderly patients found virtual consultation more convenient than face-to-face, however more than half of the participants highlighted that they encountered various issues particularly related to usability (Joughin et al., 2021). These difficulties were significant enough that they required assistance from family members to access them (Joughin et al., 2021). Turnbull et al. (2022) and Buckingham et al. (2022) explored that, 'individual resources of users' as one of the main barriers such as lack of digital literacy and financial costs of patients. In the U.K., 27% (14 million) people have the lowest digital capability, this means that even with internet connectivity and digital device, people can still experience digital exclusion if they lack digital skills and confidence (Lloyds Bank, 2022). In relation to ICSs, Voluntary, Community and Social Enterprise (VCSE) plays a key role, for the NHS in supporting its aims to tackle health inequalities, improve outcomes in population health and healthcare and others. For example, VCSE organisations are working in the community to provide digital skills training and support to the public. 'Tech to Community Connect', an initiative organised by one of the VCSEs within the Surrey ICS, led to improved digital literacy among the community and residents were more willing to invest in their own devices (NHS England, 2021a). However, The King's Fund (2023a) reported that VCSE sector faces financial and sustainable investment challenges, sharing data, intelligence and insight, service design and delivery, and commissioning. Therefore, ICB and ICP need to carefully consider avenues to equitably resource the involvement of VCSE partners in ways that respect their time and resources (NHS England, 2021b). Drawing from healthcare professionals' perspective, Patel, Loraine and Gréaux (2022) found that specialist training is most helpful in supporting the adoption of DHT, followed by access to devices. Although this study's sample was recruited digitally and potentially led to selection bias. Ross et al. (2018) also emphasise the importance of providing resources such as time, training and education sessions as part of the implementation strategy of DHT in a routine healthcare setting. Nevertheless, such enabler ('individual resources of users') is also recognised within the NHS, for example, the recent Topol Review (2019) outlined recommendations to prepare the healthcare workforce through education and training. The independent review on ICSs has put forth a recommendation stating that, alongside digital literacy training, population health, prevention, and addressing health inequalities should be integral components of training and development for all professions (The Hewitt Review, 2023). These aspects should also be incorporated into the workforce plan to ensure the acquisition of skills necessary for enhancing health equity (The Hewitt Review, 2023).

Meso-Level

In our study, at the meso-level, we have identified a range of stakeholders (refer to Table 3.). These findings align with the research conducted by author Lennon (2017) on the NHS, highlighting the consistency in recognizing the significance of involving diverse stakeholders in shaping the governance and delivering products and services within the mixed-sector digital health ecosystem in the U.K.

A total of eight studies have emphasised the significance of 'cooperation' in enabling digital transformation, this also reinforces the concept of SD logic on value cocreation through collaborative effort (Joiner and Lusch, 2016). Tolley et al. (2023) conducted a study on the utilisation of DHT in the North East and North Cumbria (NENC) integrated care system (ICS). The findings highlighted that professionals working across different care settings often need to engage with multiple IT systems as part of their daily responsibilities. The study underscored the importance of enhanced collaboration among diverse professionals across the care sector, who possess valuable information to support decision-making processes (Tolley et al.,

2023). This collaboration was identified as a key driver for transformation within the NENC ICS. However, the authors acknowledged the limited transferability of their findings due to the study's sample being confined to the NENC ICS. Similarly, Ibrahim et al. (2021) emphasised the need to raise awareness within the data and digital health communities regarding the importance of ensuring the interoperability and adaptability of digital health solutions. The authors stressed that it is crucial for funders, regulators, policymakers, and politicians to mandate that creators of digital health solutions provide assurance of their technologies' performance across diverse populations and settings. For example, within Greater Manchester collaborated with the pharmaceutical industry in adopting a machine learning algorithm in exploring the system impact of Covid-19 on the cardiometabolic pathway. This collaboration resulted in the development of a predictive tool that informs local policymaking, commissioning decisions, and service redesign efforts. (Boehringer Ingelheim, 2023; Manja, 2023). They highlighted the responsibility of health data research and digital health communities to educate these stakeholders to effectively leverage DHT in digital transformation in the NHS. In general, these studies collectively emphasise the crucial role of 'cooperation' among stakeholders in driving digital transformation in healthcare. Frame through the lens of SD logic, this synergistic interaction between stakeholders is facilitated by user engagement, which plays a fundamental role in the value co-creation process (Botti and Monda, 2020).

Below the author will outline the overlap between enablers and barriers for the theme: 'disease' and 'methodology'. Within the total of three articles that discussed 'disease' categories, two specifically pertain to mental health, while the remaining article focused on critical care. According to Bucci et al. (2019), DHT has emerged as a significant player in the mental health space, offering considerable potential to empower vulnerable individuals, particularly in the context of psychotherapy practice. Their research highlights the substantial impact of DHT in diagnosing and assessing mental health conditions, showing comparable effectiveness to traditional in-person care. This finding is further substantiated by another study that suggested DHT are not only feasible but also effective in the early intervention of psychosis, acting as a promising starting point for introducing individuals to the use of DHT services (Bucci, Schwannauer and Berry, 2019). In contrast, Twamley et al. (2022) presented a different perspective on the adoption of DHT specifically virtual reality technology, in clinical applications. Twamley and colleagues argued that a more comprehensive understanding is required to evaluate and co-create these interventions. The study highlighted the importance of considering potential side effects and adverse reactions experienced by end-users, such as dizziness among post-ICU patients. These side effects can potentially cause harm rather than provide benefits, thereby jeopardizing patient safety. In addition, our study 'methodology' is identified as an enabler. To further elaborate, this highlights the role of Health

Technology Assessment (HTA) in identifying the most clinically- and cost-effective tools based on the levels of evidence (Unsworth et al., 2021). Leigh, Ashall-Payne and Andrews (2020) found that in terms of the adoption of mobile health among healthcare professionals, an NHS stamp of approval and published studies are significant enablers of digital prescribing. However, the Organisation for the Review of Care and Health Apps (ORCHA) commissioned by NHS, reported that in 2021 out of 9,000 digital health products, only 20% met the safety and quality thresholds (Digital Health, 2021). These findings further confirmed by several scholars that digital health developers face challenges due to regulatory uncertainties and the need to demonstrate clinical and economic benefits (Kanavos et al., 2022). To improve the accessibility of applications or web-based products, it is a legal requirement to meet the Web Content Accessibility Guidelines (WCAG). However, these developers still lack awareness of the evidence required to make a robust case when approaching commissions (William et al., 2020). For example, testing for an App designed to support users with type 2 diabetes should include a diverse range of users, including older adults with sensory or cognitive impairments, to represent the intended user base accurately (Neal et al., 2022). In 2021, the National Institute for Health and Care Excellence (NICE) published an updated version of the Evidence Standards Framework (ESF) to guide developers and commissioners on the levels of evidence required for economic and clinical evaluation for DHT (Unsworth et al., 2021). In relation to the web-based product, hence, it is important for digital health companies to consider these needs, if to successfully embed DHT into NHS England.

Macro-Level

Upon reviewing our articles, in our analysis, we have identified multiple stakeholders who actively contribute to shaping healthcare policies and practices, particularly in terms of national policy or infrastructure readiness (refer to Table 3.) (Lennon et al., 2019).

A total of 10 articles have consistently highlighted common themes in the context of DHT in NHS, these themes related to ‘regulatory issues as a barrier include concerns about patient data security, trust in self-management technology, the presence of outdated regulatory procedures, and the significance of data privacy. The importance of carefully considering data privacy policies and evaluating the suitability of digital platforms for clinical use is stressed (Watson et al., 2021). Moody et al. (2022) explored the barriers to the effective use of DHT amongst the elderly cohort. Users expressed the fear of data being sold, scepticism towards big data and AI, and the anxieties associated with data privacy, all of which contribute to the reluctance in adopting digital platforms (Moody et al., 2022). Asthana et al. (2019) further elaborated that within the digital health sector, a significant presence is observed in small and medium-sized enterprises (SMEs), but a considerable number of them lack the capability to meet the technical, clinical, and cost-effectiveness standards mandated by NHS Digital and NICE. The consistent findings across these articles underscore the need to prioritize data security, trust, and regulatory compliance within the digital health sector. From the angle of SD logic, data and knowledge exchange amongst the ecosystem actors enable value co-creation and resource integration (Botti and Monda, 2020). To give an example, a case study done in Italy show that, data sharing gains valuable information that provides accuracy in diagnosing and brings benefits not just to individual patients but to the entire community (Botti and Monda, 2020). In addition, patient data holds significant value within the patient network, while the provider network's primary value lies in the knowledge derived from processing and interpreting the data.

Conversely, Ibrahim et al. (2019) recognised that digital transformation has the potential to worsen existing healthcare inequalities. To prevent a digital health divide, Ibrahim et al. (2019) argued that regulators should mandate digital health developers to increase transparency regarding the composition of training datasets in Artificial Intelligence (AI) and machine learning models. Additionally, there is a need to raise awareness and establish accountability mechanisms, as well as maintain public trust within the data and digital health communities (Subbe, et al., 2019; Sawyer, et al., 2023). Without trust, populations are less likely to agree for their health data to be used beyond their care, severely impacting available data for health care and research (NHS Confederation, 2022). In 2022, NHS published 'Data Saves Lives: Reshaping Health and Social Care with Data' reassuring that all ICSs will need to establish smart digital and data foundations in place, such as promoting interoperability, data management, and promoting trust and transparency use of data. (Department of Health & Social Care, 2022). However, each trust has place-based differences in terms of different stages of its data transformation journey. For this reason, Goldacre Review has proposed granular recommendations to mitigate and address these challenges at a national level (Goldacre and Morley, 2022).

Financial pressure on the NHS will only grow, to maintain the current level of service provided by the NHS, it is projected that there needs to be an average annual increase in spending of 3.3% over the next 15 years (The Health Foundation, 2018). In the short term, larger increases are necessary to address immediate funding issues (The Health Foundation, 2018). This would result in health spending growing at a faster rate than the national income, with the share of national income dedicated to health rising from 7.3% to 8.9% by 2033/34. In 2019, in the U.K. only spend 9.9% of Gross Domestic Product (GDP) on health, below the average for comparable countries (The King's Fund, 2023b). This further reinforces our findings where a total of five articles reported that 'funding' is a significant barrier that would hinder the progression of digital transformation in the NHS. For example, NHS has created a supportive policy context to promote and accelerate the adoption of digital transformation (Asthana et al., 2019). Such as the Accelerated Access Pathway in 2016, and Global Digital Exemplar (GDE) programme have been implemented to facilitate the integration of digital technologies in the NHS (Cresswell, Sheikh and Williams, 2021). These policy initiatives demonstrate the commitment of the NHS to embrace digital transformation. In addition, studies indicate that the distribution of financial pressures within the NHS is uneven, resulting in various concerns. Such as failing to meet its digital commitments and lack of investment in digital health infrastructures and technology, which poses significant barriers for digital health companies. These concerns encompass the absence of ring-fenced funding, insufficient financial support for training, and a tightly regulated budget when implementing projects. (O'Cathail et al., 2020; Pote et al., 2021; William et al., 2020). This further supported by another study that revealed the crucial role of adequate funding arrangements, such as a contractual framework, is vital in supporting and incentivising community pharmacists to adopt DHT. Nevertheless, this was a qualitative study with a focus on NENC's community context, thus limiting the generalisability across NHS England (Leung, 2015).

8. STRENGTHS AND LIMITATIONS

The strengths of this review include its exploration of three databases and the novel application of a theoretical framework within the context of three societal contexts of NHS England. However, its limitations must also be acknowledged. First, as a scoping review, a formal quality assessment of studies was not undertaken, which limited the assessment of the strength of evidence in this review. However, this allowed us to capture the breadth of the literature on digital facilitation in primary care. We were able to describe the breadth of the types of facilitation and provide some assessments of usefulness based on diverse evidence. It is possible that in restricting the selection of publications to 2017 onward, authors may have missed earlier publications of relevance; however, from our staged and iterative process in restricting the date, we do not anticipate that this was likely. Second, the adopted DEDHI framework was developed through an inductive approach, relying on content analysis techniques and existing justificatory knowledge (Kowatsch et al., 2019). As a result, the DEDHI framework has not been applied, validated or revised during the development and evaluation of the digital health sector. Thus, empirical evidence that supports the utility of this framework is not established yet. Furthermore, the adopted methodology carries subjective procedures. Conducting scoping reviews and qualitative content analysis is subject to limitations from the subjectivity introduced by the researchers. Nevertheless, measures were taken to minimise these biases. For instance, each step was closely supervised by 2 independent co-authors/ supervisors and any discrepancies were resolved through thorough discussion and consensus.

9. IMPLICATION TO PRACTICE

Digital healthcare companies face challenges when introducing radical innovations (e.g. digital health technology) in the product development stage into the traditional healthcare service industry. Besides that, there is also limited understanding regarding the key drivers of success during the initial growth stages of digital healthcare companies or start-ups. As noted above, our findings provide valuable insights to digital healthcare companies with respect to the ongoing digital transformation across NHS England. Through the analysis of multiple case studies on digital health service start-ups, the analysis revealed that effective network management plays an integral part of success by introducing revolutionary innovations and navigating the complex healthcare landscapes (Muhos et al., 2019). Notably, networking with funding actors (e.g., venture capitalists, private or angel investors) has proven to be a pivotal factor in the success of start-ups and the gateways into the healthcare ecosystem (Muhos et al., 2019). However, as start-ups progress into the later phases of scaling up their products or integrating them into healthcare systems like the NHS, the dynamics shift, and a more diverse range of actors becomes involved. This includes health economists, commissioners, patients, clinicians, as well as engineers or software developers, each playing unique roles in cocreating value in the healthcare ecosystem. This argument further strengthened the concepts of SD logic, such as service exchange, resource integration, value co-creation, value determination, within the health ecosystems (Vargo and Lusch, 2017).

On the micro level, its influence spans accessibility for users, the individual resources available to users, and the usability of the technology itself (refer to Table 4). On the meso level, its contributions encompass the integration of technology within the healthcare system, the imperative of interoperability, and regional infrastructure (refer to Table 5). These insights gleaned from the study provide health-tech companies with invaluable guidance on how to strategically position itself within the dynamic digital health ecosystem. Moreover, these findings serve as a compass for enhancing the company's value proposition, especially as it seeks to seamlessly embed its technology across ICSs in NHS England.

A strategy to enhance the adoption and implementation of DHT within ICSs involves a multifaceted approach. At the micro-level, the proposition is to collaboratively develop solutions by involving individuals with lived experiences, practitioners, and partners. Tailoring solutions to the unique needs and digital readiness of each ICS is pivotal, given their distinct population demands and digital maturity levels. For instance, health-tech companies' clinical engagement team could consider employing a design thinking methodology. This would facilitate a profound comprehension of organisational and user needs, acknowledging that patient-centredness is at the core of successful design thinking. By adopting this approach, usability, acceptability, and efficacy of DHT can be enhanced, aligning with patient-centric objectives. Transitioning to the meso-level, various ICSs grapple with challenges ranging from workforce shortages to insufficient bed capacity and backlogs in vital medical services like diagnostics, surgeries, and cancer care. To address these operational bottlenecks, it becomes imperative for DHT, to showcase their tangible impact. Demonstrating the ability to mitigate issues, such as reducing time expenditure and curbing referrals to secondary care, is paramount.

10. FUTURE RESEARCH AGENDA

With these in mind, this study has demonstrated that efforts should be made to incorporate the relevant stakeholders across micro-, meso- and macro-levels to achieve successful digital transformation across ICSs. Further research exploring specific DHT for different diseases and various technological tools through the SD logic (e.g. value cocreation), such as prevention, monitoring and detection, self-management and rehabilitation, would be beneficial from the perspectives of digital health companies and start-ups.

11. CONCLUSION

Drawing theoretical knowledge and practical perspective from experts, this study offers an overview of enablers and barriers across the digital health ecosystem: macro-, meso- and micro-levels. Furthermore, this review has provided deeper insights into the opportunities and barriers to the implementation of DHT in relation to the context of ICS in NHS England. The successive governments have acknowledged the significance of digitalising the NHS. ICSs are striving to improve population health and healthcare outcomes, tackle inequalities in access and experiences, and enhance productivity and cost-effectiveness. Simultaneously, the Department of Health and Social Care has prioritised the digital transformation of health services as a top agenda item for itself and NHS England (Goldacre and Morley, 2022). To effectively and sustainably integrate care into patient-centred and value-based approaches, robust digital support is essential. This necessitates adopting a comprehensive paradigm for participatory health and health informatics since digitisation cannot progress without it. Emphasising digital cooperation across the innovation space is crucial for future acceleration and seamless integration, particularly with the emergence of new care models like the hospital at home. Equally important, is safeguarding equity and inclusion in the digital age. To achieve these goals, a complete re-evaluation of interoperability, data governance, and standards adoption is indispensable. It's worth noting that the NHS's ambition for digital transformation is not new, with numerous attempts over the past two decades. The department recognises the valuable lessons learned from these endeavours and the extraordinary deployment of digital technologies during the pandemic. The National Audit Office (2020) revealed that these efforts were costly and largely unsuccessful (National Audit Office, 2020). As a consequence, digital health companies faced significant challenges in bringing radical innovations to the NHS. Literature findings support SD logic as a key concept in the digital health ecosystem, digital health companies will have to shift their perspective from solely 'making something' or 'delivering values' to 'facilitating', focusing on value cocreation through collaborative efforts (Wells et al., 2015).

In this study, we systematically listed the factors that facilitate or hinder progress at various levels (micro, meso, and macro). The insights derived from this study are intended to empower digital health companies to prioritise specific areas during their product lifecycle management, implementation, and innovation processes. By understanding the multifaceted landscape of influences, these companies can make informed decisions and strategies effectively to navigate challenges and capitalise on opportunities in their pursuit of successful development and innovation in the digital health sector.

REFERENCES

Arora, A., Wright, A., Cheng, T. K. M., Khwaja, Z., & Seah, M. (2021). Innovation pathways in the NHS: An introductory review. *Therapeutic Innovation & Regulatory Science*, *55*(5), 1045–1058. DOI: 10.1007/s43441-021-00304-w PMID: 34009551

Asthana, S., Jones, R., & Sheaff, R. (2019). Why does the NHS struggle to adopt eHealth innovations? A review of macro, meso and micro factors. *BMC Health Services Research*, *19*(984), 1–7. DOI: 10.1186/s12913-019-4790-x PMID: 31864370

Boehringer Ingelheim. (2023). Utilisation of data science to identify the system impact of COVID-19 on the cardiometabolic pathway, and identifying opportunities for transformation across Greater Manchester. https://www.boehringer-ingelheim.com/uk/partnering/working-together/partnering-interests/collaborative-working/greater-manchester-utilisation-data-science

Botti, A., & Monda, A. (2020). Sustainable value co-creation and digital health: The case of Trentino eHealth ecosystem. *Sustainability (Basel)*, *12*(13), 5263. Advance online publication. DOI: 10.3390/su12135263

Bramer, W. M., de Jonge, G. B., Rethlefsen, M. L., Mast, F., & Kleijnen, J. (2018). A systematic approach to searching: An efficient and complete method to develop literature searches. *Journal of the Medical Library Association: JMLA*, *106*(4), 531–541. DOI: 10.5195/jmla.2018.283 PMID: 30271302

Briggs, A. D. M., Göpfert, A., Thorlby, R., Allwood, D., & Alderwick, H. (2020). Integrated health and care systems in England: Can they help prevent disease? *Integrated Healthcare Journal*, *2*(11), e000013. Advance online publication. DOI: 10.1136/ihj-2019-000013 PMID: 37441304

Bucci, S., Berry, N., Morris, R., Berry, K., Haddock, G., Lewis, S., & Edge, D. (2019). "They are not hard-to-reach clients. We have just got hard-to-reach services." Staff views of digital health tools in specialist mental health services. *Frontiers in Psychiatry*, *10*, 344. Advance online publication. DOI: 10.3389/fpsyt.2019.00344 PMID: 31133906

Bucci, S., Schwannauer, M., & Berry, N. (2019). The digital revolution and its impact on mental health care. Psychology and Psychotherapy: Theory. *Psychology and Psychotherapy*, *92*(2), 277–297. DOI: 10.1111/papt.12222 PMID: 30924316

Buckingham, S. A., Walker, T., & Morrissey, K. (2022). The feasibility and acceptability of digital technology for health and wellbeing in social housing residents in Cornwall: A qualitative scoping study. *Digital Health*, *8*, 1–12. DOI: 10.1177/20552076221074124 PMID: 35096410

Cooper, R., Giangreco, A., Duffy, M., Finlayson, E., Hamilton, S., Swanson, M., Colligan, J., Gilliatt, J., McIvor, M., & Sage, E. K. (2022). Evaluation of myCOPD digital self-management technology in a remote and rural population: Real-world feasibility study. *Journal of Medical Internet Research, 10*(2), e30782. Advance online publication. DOI: 10.2196/30782 PMID: 35129453

Dave, S., Abraham, S., Ramkisson, R., Matheiken, S., Pillai, A. S., Reza, H., Bamrah, J. S., & Tracy, D. K. (2021). Digital psychiatry and Covid-19: The big bang effect for the NHS? *BJPsych Bulletin, 45*(5), 259–263. DOI: 10.1192/bjb.2020.114 PMID: 33081867

Department of Health & Social Care. (2022). Data saves lives: Reshaping health and social care with data. https://data.parliament.uk/DepositedPapers/Files/DEP2022-0485/Data_saves_lives_Reshaping_health_and_social_care_with_data.pdf

Digital Health. (2021, July). ORCHA poll reveals public are willing to embrace digital to help NHS. https://www.digitalhealth.net/2021/07/orcha-poll-digital-nhs/

Digital Health London. (2023). Rolling out a digital consent pilot for patients undergoing surgery. https://digitalhealth.london/rolling-out-a-digital-consent-pilot-for-patients-undergoing-surgery

Farabi, H., Rezapour, A., Jahangiri, R., Jafari, A., Rashki Kemmak, A., & Nikjoo, S. (2020). Economic evaluation of the utilization of telemedicine for patients with cardiovascular disease: A systematic review. *Heart Failure Reviews, 25*(6), 1063–1075. DOI: 10.1007/s10741-019-09864-4 PMID: 31760593

Goldacre, B., & Morley, J. (2022). Better, broader, safer: Using health data for research and analysis. Department of Health and Social Care. https://assets.publishing.service.gov.uk/government/uploads/system/uploads/attachment_data/file/1067058/summary-goldacre-review-using-health-data-for-research-and-analysis.pdf

Guo, C., Ashrafian, H., Ghafur, S., Fontana, G., Gardner, C., & Prime, M. (2020). Challenges for the evaluation of digital health solutions—A call for innovative evidence generation approaches. npj. *Digital Medicine, 3*(1), 110. Advance online publication. DOI: 10.1038/s41746-020-00314-2 PMID: 32904379

Gusenbauer, M., & Haddaway, N. R. (2020). Which academic search systems are suitable for systematic reviews or meta-analyses? Evaluating retrieval qualities of Google Scholar, PubMed, and 26 other resources. *Research Synthesis Methods, 11*(2), 181–217. DOI: 10.1002/jrsm.1378 PMID: 31614060

Hardyman, W., Daunt, K. L., & Kitchener, M. (2015). Value co-creation through patient engagement in health care: A micro-level approach and research agenda. *Public Management Review, 17*(1), 90–107. DOI: 10.1080/14719037.2014.881539

Harvey, J., & Powell, J. (2020). Factors influencing the implementation of self-management solutions in healthcare: An interview study with NHS managers. *British Journal of Health Care Management, 26*(3), 61–70. DOI: 10.12968/bjhc.2019.0070

Hutchings, R. (2022). The impact of Covid-19 on the use of digital technology in the NHS. Nuffield Trust. https://www.nuffieldtrust.org.uk/sites/default/files/2020-08/the-impact-of-covid-19-on-the-use-of-digital-technology-in-the-nhs-web-2.pdf

Hutchings, R., & Morris, J. (2022). Digital health care across the UK: Where are we now? Nuffield Trust. https://www.nuffieldtrust.org.uk/resource/digital-health-care-across-the-uk-where-are-we-now

Ibrahim, H., Liu, X., Zariffa, N., Morris, A. D., & Denniston, A. K. (2021). Health data poverty: An assailable barrier to equitable digital health care. *The Lancet. Digital Health, 3*(4), e260–e265. DOI: 10.1016/S2589-7500(20)30317-4 PMID: 33678589

Joiner, K. A., & Lusch, R. F. (2016). Evolving to a new service-dominant logic for health care. *Innovation and Entrepreneurship in Health, 3*, 25–33. DOI: 10.2147/IEH.S93473

Joughin, A., Ibitoye, S., Cress, A., Shipway, D., & Braude, P. (2021). Developing a virtual geriatric perioperative medicine clinic: A mixed methods healthcare improvement study. *Age and Ageing, 50*(4), 1391–1396. DOI: 10.1093/ageing/afab066 PMID: 33989380

Justinia, T. (2017). The UK's national programme for IT: Why was it dismantled? *Health Services Management Research, 30*(1), 2–9. DOI: 10.1177/0951484816662492 PMID: 28166675

Kanavos, P., Vogelsang, M., Haig, M., & Kolovou, V. (2022). Challenges for health systems seeking to embrace virtual health care for population health. *The European Journal of Health Economics : HEPAC : Health Economics in Prevention and Care, 23*(7), 1079–1083. DOI: 10.1007/s10198-022-01503-4 PMID: 35921018

Kelly, C. J., & Young, A. J. (2017). Promoting innovation in healthcare. *Future Healthcare Journal, 4*(2), 121–125. DOI: 10.7861/futurehosp.4-2-121 PMID: 31098448

Kowatsch, T., Otto, L., Harperink, S., Cotti, A., & Schlieter, H. (2019). A design and evaluation framework for digital health interventions. it - Information Technology, 61(5), 253–263. https://doi.org/DOI: 10.1515/itit-2019-0019

Kraus, S., Schiavone, F., Pluzhnikova, A., & Invernizzi, A. C. (2021). Digital transformation in healthcare: Analyzing the current state-of-research. *Journal of Business Research, 123*, 557–567. DOI: 10.1016/j.jbusres.2020.10.030

Leigh, S., Ashall-Payne, L., & Andrews, T. (2020). Barriers and facilitators to the adoption of mobile health among health care professionals from the United Kingdom: Discrete choice experiment. *JMIR mHealth and uHealth, 8*(7), e17704. Advance online publication. DOI: 10.2196/17704 PMID: 32628118

Lennon, M. R., Bouamrane, M.-M., Devlin, A. M., O'Connor, S., O'Donnell, C., Chetty, U., Agbakoba, R., Bikker, A., Grieve, E., Finch, T., Watson, N., Wyke, S., & Mair, F. S. (2017). Readiness for delivering digital health at scale: Lessons from a longitudinal qualitative evaluation of a national digital health innovation program in the United Kingdom. *Journal of Medical Internet Research, 19*(2), e6900. Advance online publication. DOI: 10.2196/jmir.6900 PMID: 28209558

Leung, L. (2015). Validity, reliability, and generalizability in qualitative research. *Journal of Family Medicine and Primary Care, 4*(3), 324–327. DOI: 10.4103/2249-4863.161306 PMID: 26288766

Lloyds Bank. (2022). 2022 consumer digital index. https://www.lloydsbank.com/assets/media/pdfs/banking_with_us/whats-happening/221103-lloyds-consumer-digital-index-2022-report.pdf

Manja, V. (2023). The power of co-creating transformation. NHS Confederation. https://www.nhsconfed.org/articles/power-co-creating-transformation

Martin, G., Clarke, J., Liew, F., Arora, S., King, D., Aylin, P., & Darzi, A. (2019). Evaluating the impact of organisational digital maturity on clinical outcomes in secondary care in England. npj. *Digital Medicine, 2*(1), 41. Advance online publication. DOI: 10.1038/s41746-019-0118-9 PMID: 31304387

Moody, L., Wood, E., Needham, A., Booth, A., Aranda, A. J., & Tindale, W. (2022). Identifying individual enablers and barriers to the use of digital technology for the self-management of long term conditions by older adults. *Journal of Medical Engineering & Technology, 46*(6), 448–461. DOI: 10.1080/03091902.2022.2089249 PMID: 35748238

Mühlensiepen, F., Kurkowski, S., Krusche, M., Mucke, J., Prill, R., Heinze, M., Welcker, M., Schulze-Koops, H., Vuillerme, N., Schett, G., & Knitza, J. (2021). Digital health transition in rheumatology: A qualitative study. *International Journal of Environmental Research and Public Health, 18*(5), 2636. Advance online publication. DOI: 10.3390/ijerph18052636 PMID: 33807952

Muhos, M., Saarela, M., Foit, D.Jr, & Rasochova, L. (2019). Management priorities of digital health service start-ups in California. *The International Entrepreneurship and Management Journal*, *15*(1), 43–62. DOI: 10.1007/s11365-018-0546-z

Munn, Z., Peters, M. D. J., Stern, C., Tufanaru, C., McArthur, A., & Aromataris, E. (2018). Systematic review or scoping review? Guidance for authors when choosing between a systematic or scoping review approach. *BMC Medical Research Methodology*, *18*(1), 143. Advance online publication. DOI: 10.1186/s12874-018-0611-x PMID: 30453902

National Audit Office. (2020). Digital transformation in the NHS. https://www.nao.org.uk/wp-content/uploads/2019/05/Digital-transformation-in-the-NHS.pdf

National Audit Office. (2022). Introducing integrated care systems: Joining up local services to improve health outcomes. https://www.nao.org.uk/wp-content/uploads/2022/10/Integrated-Care-Systems-Funding-and-accountability-for-local-health-and-care.pdf

National Health Service. (2019). The NHS Long Term Plan. https://www.longtermplan.nhs.uk/wp-content/uploads/2019/08/nhs-long-term-plan-version-1.2.pdf

Neal, D., Engelsma, T., Tan, J., Craven, M. P., Marcilly, R., Peute, L., Dening, T., Jaspers, M., & Dröes, R. (2022). Limitations of the new ISO standard for health and wellness apps. *The Lancet. Digital Health*, *4*(2), e80–e82. DOI: 10.1016/S2589-7500(21)00273-9 PMID: 35090677

Nelson, D., Inghels, M., Kenny, A., Skinner, S., McCranor, T., Wyatt, S., Phull, J., Nanyonjo, A., Yusuff, O., & Gussy, M. (2023). Mental health professionals and telehealth in a rural setting: A cross sectional survey. *BMC Health Services Research*, *23*(1), 9083. Advance online publication. DOI: 10.1186/s12913-023-09083-6 PMID: 36849933

NHS Confederation. (2022). Data and research transformation in the NHS: What must be addressed? https://www.nhsconfed.org/publications/data-and-research-transformation-nhs-what-must-be-addressed

NHS England. (2021a). Resources for integrated care: Case studies. https://www.england.nhs.uk/integratedcare/resources/case-studies/army-of-tech-angels-to-help-people-with-shopping-and-virtual-life/

NHS England. (2021b). Building strong integrated care systems everywhere. https://www.england.nhs.uk/wp-content/uploads/2021/06/B0905-vcse-and-ics-partnerships.pdf

NHS England. (2022). Digital transformation. https://www.england.nhs.uk/digitaltechnology/

Nyende, H. (2018). The role of technology in value co-creation of maternal healthcare: A service-dominant logic perspective [Doctoral dissertation, University of Agder]. CORE. https://core.ac.uk/download/pdf/301378486.pdf

O'Cathail, M., Sivanandan, A. M., Diver, C., Patel, P., & Christian, J. (2020). The use of patient-facing teleconsultations in the National Health Service: Scoping review. *JMIR Medical Informatics*, *8*(3), e15380. Advance online publication. DOI: 10.2196/15380 PMID: 32175911

Patel, R., Loraine, E., & Gréaux, M. (2022). Impact of COVID-19 on digital practice in UK paediatric speech and language therapy and implication for the future: A national survey. *International Journal of Language & Communication Disorders*, *57*(5), 1112–1119. DOI: 10.1111/1460-6984.12750 PMID: 35925005

Pote, H., Rees, A., Holloway-Biddle, C., & Griffith, E. (2021). Workforce challenges in digital health implementation: How are clinical psychology training programmes developing digital competences? *Digital Health*, *7*, 1–11. DOI: 10.1177/2055207620985396 PMID: 33628457

Richter, M., & Dragano, N. (2018). Micro, macro, but what about meso? The institutional context of health inequalities. *International Journal of Public Health*, *63*(2), 163–164. DOI: 10.1007/s00038-017-1064-4 PMID: 29250722

Ross, J., Stevenson, F., Dack, C., Pal, K., May, C., Michie, S., Barnard, M., & Murray, E. (2018). Developing an implementation strategy for a digital health intervention: An example in routine healthcare. *BMC Health Services Research*, *18*(1), 794. Advance online publication. DOI: 10.1186/s12913-018-3615-7 PMID: 30340639

Sawyer, C., Hassan, L., Sainsbury, J., Carney, R., Bucci, S., Burgess, H., Lovell, K., Torous, J., & Firth, J. (2023). Using digital technology to promote physical health in mental healthcare: A sequential mixed-methods study of clinicians' views. *Early Intervention in Psychiatry*. Advance online publication. DOI: 10.1111/eip.13441 PMID: 37318221

ScienceDirect. (2023). Cochrane Library. https://www.sciencedirect.com/topics/nursing-and-health-professions/cochrane-library

Sebastiani, R., & Anzivino, A. (2022). The long and winding road of eHealth: The service ecosystem perspective. *Journal of Business and Industrial Marketing*, *37*(10), 2036–2049. DOI: 10.1108/JBIM-02-2021-0107

Spena, T. R., & Cristina, M. (2020). Practising innovation in health ecosystem: The agency of third-party actors. *Journal of Business and Industrial Marketing*, *35*(3), 390–403. DOI: 10.1108/JBIM-01-2019-0048

Subbe, C. P., Øvretveit, J., Quinn, N., & Wyatt, J. C. (2019). Opportunities and barriers for usage of personal health records in hospital: Report from a workshop of the Health Informatics Unit at Royal College of Physicians. *Future Healthcare Journal*, *6*(1), 52–55. DOI: 10.7861/futurehosp.6-1-52 PMID: 31098587

Taquette, S. R., & Borges da Matta Souza, L. M. (2022). Ethical dilemmas in qualitative research: A critical literature review. *International Journal of Qualitative Methods*, *21*, 1–15. DOI: 10.1177/16094069221078731

Taylor, K., Hall, B., & Siegel, S. (2019). Closing the digital gap: Shaping the future of UK healthcare. Deloitte. https://www2.deloitte.com/content/dam/Deloitte/uk/Documents/life-sciences-health-care/deloitte-uk-life-sciences-health-care-closing-the-digital-gap.pdf

The Health Foundation. (2018). Cost pressures on the NHS will only grow. https://www.health.org.uk/news-and-comment/news/cost-pressures-on-the-nhs-will-only-grow-it-needs-a-long-term-funding-solution-and-that-is

The Hewitt Review. (2023). An independent review of integrated care systems. https://assets.publishing.service.gov.uk/government/uploads/system/uploads/attachment_data/file/1148568/the-hewitt-review.pdf

The King's Fund. (2023a). Actions to support partnership: Addressing barriers to working with the VCSE sector in integrated care systems. https://www.kingsfund.org.uk/sites/default/files/2023-04/Addressing_barriers_to_working_with_the_VCSE_sector_in_integrated_care_systems_0.pdf

The King's Fund. (2023b). Key facts and figures about the NHS. https://www.kingsfund.org.uk/audio-video/key-facts-figures-nhs

The Topol Review. (2019). Preparing the healthcare workforce to deliver the digital future. https://topol.hee.nhs.uk/wp-content/uploads/HEE-Topol-Review-2019.pdf

Tolley, C., Seymour, H., Watson, N., Nazar, H., Heed, J., & Belshaw, D. (2023). Barriers and opportunities for the use of digital tools in medicines optimization across the interfaces of care: Stakeholder interviews in the United Kingdom. *JMIR Medical Informatics*, *11*, e42458. Advance online publication. DOI: 10.2196/42458 PMID: 36897631

Turnbull, S., Lucas, P. J., Hay, A. D., & Cabral, C. (2021). The role of economic, educational and social resources in supporting the use of digital health technologies by people with T2D: A qualitative study. *BMC Public Health*, *21*(1), 10325. Advance online publication. DOI: 10.1186/s12889-021-10325-7 PMID: 33546661

Twamley, J., Hamer, O., Hill, J., Kenyon, R., Twamley, H., Casey, R., Zhang, J., Williams, A., & Clegg, A. (2022). Exploring the perceptions of former ICU patients and clinical staff on barriers and facilitators to the implementation of virtual reality exposure therapy: A qualitative study. *Nursing in Critical Care*. Advance online publication. DOI: 10.1111/nicc.12868 PMID: 36458458

Unsworth, H., Dillon, B., Collinson, L., Powell, H., Salmon, M., Oladapo, T., Ayiku, L., Shield, G., Holden, J., Patel, N., Campbell, M., Greaves, F., Joshi, I., Powell, J., & Tonnel, A. (2021). The NICE Evidence Standards Framework for digital health and care technologies—Developing and maintaining an innovative evidence framework with global impact. *Digital Health*, *7*, 1–20. DOI: 10.1177/20552076211018617 PMID: 34249371

Vargo, S. L., & Lusch, R. F. (2017). Service-dominant logic 2025. *International Journal of Research in Marketing*, *34*(1), 46–67. DOI: 10.1016/j.ijresmar.2016.11.001

Watson, A., Mellotte, H., Hardy, A., Peters, E., Keen, N., & Kane, F. (2022). The digital divide: Factors impacting on uptake of remote therapy in a South London psychological therapy service for people with psychosis. *Journal of Mental Health*, *31*(6), 825–832. DOI: 10.1080/09638237.2021.1952955 PMID: 34319202

Wells, R. A., Gallarza, M. G., Andreu, L., & Calero, R. (2015). Application of service dominant logic to the medical device industry. *International Review on Public and Nonprofit Marketing*, *12*(3), 207–235. DOI: 10.1007/s12208-015-0126-7

Wijk, J., Zietsma, C., Dorado, S., Bakker, F. G. A., & Martí, I. (2019). Social innovation: Integrating micro, meso, and macro level insights from institutional theory. *Business & Society*, *58*(5), 887–918. DOI: 10.1177/0007650318789104

Williams, M. G., Stott, R., Bromwich, N., Oblak, S. K., Espir, C. A., & Rose, J. B. (2020). Determinants of and barriers to adoption of digital therapeutics for mental health at scale in the NHS. *BMJ Innovations*, *6*(3), 92–98. DOI: 10.1136/bmjinnov-2019-000384

World Health Organization. (2021). Global strategy on digital health 2020–2025. https://apps.who.int/iris/bitstream/handle/10665/344249/9789240020924-eng.pdf

World Health Organization. (2023). Health system governance. https://www.who.int/health-topics/health-systems-governance#tab=tab_1

KEY TERMS AND DEFINITIONS

Design and Evaluation of Digital Health Intervention Framework: A digital health intervention framework is a structured approach that guides the design, implementation, and evaluation of technology-based solutions aimed at improving healthcare outcomes, patient experiences, and overall well-being. This framework provides a systematic way to conceptualize, develop, deploy, and assess the effectiveness of digital tools, applications, or platforms in the healthcare domain. It takes into account various factors, including user needs, technological feasibility, ethical considerations, and measurable outcomes.

Digital Health Technologies: Digital health technology refers to the application of digital and information technologies to enhance healthcare delivery, improve patient outcomes, facilitate medical research, and streamline various aspects of the healthcare ecosystem. It encompasses a wide range of technological tools, devices, platforms, and applications that leverage digital innovations to support healthcare professionals, patients, and other stakeholders in managing and accessing healthcare services and information.

National Institute for Health and Care Excellence: NICE is an organization in the United Kingdom that provides evidence-based guidance and recommendations for healthcare professionals, institutions, and policymakers to improve the quality and effectiveness of healthcare services, treatments, and interventions.

National Health Services: The NHS, or National Health Service, is the publicly funded healthcare system in the United Kingdom. Established in 1948, the NHS provides comprehensive healthcare services to residents of the UK, regardless of their ability to pay. It is known for its core principles of being free at the point of use, providing healthcare services that are based on clinical need rather than the ability to pay, and being funded through general taxation.

Service-Dominant Logic: is a theoretical framework that challenges traditional product-centred views of business and emphasizes the primacy of services in economic exchange and value creation. It represents a shift in thinking from a focus on selling tangible products to delivering value through services and collaborative interactions. S-D Logic has gained prominence in marketing and business management disciplines and has implications for how businesses design, deliver, and market their offerings.

World Health Organization: World Health Organization, a specialized agency of the United Nations responsible for international public health. The WHO's mission is to promote global health, prevent the spread of diseases, and improve the overall well-being of people around the world.

Chapter 6
Effect of Digital Mental Health Technology on Mental Healthcare Accessibility in Sub-Saharan Africa:
A Systematic Review

Dede Atsu Kobla Latey
http://orcid.org/0009-0005-5274-2764
The London School of Economics and Political Science, UK

Robert Lubajo
http://orcid.org/0009-0004-7100-6036
WHO Regional Office for Africa, South Sudan

ABSTRACT

Mental health conditions are a growing public health concern in sub-Saharan Africa (SSA), where access to care remains severely limited due to shortages of professionals, infrastructure gaps, stigma, and urban-rural disparities. Digital mental health interventions have emerged as promising tools to bridge these gaps. However, the extent to which these technologies influence access to mental healthcare in SSA has not been systematically examined. A systematic review of peer-reviewed literature published between January 2000 and June 2025 was conducted to understand digital mental health technologies and their impact on mental healthcare accessibility in Sub Saharan Africa using Levesque et al.'s healthcare access framework, which conceptualizes access across five dimensions. The dimension of Acceptability emerged

DOI: 10.4018/979-8-2600-2238-2.ch006

as the most frequently addressed access dimension. Availability and accommodation were also commonly discussed. Affordability and approachability were less frequently studied Surprisingly, only a few studies explored the dimension of appropriateness.

INTRODUCTION

Mental health conditions are an escalating global public health concern, with recent estimates indicating that nearly one in four individuals will experience a mental disorder at some point in their lives, and depression and anxiety affecting 970 million people globally (Moitra et al., 2023) (Osborn et al., 2022) (Steel et al., 2014) (Abbafati et al., 2020). Mental disorders such as depression, anxiety, bipolar disorder, and schizophrenia are linked to impaired quality of life, reduced economic productivity, and premature mortality, often due to comorbid physical illnesses and increased suicide risk (Osborn et al., 2022) (Moitra et al., 2023). The World Health Organization's 2022 World Mental Health Report emphasizes that mental health is not merely the absence of illness but a vital component of overall well-being and societal development (Osborn et al., 2022).

Traditional interventions for mental health conditions typically include pharmacotherapy, psychotherapy, and rehabilitation programs, each targeting different aspects of symptom management and recovery (Philippe et al., 2022) (Agyepong et al., 2017) Evidence suggests that combining psychotherapy with medication can lead to improved outcomes, especially for chronic or treatment-resistant depression (Philippe et al., 2022) (Agyepong et al., 2017) Rehabilitation programs, including community-based care and assertive treatment models, play a crucial role in restoring functional capacity and social integration, particularly for individuals with severe mental illness (Clausen et al., 2020) (Mudiyanselage et al., 2024).

In recent years, there has been increasing interest in Digital Mental Health Interventions entailing the use of digital technologies such as mobile phones, internet platforms, computers, and tablets to deliver mental health information, screening, treatment, and support (Torous et al., 2021) (Philippe et al., 2022). These interventions include mobile applications, web-based therapy modules, interactive tools, games, and chatbots (Agbeyangi & Lukose, 2025). One of the most prominent forms of DMHIs is telemedicine, which leverages information and communication technologies (ICTs) to provide remote mental health care. Telemedicine has enabled broader access to psychiatric consultations, psychological therapies, and follow-up services, particularly in settings with limited mental health professionals (Shigekawa et al., 2018). In parallel, mobile health (mHealth) applications have emerged as promising tools for self-monitoring symptoms, receiving cognitive behavioural therapy (CBT), and gaining personalized feedback (Dietvorst et al., 2024) (Agyepong et al.,

2017) (Naslund et al., 2017). For example, maternal mental health apps targeting perinatal depression (PPD) are helping to address this underdiagnosed condition in low-resource settings (Naslund et al., 2017).

The COVID-19 pandemic has further accelerated the adoption of DMHIs by disrupting traditional care pathways and increasing the need for remote alternatives (Galazzi et al., 2025) (Dodoo et al., 2022). In response, the World Health Organization (WHO) has recognized digital innovations in mental health as a strategic opportunity to expand access, particularly in underserved and remote areas (Galazzi et al., 2025) (Dodoo et al., 2022). (WHO, 2024). These tools are seen as scalable and cost-effective solutions to overcome geographic and systemic barriers to care.

Despite these advancements, digital inequities persist, especially in SSA (Karamagi et al., 2022) (Agbeyangi & Lukose, 2025) (Torous et al., 2021). Mental health services in SSA remain highly constrained due to shortages in infrastructure and workforce, as well as stigma and stark urban-rural disparities (Atewologun et al., 2025). The effective deployment of DMHIs in SSA is further hindered by limited internet access, low digital literacy, gender gaps in device ownership, and cost-related barriers (Naslund et al., 2017) (Galazzi et al., 2025) (Dodoo et al., 2022).

Understanding how digital tools impact access to mental health care is critical for achieving health equity, particularly in regions like SSA where disparities in mental health services remain high. This insight can inform policies and interventions that leverage technology to bridge existing gaps in care. To explore this, we draw on Levesque et al.'s access to healthcare framework, which conceptualizes access as a dynamic interaction between individual and health system characteristics (Cu et al., 2021) (Levesque et al., 2013) (Penchansky & Thomas, 1981). The model outlines five key dimensions of accessibility of approachability, acceptability, availability/accommodation, affordability, and appropriateness, and links them with individuals' abilities to perceive, seek, reach, pay for, and engage with care. Applying this framework to DMHIs offers a structured lens through which to assess the extent to which digital interventions improve equitable access to mental health services in resource-constrained environments like SSA.

METHODOLOGY

Study Design and Protocol Registration

This study employed a systematic review of peer-reviewed literature spanning the past 25 years (January 1, 2000 – June 11, 2025), focusing on how digital health technologies influence access to mental healthcare in SSA. The review followed the Preferred Reporting Items for Systematic Reviews and Meta-Analyses Protocols

(PRISMA-P) 2020 guidelines (PRISMA, 2021) (Page et al., 2021) and adhered to the PRISMA 2020 reporting checklist throughout the review process.

Search Strategy

A comprehensive literature search was conducted on June 11, 2025, across three major bibliographic databases of MEDLINE (Ovid), EMBASE (Ovid), and Global Health (CABI). The search strategy was designed using the PICO framework, with three key concepts of "Sub-Saharan Africa" for the population/setting, "Digital health technologies" for the intervention and, "Access to mental health care" for the outcome. Controlled vocabulary (e.g., MeSH and Emtree terms) and keywords were combined using Boolean operators for each concept. The full database-specific search strategies are available in table 2. The database search was supplemented by backward citation tracking (reference list screening) of included articles and forward citation searching using Google Scholar.

Eligibility Criteria

This review included peer-reviewed studies published between January 2000 and June 2025 that were conducted in SSA and examined how digital health interventions influence access to mental health services. Eligible study designs comprised systematic reviews, randomized controlled trials (RCTs), cross-sectional studies, mixed-methods studies, and qualitative descriptive studies, all of which are limited to the English language. Studies were excluded if they were non-peer-reviewed (e.g., dissertations, white papers), editorial or opinion-based articles, study protocols, narrative reviews, conference abstracts lacking full texts, or if they did not focus on digital mental health or were conducted outside SSA.

Screening and Data Extraction

All search results were imported into Rayyan, an online tool for systematic reviews, for screening and deduplication (Ouzzani et al., 2016). Duplicate articles were removed by author DL. Two reviewers (DL and RL) independently screened all titles and abstracts against the inclusion criteria. Full texts of potentially eligible articles were then retrieved by author DL and reviewed by both authors (DL and RL). Discrepancies at both stages were resolved through discussion and consensus (via WhatsApp calls), with input from a third reviewer when necessary.

A structured data extraction form was developed by DL using Microsoft Excel to systematically collect information from the included studies. Extracted variables included study ID and author(s), year of publication, country and setting, study design, sampling method and sample characteristics, type of digital intervention used, outcome(s) measured in relation to access, analytical methods, key findings, and study limitations. The initial data extraction was performed by DL and subsequently verified for accuracy by RL.

Quality Appraisal

Two reviewers (RL and ADL) independently assessed the quality of each included study using appropriate critical appraisal tools: JBI Critical Appraisal Checklist for cross-sectional and mixed-methods studies and CASP Qualitative Checklist for qualitative studies. Any disagreements in appraisal were resolved by a third person. Each study was assigned a risk of bias rating (low, moderate, or high) based on the tool used, and results of the quality appraisal are presented in **Table 1. Data Synthesis**

Given the heterogeneity of the included studies in terms of design, digital intervention types, and study contexts, a narrative synthesis was employed. We followed guidance from Popay et al. (2006) on narrative synthesis, organizing the findings thematically. Emerging themes were coded inductively and deductively and grouped under conceptual categories aligned with Levesque's healthcare access framework: Approachability, Acceptability, Availability & Accommodation, Affordability, Appropriateness and their corresponding population abilities (Cu et al., 2021).

Figure 1. Levesque conceptual framework of access to health care

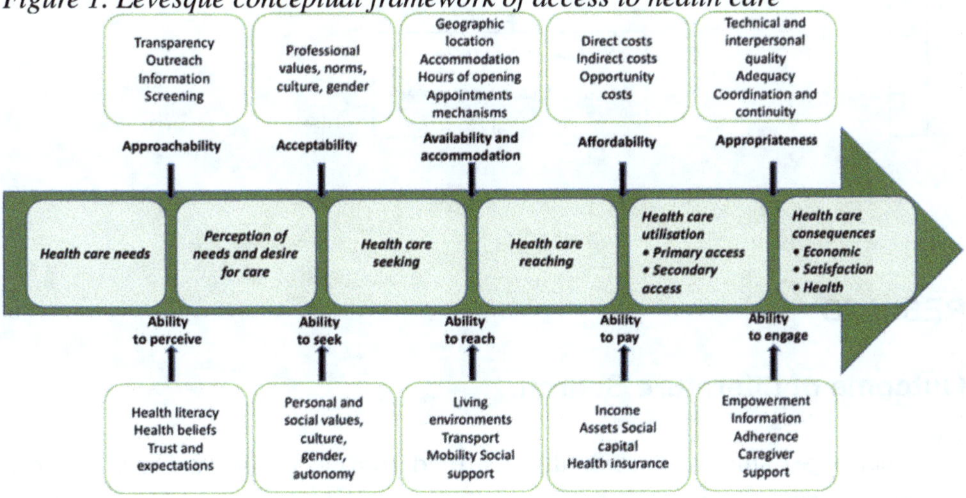

Figure 2. PRISMA 2020 Flow diagram

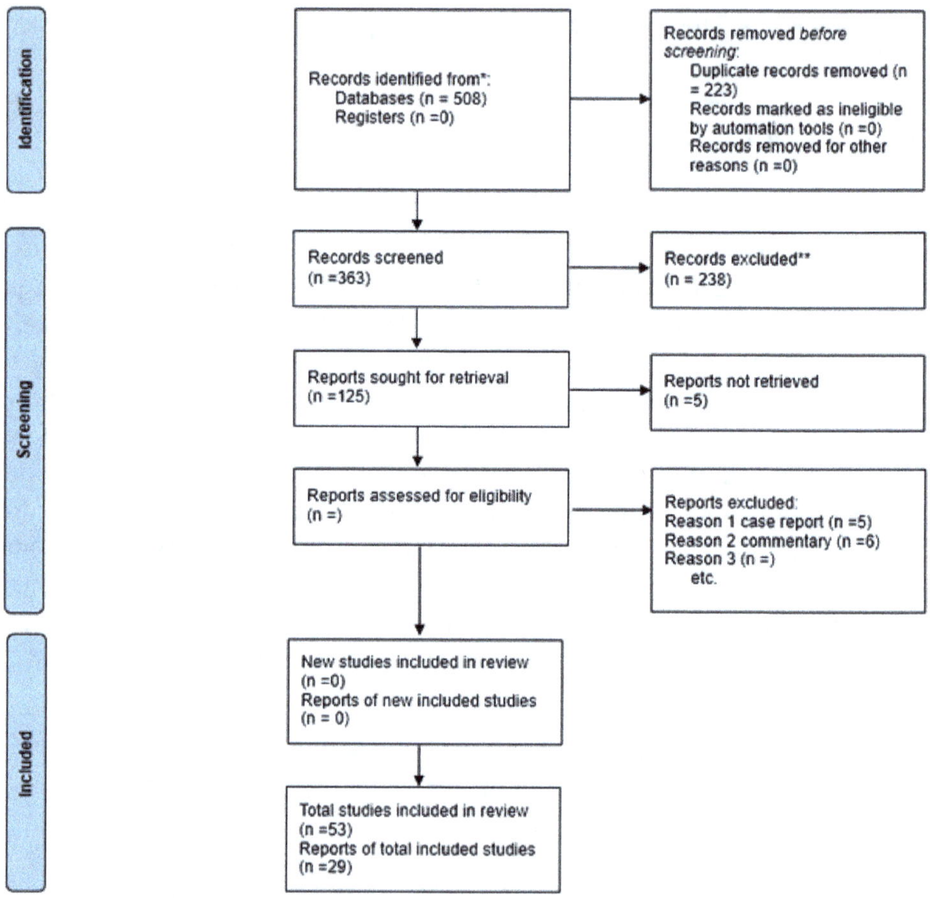

RESULTS

Outcome of Literature Search

A total of 586 studies were initially identified from electronic databases and grey literature. After removing 223 duplicates, 363 records were screened based on title, abstract, and full-text review. Of these, 238 studies were excluded, and 125 full-text articles were assessed for eligibility. Ultimately, 29 studies met the inclusion criteria and were included in this review. Details of the results are summarised on table 1 below.

Characteristics of the Included Studies

The 29 included studies were conducted across ten SSA countries. Most studies were from South Africa (8 studies) (Botes, 2025) (Chipps, Brysiewicz, et al., 2012) (Gbollie et al., 2023) (Groen et al., 2022) (Chipps & Mars, 2012) (Chipps, Ramlall, et al., 2012) (Sharma-Misra et al., 2023) (Sibeko et al., 2017), followed by Nigeria (5 studies) (Chen & Gombay, 2024) (Kola et al., 2021) (Ogundipe et al., 2025) (Adiukwu et al., 2022) (Mustafa et al., 2024), Kenya (4 studies) (Doukani et al., 2021) (Meffert et al., 2024) (Musyoka et al., 2023) (Kiburi et al., 2022), Ghana (3 studies) (Ben-Zeev et al., 2025) (Ben-Zeev et al., 2021) (Larsen et al., 2025), Ethiopia (2 studies) (Adem et al., 2023) (Sendek Anteneh et al., 2025), and Uganda (2 studies) (Kabukye et al., 2024) (Mwaka et al., 2025), with single studies each from Mozambique (O'Grady et al., 2022), Tanzania (Munishi et al., 2023), Sudan (Mustafa et al., 2024), and Malawi (Cox et al., 2024).

These studies were published between 2010 and 2025, with the majority 22/29 (76%) published from 2021onwards (Botes, 2025) (Chen & Gombay, 2024) (Chipps, Brysiewicz, et al., 2012) (Kabukye et al., 2024) (Ben-Zeev et al., 2025) (Gbollie et al., 2023) (Meffert et al., 2024) (Mustafa et al., 2024) (Larsen et al., 2025) (Munishi et al., 2023) (Mwaka et al., 2025) (Musyoka et al., 2023) (Ogundipe et al., 2025) (Adem et al., 2023) (Adiukwu et al., 2022) (Groen et al., 2022) (Cox et al., 2024) (Kaigwa et al., 2022) (Kiburi et al., 2022) (O'Grady et al., 2022) (Sendek Anteneh et al., 2025) (Sharma-Misra et al., 2023), and only 7/29 (24%) published before 2021 (Atujuna et al., 2021) (Ben-Zeev et al., 2021) (Doukani et al., 2021) (Kola et al., 2021) (Sibeko et al., 2017) (Chipps & Mars, 2012) (Chipps, Ramlall, et al., 2012) highlighting increasing interest in digital mental health solutions in the region.

Among the 29 studies, the majority employed cross-sectional methodologies (19 studies) (Atujuna et al., 2021) (Ben-Zeev et al., 2025) (Gbollie et al., 2023) (Kola et al., 2021) (Meffert et al., 2024) (Mustafa et al., 2024) (Larsen et al., 2025) (Munishi et al., 2023) (Ogundipe et al., 2025) (Sibeko et al., 2017) (Adem et al., 2023) (Adiukwu et al., 2022) (Groen et al., 2022) (Chipps & Mars, 2012) (Cox et al., 2024) (Kiburi et al., 2022) (O'Grady et al., 2022) (Sendek Anteneh et al., 2025) (Kaigwa et al., 2022), followed by qualitative studies (6) (Botes, 2025) (Chen & Gombay, 2024) (Ben-Zeev et al., 2021) (Mwaka et al., 2025) (Chipps, Ramlall, et al., 2012) (Kaigwa et al., 2022), mixed-methods approaches (3) (Kabukye et al., 2024) (O'Grady et al., 2022) (Sharma-Misra et al., 2023), and one RCT (Sibeko et al., 2017). Additionally, there was one pilot cohort study (Doukani et al., 2021). This variety of methodological designs enabled exploration of both experiences and measurable outcomes associated with digital mental health services.

The 29 included studies covered diverse population groups across various settings in SSA. Twelve studies focused on general adult populations or households (Adem et al., 2023) (Adiukwu et al., 2022) (Ben-Zeev et al., 2025) (Ben-Zeev et al., 2021) (Botes, 2025) (Chipps, Brysiewicz, et al., 2012) (Cox et al., 2024) (Kabukye et al., 2024) (Kola et al., 2021) (Meffert et al., 2024) (Ogundipe et al., 2025) (Sendek Anteneh et al., 2025). Six studies specifically targeted women, particularly pregnant or postpartum women, or those with children under five (Atujuna et al., 2021) (Chipps & Mars, 2012) (Doukani et al., 2021) (Gbollie et al., 2023) (Kaigwa et al., 2022) (Kiburi et al., 2022). Four studies sampled adolescents and youth populations (Chen & Gombay, 2024) (Chipps, Ramlall, et al., 2012) (Larsen et al., 2025) (Mwaka et al., 2025). Other studies focused on healthcare providers (Groen et al., 2022) (Munishi et al., 2023), university students (Mustafa et al., 2024) (Musyoka et al., 2023), and refugees or internally displaced persons (O'Grady et al., 2022) (Ogundipe et al., 2025) (Sharma-Misra et al., 2023) (Sibeko et al., 2017). This variation reflects the wide application of DMHIs across demographic groups.

Data collection methods ranged from structured surveys to interviews and focus group discussions, and some studies integrated telehealth usage analytics and feasibility trials while sample sizes varied greatly across studies. Quantitative surveys included anywhere from 200 to over 8,000 participants, while qualitative studies featured focused discussions with key informants, community health workers, or mental health users. Studies often targeted vulnerable groups such as youth, people with substance use disorders, and those in areas.

Most studies (n=16) reported descriptive outcomes, providing narrative or numerical summaries of findings without statistical testing (Botes, 2025) (Chen & Gombay, 2024) 28 (Chipps, Brysiewicz, et al., 2012) (Atujuna et al., 2021) (Ben-Zeev et al., 2025) (Ben-Zeev et al., 2021) (Doukani et al., 2021) (Gbollie et al., 2023) (Kola et al., 2021) (Meffert et al., 2024) (Munishi et al., 2023) (Musyoka et al., 2023) (Sibeko et al., 2017) (Adem et al., 2023) (Adiukwu et al., 2022) (Groen et al., 2022). Nine studies reported statistical significance using p-values, indicating hypothesis testing (Kabukye et al., 2024) (Mustafa et al., 2024) (Larsen et al., 2025) (Mwaka et al., 2025) (Ogundipe et al., 2025) (Cox et al., 2024) (Kaigwa et al., 2022) (Kiburi et al., 2022) (Sharma-Misra et al., 2023). One study used odds ratios as a measure of effect size (O'Grady et al., 2022). One study reported outcomes using Chi-square analysis (Sendek Anteneh et al., 2025).

Outcomes of Interest

The included studies evaluated DMHIs in relation to five dimensions of access, namely: approachability, acceptability, affordability, availability and accommodation, and appropriateness. The overall findings highlight how digital tools are influencing access to mental health care across SSA, while revealing gaps in infrastructure, equity, and contextual adaptation.

Acceptability

Acceptability was, reported in 22 studies (Adiukwu et al., 2022) (Atujuna et al., 2021) (Ben-Zeev et al., 2025) (Ben-Zeev et al., 2021) (Botes, 2025) (Chen & Gombay, 2024) (Chipps, Brysiewicz, et al., 2012) (Doukani et al., 2021) (Gbollie et al., 2023) (Kabukye et al., 2024) (Kiburi et al., 2022) (Kola et al., 2021) (Larsen et al., 2025) (Meffert et al., 2024) (Munishi et al., 2023) (Mustafa et al., 2024) (Musyoka et al., 2023) (Mwaka et al., 2025) (O'Grady et al., 2022) (Ogundipe et al., 2025) (Sendek Anteneh et al., 2025)(Sibeko et al., 2017). Across these studies, users generally viewed DMHIs as convenient, useful, and trustworthy. Acceptability was highest among young people and university students, who valued privacy, anonymity, and flexibility. Several studies highlighted how cultural and language adaptations enhanced engagement and reduced stigma. However, some users expressed concerns about confidentiality and the perceived effectiveness of digital interventions.

Affordability

Affordability was examined in studies, focusing on the cost of access to DMHIs, including the affordability of internet services, devices, and related expenditures, and how these costs influenced usage among target populations (Ben-Zeev et al., 2025) (Chen & Gombay, 2024) (Kaigwa et al., 2022) (Meffert et al., 2024).

Availability and Accommodation

Availability and Accommodation were addressed in studies, which examined system-level factors such as internet coverage, device ownership, network stability, and platform usability, affecting users' ability to access and interact with DMHIs effectively (Chipps, Ramlall, et al., 2012) (Cox et al., 2024) (Groen et al., 2022) (Kaigwa et al., 2022) (O'Grady et al., 2022) (Sharma-Misra et al., 2023) (Munishi et al., 2023).

Appropriateness

Appropriateness was reported in studies, which reflected how well the interventions were perceived to meet users' mental health needs, cultural expectations, and the suitability of the technology in the given context (Chipps, Brysiewicz, et al., 2012) (Chipps & Mars, 2012) (Chipps, Ramlall, et al., 2012) (Mustafa et al., 2024) (O'Grady et al., 2022).

Approachability

Approachability was reported in 4 studies which considered users' ability to identify and reach digital services, including awareness, digital literacy, and the clarity of information provided by platforms (Adem et al., 2023) (Adiukwu et al., 2022) (Munishi et al., 2023) (O'Grady et al., 2022).

Table 1. Study Characteristics and Findings

Author, year	Country and study design	Population	Outcome of interest	Key Findings
(Adem et al., 2023)	Cross-Sectional Study, Ethiopia	Mental health professionals in public referral hospitals	Acceptability	41 % of participants had adequate knowledge of telemental health services. Majority of the healthcare professionals (77.97%) were ready to implement telemental services.
(Adiukwu et al., 2022)	Cross-Sectional Study, Nigeria	Household members in rural Southwest Nigeria	Acceptabilty Approachability	Majority (99.4%) of the respondents knew about the two major treatment modalities available (i.e. pharmacotherapy and psychotherapy). Majority would choose telephone calls (56.3%) and instant messaging or WhatsApp (56.3%) for mental healthcare during the COVID-19 pandemic. However, they also identified stigma as a barrier in accessing telemental healthcare.
(Atujuna et al., 2021)	Cross-Sectional, South Africa	Young people (15–20 years) in South Africa	Acceptability	Bottom-up approaches, hence participatory ones used to deliver mental health support via text messaging are feasible.
(Ben-Zeev et al., 2025)	Cross-sectional Study, Ghana	200 Ghanaian women	Acceptability Affordability	Study participants prefer audio and video health modalities to others, and the interventions which have these modalities are considered more functional, accessible and affordable
(Ben-Zeev et al., 2021)	Qualitative Study, Ghana	People with mental health conditions in prayer camps	Acceptability	Mental health apps that use more animations than text are more accessible to the uneducated or those who are not used to using digital health tools.
(Botes, 2025)	Narrative Literature Review, South Africa		Acceptability	Designs that incorporate cultural nuances and adopt participatory approaches ensure reach to diverse populations. Some communities in South Africa showed reluctance to use digital mental health tools because they were concerned about stigma, trustworthiness and privacy
(Chen & Gombay, 2024)	Qualitative study, Nigeria		Acceptability Affordability	Digital mental health tools can provide free services.
(Chipps, Brysiewicz, et al., 2012)	Systematic review, South Africa		Acceptability Appropriateness	Health beliefs of the target population must be considered in managing clients from varied cultural backgrounds. Understanding culture is essential, and cultural acceptance as well, as some prefer personal interactions
(Chipps & Mars, 2012)	Cross-Sectional Survey, South Africa	District Managers in Kwa Zulu Natal South Africa	Appropriateness	Hospital and district managers did not have sufficient information and were poorly prepared about digital health projects
(Chipps, Ramlall, et al., 2012)	Narrative Literature Review, South Africa		Accommodation Availability Appropriateness	There must be adequate infrastructure to support digital mental health. Mental health facilities that are receiving referrals should be capable of accommodating the psychiatrist's recommendations.

continued on following page

Table 1. Continued

Author, year	Country and study design	Population	Outcome of interest	Key Findings
(Cox et al., 2024)	Cross-sectional Survey, Malawi		Accommodation Availability	Counselling services were significantly expanded because it could be done on the phone, and counsellors could serve multiple facilities and not just one. Also, service users did not have to commute to the facility for care.
(Doukani et al., 2021)	Pilot Cohort Study, Kenya		Acceptability	The results suggest that the participants found the intervention acceptable as reflected in their satisfaction rating of the mobile app
(Gbollie et al., 2023)	Cross-sectional study, South Africa	University students	Acceptability	Results indicate that people's intention to use digital health interventions is influenced by how they perceive technology and their attitudes towards it. Students will use such interventions if they consider them safe. When people think online therapy is less effective, they are less likely to use apps for therapy. Study participants were less familiar with chatbots as compared with other digital health interventions.
(Groen et al., 2022)	Cross-sectional Study, South Africa, Zambia	Adolescents	Availability Accommodation	Major challenges Included erratic internet connections, workforce shortage, insufficient time to use apps. Other challenges were insufficient access to smartphones, challenges with apps functions, and problems with reaching the target group because nurses did not come across any adolescents during the study period or had concerns with communicating with them successfully.
(Kabukye et al., 2024)	Mixed methods, Uganda	Members of the public who call the mental health telephone line for help	Acceptability	Majority of the callers (40.27%) who stopped at the interactive voice response even though they could opt to speak with a human agent is rather encouraging since it intimates that people are accepting IVR to an extent, and signals that they may prefer it to interacting with a human agent. Participants liked the anonymous and confidential support that the call center provided because it prevented stigma.
(Kaigwa et al., 2022)	Qualitative Study, Kenya	Patients attending a private mental health facility	Accommodation Availability Affordability	Participants indicated that digital infrastructure such as internet positively influenced their uptake of the online therapy sessions, as well as telepsychiatry costs which they perceived to be lower than in-person sessions.
(Kiburi et al., 2022)	Cross-sectional study, Kenya	People being treated for opioid use disorder	Acceptability	Majority (95%) of participants were accepting of treatment for substance use via mobile phones, as against 49.9% through computers, with receiving text messages once weekly and only a daily text message.
(Kola et al., 2021)	Cross-sectional study, Nigeria	Adolescent mothers in their perinatal or postnatal periods	Acceptability	Majority (96.2%) would like to have mental health education delivered to them, on mobile phones, and out of these, majority (50.4%) would prefer information via text messaging, 38.8% via phone calls, 10.4% via app-based short videos and 0.4% on WhatsApp and Facebook.
(Larsen et al., 2025)	Cross-sectional study, Ghana	Young adults living with early psychosis at Accra Psychiatry hospital	Acceptability	Majority of patients had access to mobile phones and are interested in using digital health interventions fort care.
(Meffert et al., 2024)	Cross-sectional study, Kenya	Outpatients in a Kisumu County Referral Hospital	Acceptability Affordability	Study participants indicated that the main 3 reasons for choosing mhealth were travel time, how affordable it was and the convenience it offered. Younger people preferred mhealth to in-person services and may reflect nuances associated with age groups, as they have had a more extensive and more complex interactions with mobile phone technology than older people have.

continued on following page

Table 1. Continued

Author, year	Country and study design	Population	Outcome of interest	Key Findings
(Munishi et al., 2023)	Cross-sectional study, Tanzania	PWDUD at Bombo Regional Hospital, Tanzania	Acceptability Approachability and availability	Majority 92% of PWDUD did no own phones due to cost of the phones and effects of drug use on their lives, although they showed readiness to access mhealth interventions.
(Mustafa et al., 2024)	Cross-sectional study, Sudan	University students in Sudan	Acceptability Appropriateness	Majority (71%) are willing to try telemental services, others prefer in person appointments. Young people and adolescence prefer face-to-face and a preferred choice for human0interfacing digital health services as compared with those without a human element.
(Musyoka et al., 2023)	Cros-sectional study, Kenya	First year peer mentors in university	Acceptability	High acceptance of mhealth based peer mentoring drug related intervention services as compared to in-person programmes, due to issues of confidentiality and stigma.
(Mwaka et al., 2025)	Qualitative Study, Uganda	Students across 9 universities	Acceptability	Majority showed positive attitude towards digital mental health initiatives due to its role in taking away stigma associated with seeking help.
(O'Grady et al., 2022)	Mixed Methods,, Mozambique		Approachability Availability Appropriateness Acceptability	Technologies that incorporate a provider-facing element show potential in supporting models which are focussed on task-shifting. This can widen access to alcohol-use interventions in LMICs. The study also showed high acceptability due to the adoption of a participatory approach when developing the mSBIRT intervention.
(Ogundipe et al., 2025)	Cross-sectional study Nigeria	Students in University	Acceptability	Many students found mhealth modalities acceptable because there was high mobile phone ownership.
(Sendek Anteneh et al., 2025)	Cross-sectional study, Ethiopia	Regular undergraduate students at University	Acceptability	Students' intention to use digitalised psychosocial counselling was 54.9%. Despite the promising findings, still, about half of the students have no intention to use digital tools for remote psycho-social support. Students' refusal could be related to digital literacy, access to digital devices, and perceived fear of information security.
(Sharma-Misra et al., 2023)	Cross-sectional study, South Africa	Patients in a psychiatric hospital in KwaZulu-Natal province	Availability and accommodation	The older people are, their less willingness to use a smart phone based mental health app. Each increase in age came with a 7% reduced odds of app utilisation.
(Sibeko et al., 2017)	South Africa, RCT	Valkenberg hospital, Cape Town	Acceptability	Results indicate that the text messaging functionality was found to be acceptable but infeasible as it were.

DISCUSSION

This systematic review is among the first to examine how DMHIs influences access to mental health services in SSA, applying a framework that includes multiple dimensions of access. The current evidence suggests a troubling paradox: while populations in SSA are highly willing to accept DMHIs, the systems are largely unavailable to accommodate them, and we know surprisingly little about whether they can afford them or if they are even appropriate.

Acceptability

Acceptability was the most frequently examined access dimension. Most studies emphasized the need for DMHIs to align with local cultural beliefs and stigmas surrounding mental illness. Participatory design approaches, where users co-create or help shape interventions were highlighted as key to ensuring engagement. These findings are consistent with research from other LMICs beyond SSA, where locally tailored, user-driven digital interventions also demonstrated higher uptake and adherence (Gonsalves et al., 2024) (Vera San Juan et al., 2024).

The involvement of traditional and faith healers, as highlighted in several SSA studies, represents not only a unique contextual insight but also a central reality of the region's mental health landscape (Berhe et al., 2024) (Nortje et al., 2016). In many communities, these practitioners are the first and often most trusted point of contact for individuals experiencing psychological distress, long before biomedical services are sought (Abbo, 2011) (Sorsdahl et al., 2009). Their role is deeply embedded in cultural and spiritual understandings of illness, making them indispensable actors in any effort to expand access to care.

Rather than viewing this reliance as a barrier, it can be reframed as an opportunity for culturally congruent integration. Emerging evidence suggests that respectful engagement with traditional and faith healers, through dialogue, co-designed training, and referral pathways, can enhance early detection, reduce stigma, and improve continuity of care (Nortje et al., 2016) (Patel et al., 2018). For example, collaborative models in Uganda and South Africa have piloted training programs where healers are equipped with basic mental health literacy, digital screening tools, and referral mechanisms to link clients with formal services when needed (Abbo, 2011) (Sorsdahl et al., 2009).

Digital platforms could further strengthen these collaborations by providing accessible training modules, decision-support tools, and secure referral systems that respect both biomedical and traditional frameworks. Such approaches not only acknowledge the pluralistic nature of health-seeking in SSA but also humanise digital interventions by embedding them within trusted community relationships. While challenges around quality control, regulation, and potential conflicts in explanatory models remain, these can be mitigated through co-creation, continuous dialogue, and culturally sensitive supervision structures (Patel et al., 2018).

Availability and Accommodation

The second most addressed dimensions were availability and accommodation. Numerous studies cited infrastructural deficits, such as unreliable electricity, limited smartphone access, and poor mobile network coverage, as major barriers. These findings reflect broader systemic challenges in SSA's digital health landscape and align with similar barriers reported in Southeast Asia (Wibowo et al., 2025) (Singh et al., 2025).

In addition, lack of national digital mental health policies or strategies emerged as a structural barrier to scalability. Without institutional frameworks to support funding, regulation, and integration of DMH services, most interventions remain pilot-based or donor-dependent. This mirrors findings from studies in Latin America, where policy fragmentation led to discontinuity in digital mental health rollouts (LeRouge et al., 2019).

Affordability

Surprisingly, affordability was rarely studied. This is problematic given that many populations in SSA face out-of-pocket payments for mobile data, device access, and related costs. Studies from the U.S. have shown that even in high-income settings, economic barriers can restrict digital access for low-income groups (Sultana & Pagán, 2023). In the African context, affordability may also intersect with gender and rural/urban disparities, limiting equity. Future studies should explore cost-effectiveness and financing models for sustained access to DMH.

Appropriateness and Quality of Care

Few studies examined the appropriateness of digital mental health tools in terms of content quality, clinical accuracy, and alignment with user needs. For example, limited evidence exists on how well current interventions address co-occurring conditions like substance use or trauma. Research from Canada warns of the potential for DMH tools to be too generic or insufficiently personalized, reducing their clinical effectiveness (Shen et al., 2022). This suggests a need for localized, evidence-based content tailored to the psychosocial contexts of SSA users.

Equity, Gender, and Digital Literacy

Cross-cutting themes such as gender disparities, digital literacy, and language barriers were infrequently discussed in the reviewed SSA studies, yet they represent fundamental equity challenges that cut across all five dimensions of access and must be addressed from the outset. Global reviews indicate that women are less likely to own smartphones or use mobile data for health purposes (Groupe Speciale Mobile Association, 2021). This is reinforced by GSMA's Mobile Gender Gap Report 2025 (Jeffrie Nadia et al., 2025), which found that across low- and middle-income countries, women are 14% less likely than men to use mobile internet, and 8% less likely to own a mobile phone. These disparities are more pronounced in rural areas and among older or less-educated populations. These inequities highlight the need for intentional, equity-driven design strategies, such as voice-based interfaces, community digital health training, and gender-sensitive approaches that ensure women, older adults, and low-literacy populations are not left behind.

AI and Innovation

None of the reviewed studies examined the use of artificial intelligence (AI) or advanced chatbots, despite their growing global presence. AI enabled tools like Woebot or Wysa have shown promise in delivering scalable, evidence-based mental health support in low-resource settings (Abd-Alrazaq et al., 2020). Their potential in SSA is considerable, particularly for addressing the severe human resource gaps in mental health services by offering low-cost, on-demand, and personalized support.

However, their application in SSA raises unique ethical and practical challenges that must be carefully considered. Data bias is a central concern, as most AI models are trained on datasets from high-income countries, which may not capture the cultural, linguistic, and contextual realities of African populations (Birhane, 2021). The region's linguistic diversity further complicates natural language processing, requiring locally adapted models to ensure inclusivity and effectiveness (Orife et al., 2020). In addition, issues of digital literacy, infrastructure reliability, and data governance are critical to ensuring equitable access and safeguarding against unintended harms (CEPAL, 2022). Future research should therefore explore both the opportunities and risks of integrating AI-driven mental health interventions in SSA, with particular attention to equity, cultural relevance, and ethical governance frameworks.

The Impact of COVID-19 on Digital Health

Many studies were conducted post-COVID-19, reflecting a global trend toward rapid adoption of digital solutions during the pandemic. The crisis both highlighted and exacerbated existing mental health service gaps while accelerating innovation. However, as seen globally, pandemic-driven innovations often lacked long-term sustainability plans (Torous et al., 2020). There is an urgent need to transition from reactive pilots to integrated, system-wide digital mental health programs. Torous et al. (2020) emphasize that lessons from this period can guide the integration of digital mental health tools to expand access and improve quality beyond the pandemic.

Strengths and Limitations

This study has several strengths. First, it is among the first systematic reviews to comprehensively explore how digital mental health technologies influence access to mental healthcare in SSA, addressing the multiple dimensions of accessibility such as acceptability, availability, affordability, and approachability. The review synthesizes findings across a range of study designs and countries, providing a broad perspective on this emerging field. Moreover, by applying a clear conceptual framework of access, the study offers a structured understanding of the complex factors influencing digital mental health uptake in the region. The inclusion of recent studies, especially from the post-COVID-19 era, reflects the rapidly evolving digital health landscape.

However, this study also has several limitations. First, only English language studies were included which limit the coverage of francophone and Lusophone SSA. Findings are therefore likely most representative of Anglophone contexts. This omission reduces the geographic and cultural representativeness of the findings and may exclude valuable insights from culturally and linguistically diverse populations within the region. Future reviews should actively incorporate French- and Portuguese-language databases to improve representativeness.

Second, many included studies were conducted during the post-COVID-19 period, a time when digital health modalities were rapidly scaled and normalized due to safety protocols and urgent mental health needs. This timing may have masked more nuanced or longer-term barriers and facilitators to accessibility, potentially overestimating acceptance or availability in normal circumstances.

Third, none of the reviewed studies explicitly examined the role of artificial intelligence (AI)-embedded digital mental health interventions. Given AI's growing role in healthcare, this gap limits our understanding of how emerging technologies might uniquely influence accessibility in Sub-Saharan Africa.

Fourth, the review only considered peer-reviewed published articles, excluding grey literature, case reports, conference proceedings, and non-peer-reviewed studies that might contain important practical information or innovative interventions. This may have narrowed the scope of evidence and missed emerging trends or unpublished challenges in digital mental health accessibility. Future iterations should include a targeted search of grey literature from major institutions like WHO, UNICEF, Africa CDC and government health ministries to capture implementation reports and pilot study findings that haven't yet made it to peer-reviewed publication.

Finally, the heterogeneity of study designs, populations, and settings posed challenges for synthesis, limiting the ability to perform meta-analyses or quantify effect sizes. Although a narrative synthesis was appropriate, the diversity of methodologies means findings should be interpreted cautiously, recognizing contextual differences.

CONCLUSION AND RECOMMENDATIONS

This systematic review provides a comprehensive synthesis of the current evidence on how digital health technologies influence access to mental healthcare in SSA. Findings reveal that digital interventions such as mHealth, telepsychiatry, and digital decision-support tools have demonstrated significant potential in improving the accessibility of mental health services across the region. These technologies enhance approachability through mental health awareness campaigns, improve acceptability by reducing stigma via anonymous engagement, and increase availability by bridging the geographical and human resource gaps prevalent in many low-resource settings. However, challenges such as limited digital literacy, unreliable internet connectivity, infrastructure gaps, and concerns about data privacy continue to hinder full realization of these benefits.

The review underscores the need for context-specific, equity-focused digital health interventions supported by strong health systems, enabling and supportive policy frameworks, and community engagement. Investments in digital infrastructure, capacity building, and cross-sectoral collaboration are essential to sustain and scale up successful innovations. To support this transition from pilot projects to large-scale implementation, future efforts would benefit from the application of established implementation science frameworks, such as the Consolidated Framework for Implementation Research (CFIR) (Damschroder et al., 2022) and the RE-AIM framework (Holtrop et al., 2021), which provide structured approaches to evaluating reach, adoption, implementation, and sustainability.

Future research should explore implementation outcomes and cost-effectiveness of DMHIs to inform policy and practice and should incorporate policy analysis to examine how enabling environments can be created and sustained for digital mental health integration in SSA. Ultimately, while digital health technologies are not a panacea, they represent a transformative tool to advance equitable access to mental healthcare in SSA when integrated thoughtfully within the broader health system.

REFERENCES

Abbafati, C., Abbas, K. M., Abbasi, M., Abbasifard, M., Abbasi-Kangevari, M., Abbastabar, H., Abd-Allah, F., Abdelalim, A., Abdollahi, M., Abdollahpour, I., Abedi, A., Abedi, P., Abegaz, K. H., Abolhassani, H., Abosetugn, A. E., Aboyans, V., Abrams, E. M., Abreu, L. G., Abrigo, M. R. M., & Murray, C. J. L. (2020). Global burden of 369 diseases and injuries in 204 countries and territories, 1990–2019: A systematic analysis for the Global Burden of Disease Study 2019. *Lancet, 396*(10258), 1204–1222. DOI: 10.1016/S0140-6736(20)30925-9

Abbo, C. (2011). Profiles and outcome of traditional healing practices for severe mental illnesses in two districts of Eastern Uganda. *Global Health Action, 4*. Advance online publication. DOI: 10.3402/gha.v4i0.7117

Abd-Alrazaq, A. A., Rababeh, A., Alajlani, M., Bewick, B. M., & Househ, M. (2020). Effectiveness and safety of using chatbots to improve mental health: Systematic review and meta-analysis. *Journal of Medical Internet Research, 22*(7), 1–17. DOI: 10.2196/16021

Adem, J. B., Zeleke, T., Walle, A. D., Atinafu, W. T., Tilahun, K. N., Melaku, M. S., & Kebede, S. D. (2023). Awareness and readiness of mental healthcare providers to implement telemental health services and associated factors at public referral hospitals in Addis Ababa City, Ethiopia. *BMJ Open, 13*(7), 1–13. DOI: 10.1136/bmjopen-2022-069671

Adiukwu, F., Ojeahere, M., Adesokun, O., & Babalola, G. (2022). Mental health distress during the COVID-19 pandemic in Nigeria: Need for psychological intervention. *South African Journal of Psychiatry, 28*, 1–6. DOI: 10.4102/sajpsychiatry.v28i0.1550

Agbeyangi, A. O., & Lukose, J. M. (2025). Telemedicine Adoption and Prospects in Sub-Sahara Africa: A Systematic Review with a Focus on South Africa, Kenya, and Nigeria. *Healthcare (Switzerland), 13*(7), 1–25. DOI: 10.3390/healthcare13070762

Agyepong, I. A., Sewankambo, N., Binagwaho, A., Coll-Seck, A. M., Corrah, T., Ezeh, A., Fekadu, A., Kilonzo, N., Lamptey, P., Masiye, F., Mayosi, B., Mboup, S., Muyembe, J. J., Pate, M., Sidibe, M., Simons, B., Tlou, S., Gheorghe, A., Legido-Quigley, H., & Piot, P. (2017). The path to longer and healthier lives for all Africans by 2030: The Lancet Commission on the future of health in sub-Saharan Africa. *Lancet, 390*(10114), 2803–2859. DOI: 10.1016/S0140-6736(17)31509-X

Atewologun, F., Adigun, O. A., Okesanya, O. J., Hassan, H. K., Olabode, O. N., Micheal, A. S., Ahmed, M. M., Ukoaka, B. M., Idris, N. B., Oso, T. A., & Lucero-Prisno, D. E. (2025). A comprehensive review of mental health services across selected countries in sub-Saharan Africa: Assessing progress, challenges, and future direction. *Discover Mental Health, 5*(1). Advance online publication. DOI: 10.1007/s44192-025-00177-7

Atujuna, M., Simpson, N., Ngobeni, M., Monese, T., Giovenco, D., Pike, C., Figerova, Z., Visser, M., Biriotti, M., Kydd, A., & Bekker, L. G. (2021). Khuluma: Using Participatory, Peer-Led and Digital Methods to Deliver Psychosocial Support to Young People Living With HIV in South Africa. *Frontiers in Reproductive Health, 3*(July). Advance online publication. DOI: 10.3389/frph.2021.687677

Ben-Zeev, D., Agorinya, J., Beaulieu, A., Sottie, E. Q., Larsen, A., Attah, D. A., Bedard-Gilligan, M., Ohene, S., Collins, P. Y., Lindgren, K. P., Ofori-Atta, A., Kaysen, D., & Obeng, K. (2025). Sexual trauma and interest in mobile health among women with mental illness in Ghana. Internet Interventions, 40(October 2024), 100829. DOI: 10.1016/j.invent.2025.100829

Ben-Zeev, D., Meller, S., Snyder, J., Attah, D. A., Albright, L., Le, H., Asafo, S. M., Collins, P. Y., & Ofori-Atta, A. (2021). A digital toolkit (m-healer) to improve care and reduce human rights abuses against people with mental illness in west africa: User-centered design, development, and usability study. *JMIR Mental Health, 8*(7). Advance online publication. DOI: 10.2196/28526

Berhe, K. T., Gesesew, H. A., & Ward, P. R. (2024). Traditional healing practices, factors influencing to access the practices and its complementary effect on mental health in sub-Saharan Africa: A systematic review. *BMJ Open, 14*(9). Advance online publication. DOI: 10.1136/bmjopen-2023-083004

Birhane, A. (2021). Algorithmic injustice: A relational ethics approach. *Patterns (New York, N.Y.), 2*(2), 100205. DOI: 10.1016/j.patter.2021.100205

Botes, M. (2025). Regulatory challenges of digital health: The case of mental health applications and personal data in South Africa. *Frontiers in Pharmacology, 16*(April), 1–7. DOI: 10.3389/fphar.2025.1498600

CEPAL. (2022). Closing the Digital Divide: More and Better Funding for the Digital Transformation of Health in Latin America and the Caribbean. Transform Health, November, 1–5. https://transformhealthcoalition.org/wp-content/uploads/2023/08/Latin-America-Regional-Brief-English-v2.pdf?

Chen, T., & Gombay, C. (2024). Advantages and disadvantages of digital mental health initiatives in Nigeria - a qualitative interview study. *Journal of Mental Health (Abingdon, England), 33*(5), 613–618. DOI: 10.1080/09638237.2024.2361234

Chipps, J., Brysiewicz, P., & Mars, M. (2012). Effectiveness and feasibility of telepsychiatry in resource constrained environments? A systematic review of the evidence. *African Journal of Psychiatry (South Africa), 15*(4), 235–243. DOI: 10.4314/ajpsy.v15i4.30

Chipps, J., & Mars, M. (2012). Readiness of health-care institutions in KwaZulu-Natal to implement telepsychiatry. *Journal of Telemedicine and Telecare, 18*(3), 133–137. DOI: 10.1258/jtt.2012.SFT103

Chipps, J., Ramlall, S., & Mars, M. (2012). A telepsychiatry model to support psychiatric outreach in the public sector in South Africa. *African Journal of Psychiatry (South Africa), 15*(4), 264–270. DOI: 10.4314/ajpsy. v15i4.34

Clausen, H., Ruud, T., Odden, S., Benth, J. Š., Heiervang, K. S., Stuen, H. K., & Landheim, A. (2020). Improved Rehabilitation Outcomes for Persons With and Without Problematic Substance Use After 2 Years With Assertive Community Treatment—A Prospective Study of Patients With Severe Mental Illness in 12 Norwegian ACT Teams. *Frontiers in Psychiatry, 11*(December), 1–11. DOI: 10.3389/fpsyt.2020.607071

Cox, C. M., Masiano, S., Mazenga, A., Stark, M., Udedi, M., Simon, K. R., Ahmed, S., Nyasulu, P., & Kim, M. H. (2024). Phone-based psychosocial counseling for people living with HIV: Feasibility, acceptability and impact on uptake of psychosocial counseling services in Malawi. *Global Mental Health (Cambridge, England), 11*. Advance online publication. DOI: 10.1017/gmh.2023.84

Cu, A., Meister, S., Lefebvre, B., & Ridde, V. (2021). Assessing healthcare access using the Levesque's conceptual framework– a scoping review. *International Journal for Equity in Health, 20*(1), 1–14. DOI: 10.1186/s12939-021-01416-3

Damschroder, L. J., Reardon, C. M., Widerquist, M. A. O., & Lowery, J. (2022). The updated Consolidated Framework for Implementation Research based on user feedback. *Implementation Science : IS, 17*(1), 1–16. DOI: 10.1186/s13012-022-01245-0

Dietvorst, E., Hillegers, M. H. J., Legerstee, J. S., De Vries, L. P., Vreeker, A., & Keijsers, L. (2024). Real-time personalized feedback in mHealth for adolescents. *Digital Health, 10*. Advance online publication. DOI: 10.1177/20552076241247937

Dodoo, J. E., Al-Samarraie, H., & Alsswey, A. (2022). The development of telemedicine programs in Sub-Saharan Africa: Progress and associated challenges. *Health and Technology, 12*(1), 33–46. DOI: 10.1007/s12553-021-00626-7

Doukani, A., van Dalen, R., Valev, H., Njenga, A., Sera, F., & Chibanda, D. (2021). A community health volunteer delivered problem-solving therapy mobile application based on the Friendship Bench 'Inuka Coaching' in Kenya: A pilot cohort study. *Global Mental Health (Cambridge, England), 8*. Advance online publication. DOI: 10.1017/gmh.2021.3

Galazzi, A., Fonda, F., Chiappinotto, S., Justi, L., Sønderskov Frydensberg, M., Lehmann Boesen, R., Macur, M., de San Pedro, M., Reixach Espaulella, E., & Palese, A. (2025). Recommendations to promote the digital healthcare transformation in the clinical practice: Findings from an international consensus development method. *BMC Health Services Research*, *25*(1). Advance online publication. DOI: 10.1186/s12913-025-13079-9

Gbollie, E. F., Bantjes, J., Jarvis, L., Swandevelder, S., du Plessis, J., Shadwell, R., Davids, C., Gerber, R., Holland, N., & Hunt, X. (2023). Intention to use digital mental health solutions: A cross-sectional survey of university students attitudes and perceptions toward online therapy, mental health apps, and chatbots. *Digital Health*, *9*. Advance online publication. DOI: 10.1177/20552076231216559

Gonsalves, P. P., Ansari, S., Berry, C., Gonsalves, F., Iyengar, S., Kashyap, P., Mittal, D., Pal, S., Razdan, E., & Michelson, D. (2024). Co-designing digital mental health interventions with young people: 10 recommendations from lessons learned in low-and-middle-income countries. *Health Education Journal*, *84*(4), 373–384. DOI: 10.1177/00178969241297821

Groen, G., Jörns-Presentati, A., Dessauvagie, A., Seedat, S., van den Heuvel, L. L., Suliman, S., Grobler, G., Jansen, R., Mwape, L., Mukwato, P., Chapima, F., Korhonen, J., Stein, D. J., Jonker, D., Mudenda, J., Turunen, T., Valtiņš, K., Beinaroviča, A., Grada, L., & Lahti, M. (2022). Development of a Mobile Application for Detection of Adolescent Mental Health Problems and Feasibility Assessment with Primary Health Care Workers. *Issues in Mental Health Nursing*, *43*(11), 1046–1055. DOI: 10.1080/01612840.2022.2124003

Groupe Speciale Mobile Association. (2021). Connected Women. The Mobile Gender Gap Report 2021. 65. https://www.gsma.com/r/wp-content/uploads/2021/07/The-Mobile-Gender-Gap-Report-2021.pdf

Holtrop, J. S., Estabrooks, P. A., Gaglio, B., Harden, S. M., Kessler, R. S., King, D. K., Kwan, B. M., Ory, M. G., Rabin, B. A., Shelton, R. C., & Glasgow, R. E. (2021). Understanding and applying the RE-AIM framework: Clarifications and resources. *Journal of Clinical and Translational Science*, *5*(1). Advance online publication. DOI: 10.1017/cts.2021.789

Nadia, J., Kalvin, B., Abi, G., Simran, J., Boraiba, K., Rosie, L., Dominca, L., Jakub, Z., & Claire, S. (2025). GSMA - The Mobile Gender Gap Report 2025. 1–72. www.gsmaintelligence.com

Kabukye, J. K., Nakku, J., Niwemuhwezi, J., Nsereko, J., Namagembe, R., Groen, I. D. E., Neumbe, R., Mubiru, D., Kisakye, C., Nanyonga, R., Sjölinder, M., Nilsson, S., & Wamala-Larsson, C. (2024). Assessing the Usage and Usability of a Mental Health Advice Telephone Service in Uganda: Mixed Methods Study. *Journal of Medical Internet Research, 26*, e65692. DOI: 10.2196/65692

Kaigwa, L. C., Njenga, F., Ongeri, L., Nguithi, A., Mugane, M., Mbugua, G. M., Anundo, J., Kimari, M. Z., & Onono, M. (2022). Implementation of telepsychiatry in Kenya: Acceptability study. *BJPsych Open, 8*(3), 1–6. DOI: 10.1192/bjo.2022.53

Karamagi, H. C., Muneene, D., Droti, B., Jepchumba, V., Okeibunor, J. C., Nabyonga, J., Asamani, J. A., Traore, M., & Kipruto, H. (2022). eHealth or e-Chaos: The use of Digital Health Interventions for Health Systems Strengthening in sub-Saharan Africa over the last 10 years: A scoping review. *Journal of Global Health, 12*, 04090. DOI: 10.7189/jogh.12.04090

Kiburi, S. K., Paruk, S., & Chiliza, B. (2022). Mobile phone ownership, digital technology use and acceptability of digital interventions among individuals on opioid use disorder treatment in Kenya. *Frontiers in Digital Health, 4.* Advance online publication. DOI: 10.3389/fdgth.2022.975168

Kola, L., Abiona, D., Adefolarin, A. O., & Ben-Zeev, D. (2021). Mobile phone use and acceptability for the delivery of mental health information among perinatal adolescents in Nigeria: Survey study. In JMIR Mental Health (Vol. 8, Issue 1). JMIR Publications Inc. DOI: 10.2196/20314

Larsen, A., Agorinya, J., Beaulieu, A., Sottie, E. Q., Buck, B., Obeng, K., Kyeremeh, B., Dogbe, F. K., Iddrisu, M. I., Dowuona, P. E. O., Tetteh, O. O. A., Emmanuel, O. B., Ofori-Atta, A., & Ben-Zeev, D. (2025). Digital health for early psychosis in Ghana: Patient and caregiver needs and preferences. *Schizophrenia, 11*(1), 1–7. DOI: 10.1038/s41537-025-00554-9

LeRouge, C. M., Gupta, M., Corpart, G., & Arrieta, A. (2019). Health system approaches are needed to expand telemedicine use across nine latin american nations. *Health Affairs, 38*(2), 212–221. DOI: 10.1377/hlthaff.2018.05274

Levesque, J. F., Harris, M. F., & Russell, G. (2013). Patient-centred access to health care: Conceptualising access at the interface of health systems and populations. *International Journal for Equity in Health, 12*(1), 1. DOI: 10.1186/1475-9276-12-18

Meffert, S., Mathai, M., Neylan, T., Mwai, D., Onyango, D. O., Rota, G., Otieno, A., Obura, R. R., Wangia, J., Opiyo, E., Muchembre, P., Oluoch, D., Wambura, R., Mbwayo, A., Kahn, J. G., Cohen, C. R., Bukusi, D., Aarons, G. A., Burger, R. L., & Ongeri, L. (2024). Preference of mHealth versus in-person treatment for depression and post-traumatic stress disorder in Kenya: Demographic and clinical characteristics. *BMJ Open*, *14*(11), 1–9. DOI: 10.1136/bmjopen-2023-083094

Moitra, M., Owens, S., Hailemariam, M., Wilson, K. S., Mensa-Kwao, A., Gonese, G., Kamamia, C. K., White, B., Young, D. M., & Collins, P. Y. (2023). Global Mental Health: Where We Are and Where We Are Going. *Current Psychiatry Reports*, *25*(7), 301–311. DOI: 10.1007/s11920-023-01426-8

Mudiyanselage, K. W. W., De Santis, K. K., Jörg, F., Saleem, M., Stewart, R., Zeeb, H., & Busse, H. (2024). The effectiveness of mental health interventions involving non-specialists and digital technology in low-and middle-income countries – a systematic review. *BMC Public Health*, *24*(1). Advance online publication. DOI: 10.1186/s12889-023-17417-6

Munishi, C., Ndumwa, H. P., Massawe, J. E., Njiro, B. J., Ngowi, J., Suhartono, S., Busse, A., Campello, G., Garofalo, G., Cipolla, P., Nyandindi, C., Ubuguyu, O., & Sunguya, B. (2023). Acceptability of using mobile Health (mHealth) as an intervention tool for people with drug use disorders in Tanga, Tanzania. PLOS Digital Health, 2(9 September). DOI: 10.1371/journal.pdig.0000257

Mustafa, S. H., Mohammed, E. A., Makkawi, S. T., & Mohammed, Y. Y. (2024). Attitudes of university students in Sudan towards digital mental health. *South Sudan Medical Journal*, *17*(4), 185–189. DOI: 10.4314/ssmj.v17i4.6

Musyoka, C. M., Mbwayo, A., Donovan, D. M., & Mathai, M. (2023). Student peer mentoring: Feasibility and acceptability of mHealth-based tool for alcohol and substance abuse prevention by peer mentors at a university in Kenya. *PLOS Digital Health*, *2*(1). Advance online publication. DOI: 10.1371/journal.pdig.0000177

Mwaka, E. S., Bazzeketa, D., Mirembe, J., Emoru, R. D., Twimukye, A., & Kivumbi, A. (2025). Barriers to and enhancement of the utilization of digital mental health interventions in low-resource settings: Perceptions of young people in Uganda. *Digital Health*, *11*, 20552076251321696. DOI: 10.1177/20552076251321698

Naslund, J. A., Aschbrenner, K. A., Araya, R., Marsch, L. A., Unützer, J., Patel, V., & Bartels, S. J. (2017). Digital technology for treating and preventing mental disorders in low-income and middle-income countries: A narrative review of the literature. *The Lancet. Psychiatry*, *4*(6), 486–500. DOI: 10.1016/S2215-0366(17)30096-2

Nortje, G., Oladeji, B., Gureje, O., & Seedat, S. (2016). Effectiveness of traditional healers in treating mental disorders: A systematic review. *The Lancet. Psychiatry, 3*(2), 154–170. DOI: 10.1016/S2215-0366(15)00515-5

O'Grady, M. A., Mootz, J., Suleman, A., Sweetland, A., Teodoro, E., Anube, A., Feliciano, P., Bezuidenhout, C., Dos Santos, P. F., Fumo, W., Gouveia, L., Pinsky, I., Mello, M., Kann, B., & Wainberg, M. L. (2022). Mobile technology and task shifting to improve access to alcohol treatment services in Mozambique. *Journal of Substance Abuse Treatment, 134*. Advance online publication. DOI: 10.1016/j.jsat.2021.108549

Ogundipe, R. O., Omotosho, O. E., & John-Akinola, Y. O. (2025). Perception, attitude and use of digital health platforms for mental health promotion among students in a national university in the south-western part of Nigeria: A cross-sectional study. *Digital Health, 11*. Advance online publication. DOI: 10.1177/20552076251331841

Orife, I., Kreutzer, J., Sibanda, B., Whitenack, D., Siminyu, K., Martinus, L., Ali, J. T., Abbott, J., Marivate, V., Kabongo, S., Meressa, M., Murhabazi, E., Ahia, O., van Biljon, E., Ramkilowan, A., Akinfaderin, A., Öktem, A., Akin, W., Kioko, G., & Bashir, A. (2020). Masakhane — Machine Translation For Africa. 1–4. https://arxiv.org/abs/2003.11529

Osborn, T. L., Wasanga, C. M., & Ndetei, D. M. (2022). Transforming mental health for all. In The BMJ. DOI: 10.1136/bmj.o1593

Ouzzani, M., Hammady, H., Fedorowicz, Z., & Elmagarmid, A. (2016). Rayyan-a web and mobile app for systematic reviews. *Systematic Reviews, 5*(1), 1–10. DOI: 10.1186/s13643-016-0384-4

Page, M. J., McKenzie, J. E., Bossuyt, P. M., Boutron, I., Hoffmann, T. C., Mulrow, C. D., Shamseer, L., Tetzlaff, J. M., Akl, E. A., Brennan, S. E., Chou, R., Glanville, J., Grimshaw, J. M., Hróbjartsson, A., Lalu, M. M., Li, T., Loder, E. W., Mayo-Wilson, E., McDonald, S., & Moher, D. (2021). The PRISMA 2020 statement: An updated guideline for reporting systematic reviews. *BMJ (Clinical Research Ed.), 372*. Advance online publication. DOI: 10.1136/bmj.n71

Patel, V., Saxena, S., Lund, C., Thornicroft, G., Baingana, F., Bolton, P., Chisholm, D., Collins, P. Y., Cooper, J. L., Eaton, J., Herrman, H., Herzallah, M. M., Huang, Y., Jordans, M. J. D., Kleinman, A., Medina-Mora, M. E., Morgan, E., Niaz, U., & Omigbodun, O. UnÜtzer, Jü. (2018). The Lancet Commission on global mental health and sustainable development. *Lancet, 392*(10157), 1553–1598. DOI: 10.1016/S0140-6736(18)31612-X

Penchansky, R., & Thomas, J. W. (1981). The Concept of Access: Definition and Relationship to Consumer Satisfaction. *Medical Care, 19*(2). https://journals.lww.com/lww-medicalcare/fulltext/1981/02000/the_concept_of_access__definition_and_relationship.1.aspx

Philippe, T. J., Sikder, N., Jackson, A., Koblanski, M. E., Liow, E., Pilarinos, A., & Vasarhelyi, K. (2022). Digital Health Interventions for Delivery of Mental Health Care: Systematic and Comprehensive Meta-Review. *JMIR Mental Health, 9*(5). Advance online publication. DOI: 10.2196/35159

Popay, J., Roberts, H., Sowden, A., Petticrew, M., Arai, L., Rodgers, M., & Britten, N. (2006). Narrative Synthesis in Systematic Reviews: A Product from the ESRC Methods Programme. ESRC Methods Programme, 2006, 93. DOI: 10.13140/2.1.1018.4643

PRISMA. (2021). PRISMA_2020_expanded_checklist.pdf.

Sendek Anteneh, D., Kelkay, J. M., Wubneh, H. D., Beshir, M. A., & Gashu, K. D. (2025). Intention to use digital-based psychosocial counseling and its predictors among students in University of Gondar, Northwest Ethiopia, 2023: Using modified unified theory of acceptance and use of technology model. *SAGE Open Medicine, 13*. Advance online publication. DOI: 10.1177/20503121241307136

Sharma-Misra, S., Maru, M., Tomita, A., & Paruk, S. (2023). Access and use of digital technology by patients with psychosis at a hospital in South Africa. *South African Journal of Psychiatry, 29*. Advance online publication. DOI: 10.4102/sajpsychiatry.v29i0.2151

Shen, N., Kassam, I., Chen, S., Ma, C., Wang, W., Boparai, N., Jankowicz, D., & Strudwick, G. (2022). Canadian perspectives of digital mental health supports: Findings from a national survey conducted during the COVID-19 pandemic. *Digital Health, 8*. Advance online publication. DOI: 10.1177/20552076221102253

Shigekawa, E., Fix, M., Corbett, G., Roby, D. H., & Coffman, J. (2018). The current state of telehealth evidence: A rapid review. *Health Affairs, 37*(12), 1975–1982. DOI: 10.1377/hlthaff.2018.05132

Sibeko, G., Temmingh, H., Mall, S., Williams-Ashman, P., Thornicroft, G., Susser, E. S., Lund, C., Stein, D. J., & Milligan, P. D. (2017). Improving adherence in mental health service users with severe mental illness in South Africa: A pilot randomized controlled trial of a treatment partner and text message intervention vs. treatment as usual PACTR201610001830190 PACTR. *BMC Research Notes, 10*(1). Advance online publication. DOI: 10.1186/s13104-017-2915-z

Singh, V., Johnson, K. R., Jacob, A. G., & John, O. (2025). The potential of digital health interventions to address health system challenges in Southeast Asia: A scoping review. *Digital Health, 11*. Advance online publication. DOI: 10.1177/20552076241311062

Sorsdahl, K., Stein, D. J., Grimsrud, A., Seedat, S., Flisher, A. J., Williams, D. R., & Myer, L. (2009). Traditional Healers in the Treatment of Common Mental Disorders in South Africa. *The Journal of Nervous and Mental Disease, 197*(6). https://journals.lww.com/jonmd/fulltext/2009/06000/traditional_healers_in_the_treatment_of_common.9.aspx

Steel, Z., Marnane, C., Iranpour, C., Chey, T., Jackson, J. W., Patel, V., & Silove, D. (2014). The global prevalence of common mental disorders: A systematic review and meta-analysis 1980-2013. *International Journal of Epidemiology, 43*(2), 476–493. DOI: 10.1093/ije/dyu038

Sultana, S., & Pagán, J. A. (2023). Use of Telehealth to Address Depression and Anxiety in Low-income US Populations: A Narrative Review. *Journal of Primary Care & Community Health, 14*. Advance online publication. DOI: 10.1177/21501319231168036

Torous, J., Bucci, S., Bell, I. H., Kessing, L. V., Faurholt-Jepsen, M., Whelan, P., Carvalho, A. F., Keshavan, M., Linardon, J., & Firth, J. (2021). The growing field of digital psychiatry: Current evidence and the future of apps, social media, chatbots, and virtual reality. *World Psychiatry; Official Journal of the World Psychiatric Association (WPA), 20*(3), 318–335. DOI: 10.1002/wps.20883

Torous, J., Myrick, K. J., Rauseo-Ricupero, N., & Firth, J. (2020). Digital mental health and COVID-19: Using technology today to accelerate the curve on access and quality tomorrow. *JMIR Mental Health, 7*(3), 1–6. DOI: 10.2196/18848

Vera San Juan, N., Martin, S., Barnett, P., Chandrasekar, A., Makhmud, A., & Palacios, J. (2024). Digital Mental Health Landscaping in Low-and Middle-Income Countries Rapid Research Evaluation and Appraisal Lab (Rreal). *Wellcome Open Research, 9*(383). https://www.rapidresearchandevaluation.com/

WHO. (2024). Digital Health and Innovation Achieving health for all through innovation and digital transformation. www.who.int/teams/digital-health-and-innovation/digital-channels/fides

Wibowo, M. F., Pyle, A., Lim, E., Ohde, J. W., Liu, N., & Karlström, J. (2025). Insights Into the Current and Future State of AI Adoption Within Health Systems in Southeast Asia: Cross-Sectional Qualitative Study. *Journal of Medical Internet Research, 27*. Advance online publication. 10.2196/71591

APPENDIX

Table 2. Study Characteristics and Findings

#	Title	Author, year	Country	Study design	Study population	Outcome of interest	Quality appraisal	Findings	Outcome measure
1	Awareness and readiness of mental healthcare providers to implement telemental health services and associated factors at public referral hospitals in Addis Ababa City, Ethiopia	Adem et al, 2023 (Adem et al., 2023)	Ethiopia	Cross-sectional study	Mental health professionals in public referral hospitals	Approachability	High	41 % of participants had adequate knowledge of telemental health services. Majority of the healthcare professionals (77.97%) were ready to implement telemental services.	Odds ratio
2	Mental health distress during the COVID-19 pandemic in Nigeria: Need for psychological intervention	Aduikwu et al, 2022 (Adiukwu et al., 2022)	Nigeria	Cross-sectional study	Household members in rural Southwest Nigeria	Approachability Acceptability	Medium	Majority (99.4%) of the respondents knew about the two major treatment modalities available (i.e. pharmacotherapy and psychotherapy). Majority would choose telephone calls (56.3%) and instant messaging or WhatsApp (56.3%) for mental healthcare during the COVID-19 pandemic. However, they also identified stigma as a barrier in accessing telemental healthcare.	Description
3	Khuluma: Using Participatory, Peer-Led and Digital Methods to Deliver Psychosocial Support to Young People Living With HIV in South Africa	Atujuna et al, 2021 (Atujuna et al., 2021)	South Africa	Descriptive cross sectional study	Young people (15–20 years) in South Africa	Acceptability	Medium	Bottom-up approaches, hence participatory ones used to deliver mental health support via text messaging are feasible.	Descriptive
4	Sexual trauma and interest in mobile health among women with mental illness in Ghana	Ben-Zeev et al, 2025 (Ben-Zeev et al., 2025)	Ghana	Cross-sectional survey	200 Ghanaian women	Acceptability Affordability	Medium	Study participants prefer audio and video health modalities to others, and the interventions which have these modalities are considered more functional, accessible and affordable.	
5	A Digital Toolkit (M-Healer) to Improve Care and Reduce Human Rights Abuses Against People With Mental Illness in West Africa: User-Centered Design, Development, and Usability Study	Ben-Zeev et al, 2021 (Ben-Zeev et al., 2021)	Ghana	Qualitative	People with mental health conditions in prayer camps	Acceptability	High	Mental health apps that use more animations than text are more accessible to the uneducated or those who are not used to using digital health tools.	
6	Regulatory challenges of digital health; the case of mental; health applications and personal data in SSA	Maruetje Bote, 2025 (Botes, 2025)	South Africa	Narrative literature review (Qual)		Acceptability	Medium	Designs that incorporate cultural nuances and adopt participatory approaches ensure reach to diverse populations. Some communities in South Africa showed reluctance to use digital mental health tools because they were concerned about stigma, trustworthiness and privacy.	Description

continued on following page

Table 2. Continued

#	Title	Author, year	Country	Study design	Study population	Outcome of interest	Quality appraisal	Findings	Outcome measure
7	Advantages and disadvantages of digital mental health initiatives in Nigeria – a qualitative interview study	Tiffany Chen & Christy Gombay, 2024 (Chen & Gombay, 2024)	Nigeria	Qualitiative interview		Acceptability Affordability	High	Digital mental health tools can provide free services.	
8	Effectiveness and feasibility of telepsychiatry in resource constrained environments? A systematic review of the evidence	J Chipps, P Brysiewicz, Mars, 2022 (Chipps, Brysiewicz, et al., 2012)	South Africa	Systematic review		Acceptability	Medium	Health beliefs of the target population must be considered in managing clients from varied cultural backgrounds. Understanding culture is essential, and cultural acceptance as well, as some prefer personal interactions.	
9	Readiness of health-care institutions in KwaZulu-Natal to implement telepsychiatry	Jennifer Chipps and Maurice Mars, 2012 (Chipps & Mars, 2012)	South Africa	Cross-sectional survey	District Managers in Kwa Zulu Natal South Africa		Medium	Hospital and district managers did not have sufficient information and were poorly prepared about digital health projects.	
10	A telepsychiatry model to support psychiatric outreach in the public sector in South Africa	J Chipps , S Ramlall, M Mars, 2012 (Chipps, Ramlall, et al., 2012)	South Africa	Narrative review			Medium	There must be adequate infrastructure to support digital mental health. Mental health facilities that are receiving referrals should be capable of accommodating the psychiatrist's recommendations.	Description
11	Phone-based psychosocial counseling for people living with HIV: Feasibility, acceptability and impact on uptake of psychosocial counseling services in Malawi	Cox et al, 2024 (Cox et al., 2024)	Malawi	Cross-sectional survey			High	Counselling services were significantly expanded because it could be done on the phone, and counsellors could serve multiple facilities and not just one. Also, service users did not have to commute to the facility for care.	
12	A community health volunteer delivered problem-solving therapy mobile application based on the Friendship Bench 'Inuka Coaching' in Kenya: A pilot cohort study	Doukane et al, 2021 (Doukani et al., 2021)	Kenya	Pilot cohort study (Observational Study)		Acceptability	Not done	The results suggest that the participants found the intervention acceptable as reflected in their satisfaction rating of the mobile app.	

continued on following page

Table 2. Continued

#	Title	Author, year	Country	Study design	Study population	Outcome of interest	Quality appraisal	Findings	Outcome measure
13	Intention to use digital mental health solutions: A cross-sectional survey of university students attitudes and perceptions toward online therapy, mental health apps, and chatbots	Gboliie et al, 2023 (Gbollie et al., 2023)	South Africa	Cross-sectional	University students from 4 Southern universities	Acceptability	Medium	Results indicate that people's intention to use digital health interventions is influenced by how they perceive technology and their attitudes towards it. Students would use such interventions if they consider them safe. When people think online therapy is less effective, they are less likely to use apps for therapy. Study participants were less familiar with chatbots as compared with other digital health interventions.	Description
14	Development of a Mobile Application for Detection of Adolescent Mental Health Problems and Feasibility Assessment with Primary Health Care Workers	Groen et al, 2022 (Groen et al., 2022)	South Africa Zambia	Cross-sectional	Adolescents in Zambia and South Africa	Availability and	Medium	Major challenges Included erratic internet connections, workforce shortage, insufficient time to use apps. Other challenges were insufficient access to smartphones, challenges with apps functions, and problems with reaching the target group because nurses did not come across any adolescents during the study period or had concerns with communicating with them successfully.	
15	Assessing the Usage and Usability of a Mental Health Advice Telephone Service in Uganda: Mixed Methods Study	Kabukye et al, 2024 (Kabukye et al., 2024)	Uganda	Mixed methods (qual and quant)	Members of the public in Uganda who call the mental health telephone line for help	Acceptability	Medium	Majority of the callers (40.27%) who stopped at the interactive voice response even though they could opt to speak with a human agent is rather encouraging since it intimates that people are accepting IVR to an extent, and signals that they may prefer it to interacting with a human agent. Participants liked the anonymous and confidential support that the call center provided because it prevented stigma.	P value
16	Implementation of telepsychiatry in Kenya: acceptability study	Kaigwa et al, 2022 (Kaigwa et al., 2022)	Kenya	Qualitative	Patients attending a private mental health facility in Nairobi, Kenya.		High	Participants indicated that digital infrastructure such as internet positively influenced their uptake of the online therapy sessions, as well as telepshychairty costs which they perceived to be lower than in-person sessions.	Description

continued on following page

Table 2. Continued

#	Title	Author, year	Country	Study design	Study population	Outcome of interest	Quality appraisal	Findings	Outcome measure
17	Mobile phone ownership. Digital technology use and acceptability of digital interventions among individuals on opioid use disorder treatment in Kenya	Kiburi, Saeeda and Chilioza, 2022 (Kiburi et al., 2022)	Kenya	Cross sectional	People being treated for opioid use disorder in Kenya at Ngara methadone clinic	Acceptability	Medium	Majority (95%) of participants were accepting of treatment for substance use via mobile phones, as against 49.9% through computers, with receiving text messages once weekly and only a daily text message.	P value
18	Mobile Phone Use and Acceptability for the Delivery of Mental Health Information Among Perinatal Adolescents in Nigeria: Survey Study	Kola et al, 2021 (Kola et al., 2021)	Nigeria	Cross-sectional study	Adolescent mothers in their perinatal or postnatal periods in 313 primary health clinics in Ibadan.	Acceptability	Medium	Majority (96.2%) would like to have mental health education delivered to them, on mobile phones, and out of these, majority (50.4%) would prefer information via text messaging, 38.8% via phone calls, 10.4% via app-based short videos and 0.4% on WhatsApp and facebook.	Description
19	Digital health for early psychosis in Ghana: patient and caregiver needs and preferences	Larsen et al, 2025 (Larsen et al., 2025)	Ghana	Cross-sectional study	Young adults living with early psychosis at Accra Psychiatry hospital	Acceptability	Medium	Majority of patients had access to mobile phones and are interested in using digital health interventions fort care.	P-value
20	Preference of mHealth versus in-person treatment for depression and post-traumatic stress disorder in Kenya: demographic and clinical characteristics	Meffert et al, 2024 (Meffert et al., 2024)	Kenya	Cross-sectional study	Outpatients in a Kisumu County Referral Hospital	Acceptability Affordability	Medium	Study participants indicated that the main 3 reasons for choosing mhealth were travel time, how affordable it was and the convenience it offered. Younger people preferred mhealth to in-person services and may reflect nuances associated with age groups, as they have had a more extensive and more complex interactions with mobile phone technology than older people have.	
21	Acceptability of using mobile Health (mHealth) as an intervention tool for people with drug use disorders in Tanga, Tanzania	Munishi et al, 2023 (Munishi et al., 2023)	Tanga, Tanzania	Cross-sectional study	PWDUD at bombo Regional Hospital, Tanzania	Acceptability Approachability and availability	Medium	Majority 92/3) of PWDUD did no own phones due to cost of the phones and effects of drug use on their lives, although they showed readiness to access mhealth interventions.	P value

continued on following page

Table 2. Continued

#	Title	Author, year	Country	Study design	Study population	Outcome of interest	Quality appraisal	Findings	Outcome measure
22	Attitudes of university students in Sudan towards digital mental health towards digital mental health	Mustafa et al, 2024 (Mustafa et al., 2024)	Sudan	Cross-sectional study	University students in Sudan	Acceptability	Medium	Majority (71%) are willing to trey telemental services, others prefer in person appointments. Young people and adolescence prefer face-to-face and a preferred choice for human0interfacing digital health services as compared with those without a human element.	P-value
23	Student peer mentoring: Feasibility and acceptability of mHealth-based tool for alcohol and substance abuse prevention by peer mentors at a university in Kenya	Musyoka et al, 2022 (Musyoka et al., 2023)	Kenya	Cross sectional study	First year peer mentors in university in kenya	Acceptability	High	High acceptance of mhealth based peer mentoring drug related intervention services as compared to in-person programmes, due to issues of confidentiality and stigma.	P-value
24	Barriers to and enhancement of the utilization of digital mental health interventions in low-resource settings: Perceptions of young people in Uganda	Mwaka et al, 2025 (Mwaka et al., 2025)	Uganda	Qualitative	Students across 9 universities in Uganda	Acceptability	Medium	Majority showed positive attitude towards digital mental health initiatives due to its role in taking away stigma associated with seeking help.	Description
25	Mobile Technology and Task Shifting to Improve Access to Alcohol Treatment Services in Mozambique	O'Grady et al, 2022 (O'Grady et al., 2022)	Mozambique	Mixed methods		Approachability and availability	Medium	Technologies that incorporate a provider-facing element show potential in supporting models which are focussed on task-shifting. This can widen access to alcohol-use interventions in LMICs. The study also showed high acceptability due to the adoption of a participatory approach when developing the mSBIRT intervention.	Description
26	Perception, attitude and use of digital health platforms for mental health promotion among students in a national university in the south-western part of Nigeria: A cross-sectional study	Ogundipe et a, 2025 (Ogundipe et al., 2025)	Nigeria	Cross-sectional	Students in University of Ibadan, Nigeria	Acceptability	High	Many students found mhealth modalities acceptable because there was high mobile phone ownership.	P-value

continued on following page

Table 2. Continued

#	Title	Author, year	Country	Study design	Study population	Outcome of interest	Quality appraisal	Findings	Outcome measure
27	Intention to use digital-based psychosocial counseling and its predictors among students in University of Gondar, Northwest Ethiopia, 2023: Using modified unified theory of acceptance and use of technology model	Anteneh et al, 2024 (Sendek Anteneh et al., 2025)	Ethiopia	Cross-sectional study	Regular undergraduate students at University of Gondar	Acceptability	Medium	Students' intention to use digitalised psychosocial counselling was 54.9%. Despite the promising findings, still, about half of the students have no intention to use digital tools for remote psycho-social support. Students' refusal could be related to digital literacy, access to digital devices, and perceived fear of information security.	Chi square
28	Access and use of digital technology by patients with psychosis at a hospital in South Africa	Sharma-Misra et al, 2023 (Sharma-Misra et al., 2023)	South Africa	Cross-sectional study	Patients in a psychiatric hospital in KwaZulu-Natal province	Availability and accommodation	High	The older people are, their less willingness to use a smart phone based mental health app. Each increase in age came with a 7% reduced odds of app utilisation.	P-value
29	Improving adherence in mental health service users with severe mental illness in South Africa: a pilot randomized controlled trial of a treatment partner and text message intervention vs. treatment as usual	Sibeko et al, 2017 (Sibeko et al., 2017)	South Africa	RCT	Folders from Valkenberg hospital, Cape Town	Acceptability		Results indicate that the text messaging functionality was found to be acceptable but infeasible as it were.	p-value

Table 3. Search strategy

S.No.	Key Concept	MEDLINE SEARCH TERMS	RESULTS
1	digital health	exp Digital Health/	899
2		exp Telemedicine/	52901
3		(ehealth* or "e-health*" or electronic health* or "electronic care" or (digital health* or "digital care" or digital technolog* or "digital intervention") or ("tele medicine" or tele health* or "tele care" or telecare or tele monitor* or tele consult* or video consult*)).mp. or (mobile health* or "mobile care" or mhealth or "m health").tw. [mp=title, book title, abstract, original title, name of substance word, subject heading word, floating sub-heading word, keyword heading word, organism supplementary concept word, protocol supplementary concept word, rare disease supplementary concept word, unique identifier, synonyms, population supplementary concept word, anatomy supplementary concept word]	103674
4		1 or 2 or 3	142451
5	mental health	exp Mental Health/	73109
6		exp Mental Disorders/	1549370
7		((mental* adj (health or disease* or disorder* or ill* or wellbeing or well-being or "wellbeing" or disabilit*)) or (depress* or anxi* or schizophreni* or psych*)).tw.	1867378
8		5 or 6 or 7	2771530
9	SSA	exp "Africa South of the Sahara"/	283959
10		("Sub-Saharan Africa" or Angola or Benin or Botswana or "Burkina Faso" or Burundi or Cameroon or "Cape Verde" or "Central African Republic" or Chad or Comoros or "Ivory Coast" or Congo or "Equatorial Guinea" or Eritrea or Ethiopia or Gabon or Gambia or Ghana or Guinea or "Guinea Bissau" or Kenya or Lesotho or Liberia or Madagascar or Malawi or Mali or Mauritania or Mauritius or Mozambique or Namibia or Niger or Nigeria or Rwanda or "Sao Tome" or Senegal or Seychelles or "Sierra Leone" or "South Africa" or Swaziland or Tanzania or Togo or Uganda or Zambia or Zimbabwe).tw.	430851
11		(("Sub-Sahara" and Africa*) or "africa south of the sahara" or (Africa* and (south* or west* or east* or central*) and sahara*) or ("africa south of the sahara" or ("sub" and sahara* and Africa*)) or ("sub saharan africa" or ("Sub-Saharan" and (Africa* or black*)))).mp. or ("east africa*" or "west Africa*" or "central Africa*" or "south Africa*").tw.	134265
12		9 or 10 or 11	526422
13		4 and 8 and 12	206

continued on following page

Table 3. Continued

S.No.	Key Concept	MEDLINE SEARCH TERMS	RESULTS
14	Limits	Letter/ or editorial/ or news/ or exp historical article/ or anecdotes as topic/ or comment/ or (comment or editorial or letter or "case report*").pt.	5176892
15		13 not 14	155
16		(exp animals/ or exp animals, laboratory/ or exp animal experimentation/ or exp models, animal/ or exp rodentia/ or (rat or rats or mouse or mice).ti.) not humans/	5445642
17		**15 not 16**	**155**

Table 4.

S.No.	Key Concept	EMBASE SEARCH TERMS	RESULTS
1	digital health	exp Digital Health/	4898
2		exp Telemedicine/	88263
3		(ehealth* or "e-health*" or electronic health* or "electronic care" or (digital health* or "digital care" or digital technolog* or "digital intervention") or ("tele medicine" or tele health* or "tele care" or telecare or tele monitor* or tele consult* or video consult*)).mp. or (mobile health* or "mobile care" or mhealth or "m health").tw. [mp=title, book title, abstract, original title, name of substance word, subject heading word, floating sub-heading word, keyword heading word, organism supplementary concept word, protocol supplementary concept word, rare disease supplementary concept word, unique identifier, synonyms, population supplementary concept word, anatomy supplementary concept word]	140080
4		1 or 2 or 3	212195
5	mental health	exp Mental Health/	300946
6		exp mental disease/	3113738
7		((mental* adj (health or disease* or disorder* or ill* or wellbeing or well-being or "wellbeing" or disabilit*)) or (depress* or anxi* or schizophreni* or psych*)).tw.	2463798
8		5 or 6 or 7	4261550

continued on following page

Table 4. Continued

S.No.	Key Concept	EMBASE SEARCH TERMS	RESULTS
9	SSA	exp "Africa South of the Sahara"/	350993
10		("Sub-Saharan Africa" or Angola or Benin or Botswana or "Burkina Faso" or Burundi or Cameroon or "Cape Verde" or "Central African Republic" or Chad or Comoros or "Ivory Coast" or Congo or "Equatorial Guinea" or Eritrea or Ethiopia or Gabon or Gambia or Ghana or Guinea or "Guinea Bissau" or Kenya or Lesotho or Liberia or Madagascar or Malawi or Mali or Mauritania or Mauritius or Mozambique or Namibia or Niger or Nigeria or Rwanda or "Sao Tome" or Senegal or Seychelles or "Sierra Leone" or "South Africa" or Swaziland or Tanzania or Togo or Uganda or Zambia or Zimbabwe).tw.	481611
11		(("Sub-Sahara" and Africa*) or "africa south of the sahara" or (Africa* and (south* or west* or east* or central*) and sahara*) or ("africa south of the sahara" or ("sub" and sahara* and Africa*)) or ("sub saharan africa" or ("Sub-Saharan" and (Africa* or black*)))).mp. or ("east africa*" or "west Africa*" or "central Africa*" or "south Africa*").tw.	47487
12		9 or 10 or 11	554228
13		4 and 8 and 12	333
14	Limits	Letter/ or editorial/ or news/ or exp historical article/ or anecdotes as topic/ or comment/ or (comment or editorial or letter or "case report*"). pt.	2300511
15		13 not 14	323
16		(exp animals/ or exp animals, laboratory/ or exp animal experimentation/ or exp models, animal/ or exp rodentia/ or (rat or rats or mouse or mice).ti.) not humans/	6171311
17		**15 not 16**	**323**

Table 5.

S.No.	Key Concept	Global Health SEARCH TERMS	RESULTS
1	Digital Health	exp telemedicine/	5320
2		(ehealth* or "e-health*" or electronic health* or "electronic care" or (digital health* or "digital care" or digital technolog* or "digital intervention") or ("tele medicine" or tele health* or "tele care" or telecare or tele monitor* or tele consult* or video consult*)).mp. or (mobile health* or "mobile care" or mhealth or "m health").tw.	140080
3		1 or 2	212195

continued on following page

Table 5. Continued

S.No.	Key Concept	Global Health SEARCH TERMS	RESULTS
4	Mental Health	exp mental health/	62096
5		exp mental disorders/	141528
6		((mental* adj (health or disease* or disorder* or ill* or wellbeing or well-being or "wellbeing" or disabilit*)) or (depress* or anxi* or schizophreni* or psych*)).tw.	297646
7		4 or 5 or 6	316423
8	SSA	exp "Africa South of the Sahara"/	442300
9		("Sub-Saharan Africa" or Angola or Benin or Botswana or "Burkina Faso" or Burundi or Cameroon or "Cape Verde" or "Central African Republic" or Chad or Comoros or "Ivory Coast" or Congo or "Equatorial Guinea" or Eritrea or Ethiopia or Gabon or Gambia or Ghana or Guinea or "Guinea Bissau" or Kenya or Lesotho or Liberia or Madagascar or Malawi or Mali or Mauritania or Mauritius or Mozambique or Namibia or Niger or Nigeria or Rwanda or "Sao Tome" or Senegal or Seychelles or "Sierra Leone" or "South Africa" or Swaziland or Tanzania or Togo or Uganda or Zambia or Zimbabwe).tw.	469495
10		(("Sub-Sahara" and Africa*) or "africa south of the sahara" or (Africa* and (south* or west* or east* or central*) and sahara*) or ("africa south of the sahara" or ("sub" and sahara* and Africa*)) or ("sub saharan africa" or ("Sub-Saharan" and (Africa* or black*)))).mp. or ("east africa*" or "west Africa*" or "central Africa*" or "south Africa*").tw.	446928
11		9 or 10 or 11	490476
12		**4 and 8 and 12**	**108**

Chapter 7
Mapping Online Patient Narratives in China's Private Healthcare: A Semantic Network Approach

Yufeng Xue
Southern Medical University, China & ISCTE, University Institute of Lisbon, Portugal

Ana Brochado
http://orcid.org/0009-0009-7407-3695
Universidade Aberta, Portugal & Dinâmia'CET-Iscte, Portugal

ABSTRACT

This study sought to identify the main dimensions of narratives shared online by consumers of physical examination services provided by a private hospital in China, as well as the main themes associated with clients' satisfaction and unsatisfaction. The research relied on secondary data (satisfaction ratings and Web reviews). Content analyses were conducted with Leximancer and Regional Operations Support Team Content Mining software. The reviews cover all phases of patients' experiences. The main dimensions of physical examination services are linked with the themes of staff attitude, medical check-up, hospital environment, price, procedure, and consultation. Satisfied patients are more likely to share narratives about core services (imedical check-ups, procedures, and examinations), while unsatisfied clients focus on staff attitudes and prices. The findings add to the knowledge about physical examinations' service quality dimensions and confirm the usefulness of online review content analysis to healthcare management practitioners and researchers.

DOI: 10.4018/979-8-2600-2238-2.ch007

INTRODUCTION

China's government has recently made promoting healthcare an important national strategy (The General Office of the State Council of the People's Republic of China, 2015). Underpinned by the "big health" paradigm, China's healthcare service sector has been positioned as a driver of national economic growth (Luo, 2016). More recently, healthcare reforms have been implemented in response to increasing epidemiological, demographic, and socioeconomic pressures (Rao et al., 2000; Hu et al., 2016). These initiatives align with the national "Healthy China 2030" strategy, which emphasizes prevention, equity, and overall population well-being (Luo, 2016).

In the context of China's rapid economic development, health management and the application of concepts such as early disease prevention, proactive treatment, and physical examination have become increasingly important. The new healthcare reform's main objective has been to offer Chinese citizens universal, equitable, and high-quality access to healthcare.5 Thus, a major effort has been made to develop primary care and general practice and "shift from a disease-centered biomedical model dominated by specialist medical services to a bio-psycho-social medical model (Xu et al., 2019)."

Primary healthcare offers individuals and families a first level of contact with the national health system (Li et al., 2017), providing generalist healthcare that includes diagnosis, treatment, prescription, and chronic disease management (Li et al., 2017, Li et al., 2020) . The recent reforms have promoted vertical integration in the healthcare system (Cao et al., 2024), which strengthens and prioritizes primary care and makes the foundation for a more coordinated healthcare approach. Health system reforms have also encouraged the opening of private hospitals (The General Office of the State Council of the People's Republic of China, 2015; Yip & Hsiao, 2015), so an increasing number of public and private healthcare facilities offer consumers more opportunities. Together, these changes reflect the policy shift toward a mixed public–private healthcare model promoted under the Healthy China 2030 strategy. This shift - from public dominance to a hybrid arrangement in which private operators play a supporting role - is, however, far from frictionless for private hospitals (Feng & Zhang, 2009). In practice, Chinese private health management firms continue to operate under considerable competitive strain from well-established public providers.

Sustained growth in this segment will therefore depend on how effectively private operators learn to navigate such competitive headwinds. Private hospitals must understand their patients' experiences more fully (Frampton & Guastellos, 2008) and offer quality services to clients (Swain & Kar, 2018). Service quality and patient satisfaction are seen as key criteria in China's healthcare reform (Hu et al., 2020).

Despite service quality's importance, yhe quality of primary health care in China is not well characterized and Xu et al. (2019) suggest that more research is needed on how to improve Chinese patients' experiences of primary healthcare.

Healthcare services can be categorized as customer-intensive services (Wang et al., 2021) so the relevant organizations need to examine patients' perceptions of service quality in order to identify areas requiring further improvement and generate more positive behavioral responses among clients (Raposo et al., 2009; Meesala & Paul, 2018). The healthcare industry is thus fundamentally a service industry. Hospitals provide not only medical treatments but also comprehensive experiences that ensure quality care, comfort, and patient satisfaction (Zhang et al., 2018). Clients' assessment of the services provided, therefore, comprise a performance outcome for hospitals (Aljafari et al., 2023).

According to Um and Lau (2018), researchers must study drivers of not only service quality but also healthcare service failure. The cited authors found that dissatisfied patients adopt behaviors such as spreading negative word-of-mouth, switching, and complaining. Zhang et al. (2019), in turn, argue that negative comments shared online are more influential than positive ones.

Sharing healthcare experiences in social media platforms has become a popular practice (Zhang et al., 2018; Zhang et al., 2019). As a result, online reviews have been increasingly used in healthcare service quality studies (Zhang et al., 2018). These reviews allow researchers to overcome the limitations associated with surveys, such as poor response rates, information that cannot be further explored by investigators, and high fieldwork costs when data needs to be gathered from different locations (Brochado et al., 2025).

Recent studies have identified dimensions of healthcare service quality based on patients' reviews of online doctors' (Dhakate & Joshi, 2023) and hospitals' services (AlNasser & AlMuhaideb, 2024). After examining China's primary healthcare system, Li et al. (2020) and Li et al. (2017) recommended that researchers should use digital data and innovative technologies, especially when the goal is to strengthen quality control.

To address these calls for additional studies (Li et al., 2020) the present research set as its primary objective the identification of the main dimensions of Chinese patients' experiences shared in social media platforms regarding physical examination services. As previous studies conducted in China have targeted public hospitals (e.g., Fan et al., 2017, Tam, 2019), the current investigation focused on private hospitals, whose development has also been promoted by recent healthcare reform. Thus, this study addressed two research questions:

- What are the main dimensions of narratives about physical examination services shared by Chinese private hospitals' patients online?

- Do these main dimensions vary by satisfied and dissatisfied patients?

This paper is structured as follows. After the introduction, the second section provides an overview of China's healthcare system and discusses the main dimensions of healthcare service quality. Next, the methodology section describes the research context, data collection procedures, and content analysis methods. The results section then presents the main findings of the content analyses of satisfied and dissatisfied patients' online narratives. Finally, the conclusion discusses the findings, theoretical and managerial implications, limitations, and avenues for future research.

LITERATURE REVIEW

China's Healthcare Industry

According to the World Health Organization World Health Organization (2006), health systems should combine various characteristics that improve the quality of healthcare, including, among others, efficiency, effectiveness, accessibility, patient-centered care, equitability, and safeness. At its core, health management refers to a set of practices aimed at containing healthcare costs while simultaneously improving patients' well-being and overall health outcomes (Fu et al., 2011; Liu & Wang, 2016). The approach is inherently cyclical: risk factors are tracked, interventions are introduced, outcomes are reassessed, and the cycle restarts as needed (Chen et al., 2016).

Although many ideas about health management are found in traditional Chinese medicine Peng & Lin (2009) this concept only began to spread throughout China in the 1990s (Liu & Wang, 2016).

To promote the development of the health management service industry, the Chinese government has, in recent years, formulated many policies related to this industry (Yip & Hsiao, 2015). China introduced the "Healthy China" strategy with the National Thirteenth Five-Year Plan (Liu & Wang, 2016).

This recent health reform has focused on patients and defined ways to improve their medical experiences (National Health and Family Planning Commission of the People's Republic of China, 2015).

China's healthcare system is structured as a three-tiered system (Swain & Kar, 2018): tertiary medical centers (Level 3), secondary hospitals (Level 2), and primary hospitals (Level 1) (Hu et al., 2016). Overall, primary care facilities comprise not only Level 1 hospitals but also unrated healthcare services, village clinics in rural areas, and community health stations in urban areas (Liu et al., 2018). A study by Hu et al. (2016) revealed that, from the patients' perspective, community health centers offer better quality healthcare in terms of primary care than secondary and tertiary care facilities do.

The healthcare reform launched in 2009 sought to strengthen primary care and upgrade community health centers (Chen, 2009) in order to develop a sustainable health system (Liu et al., 2018).

Primary care facilitates healthcare provision from locations closer to the relevant populations and thus minimizes transportation costs for patients accessing health services (Hu et al., 2016). Recent healthcare reforms recognize that a hospital-centric system is costly and that it does not address citizens' needs (Li et al., 2020). Primary care can thus contribute to a balanced use of healthcare facilities at different levels (Miao et al., 2019) and foster better management of chronic and infectious diseases (Li et al., 2020).

However, some researchers have shown that the Chinese still do not trust the quality of services offered by community healthcare (Yip & Hsiao, 2015).

In addition, Liu et al.'s study (Liu et al., 2018) revealed that provider factors such as perceived poor quality, obsolete equipment, and a lack of variety in drugs has strengthened patients' preferences for Level 2 and Level 3 hospitals. This preference for higher level facilities has resulted in overcrowding, which creates challenges for those seeking to provide quality services (Li et al., 2015). The phenomenon has been labeled "three longs and one short" (Chao et al., 2017): long waiting periods for appointments, registration, and prepayments of charges followed by short appointments. As a result, healthcare reform in China has promoted a referral-based healthcare system and vertical integration (Cao et al., 2024).

In terms of ownership, major medical facilities can be divided into public and private hospitals (Feng & Zhang, 2009).

Within China's medical services market, public hospitals remain the dominant force. Yet the central government has been actively encouraging the growth of private providers as part of a broader push to lift living standards and strengthen public health awareness (The General Office of the State Council of the People's Republic of China, 2015). The result is a healthcare landscape in which both supply and demand have become noticeably more stratified and diverse.

Even so, the rebalancing toward a public-led, privately-supplemented model is not without friction for private hospitals (Yip & Hsiao, 2015). One persistent barrier is consumer loyalty to state-owned institutions, which constrains the expansion of private health management firms. Trust plays a parallel role: the profit-seeking nature of private operators tends to attract greater scepticism than the perceived public-service ethos of state hospitals. Combined with the lower fees charged by public providers, this scepticism translates into a reduced willingness to pay for private care. Rising expectations around service quality add a further layer of difficulty, pushing customer satisfaction further out of reach (Wagstaff et al., 2009).

Service Quality Measurement in the Healthcare Industry

Healthcare service quality has attracted increasing interest among researchers (Valencia-Arias et al., 2018). The measurement of healthcare service quality is made more challenging by healthcare's complexity due to diverse and unpredictable customer needs, intangibility, and co-production with patients. The human, financial, and social consequences of low healthcare quality are, however, known to be high (Vogus & McClelland, 2016).

Because patients rarely possess the expertise to assess the clinical side of their care, their judgements of service quality tend to rest on more accessible cues: the way they are treated by staff and the broader feel of the facility, among other process-related signals (Bowers et al., 1994). To deal with this complex context, researchers have proposed various measurement instruments in the form of surveys to assess medical service quality (see Fatima et al., 2018 and Swain and Kar (2018) for a review of the relevant literature). Healthcare service quality has been conceptualized as a multidimensional construct and as patients' perceptions of a bundle of service quality dimensions (Zhang et al., 2018, Giovanis et al., 2018).

Many studies have applied the service quality (i.e., SERVQUAL) (Parasuraman, et al., 1988) or service performance (i.e., SERVPERF) model (Cronin & Taylor, 1994), using five dimensions to describe service quality in hospitals: reliability, assurance, tangibles, empathy, and responsiveness (e.g., Moghadam & Amiresmaili, 2009; Alborie & Damanhouri, 2013; Akdere et al., 2020; Altuntas et al., 2020). For example, Shafei et al. (2019) compared the psychometric properties of SERVQUAL and SERVPERF's weighted versions and concluded a weighted SERVQUAL model is the best approach to assessing healthcare service quality. Zhang et al. (2018) adapted SERVQUAL to fit Asian contexts. Drawing on social identity theory, the cited authors concluded that service quality has a positive effect on patient loyalty when the latter is mediated by providers' level of empathy.

Researchers have also modified the SERVQUAL scale by adding new dimensions to cope with the specificities of healthcare settings. For example, Rashid and Jusoff (2009) proposed a conceptual model of hospital service quality in which they added five more dimensions to the SERVQUAL scale (i.e., access, choice, information, redress, and representation) for a total of 10 dimensions contributing to service quality. Eleuch (2011) in turn, maintains that service quality in healthcare includes not only functional quality, which is measured by the five SERVQUAL dimensions, but also technical quality consisting of doctors' services, adequate diagnostic tests, and appropriate treatments.

Despite SERVQUAL's popularity, researchers have also expressed concerns about the dimensions' stability and the measurement of service quality as the gap between expectations and perceptions (Miranda et al., 2012). Consequently, some studies have developed new scales to evaluate healthcare service quality (Swain & Kar, 2018). In a similar vein, Raposo et al. (2009) single out medical care, nursing, administrative support, personnel, and facilities as the building blocks of service quality at the primary care level. Miranda et al. (2012) found that service quality can be defined according to four dimensions: facilities' condition, health staff quality, other staff quality, and operational efficiency. In addition, Zarei (2015) identified key dimensions of service quality in healthcare as physical environment, service cost, physician consultation, information provided to patients, waiting time, admission process, and appointment accessibility.

Giovanis et al. (2018) in turn, concluded that service quality perceptions in primary care are linked with medical care, nursing care, administrative services, staff, and facilities' condition. Shabbir et al. (2016) used five dimensions to measure service quality perceptions both in public and private hospitals: physician care, nurse care, support staff, operational activities, and physical maintenance. Trivedi and Jagani (2018) also evaluated health service quality using the following dimensions: experiences with doctors, physical environment, nursing staff, hospital pharmacy, laboratory and x-ray technical services, and experiences with administrators and patient-relations officers.

In addition, Fatima et al. (2018) considered several service quality dimensions when measuring service quality perceptions of private hospitals, that is, physical environment, customer-friendly environment, responsiveness, communication, and privacy and safety. Swain and Kar (2018) conducted a literature review of research on healthcare service quality and then proposed a model to measure perceived service quality in hospitals based on six main areas: technical features, procedures, infrastructure, interactions, personnel, and social support quality.

Recent studies have further highlighted the importance of patients' reviews of service quality (Rodrigues et al., 2017). For instance, Rodrigues et al.'s research (2017) revealed that medical tourists (e.g., cosmetic surgery and dentistry treatments) share online their evaluations of cost, treatment effectiveness, and time spent (Dhakate & Joshi, 2023, AlNasser & AlMuhaideb, 2024).

Dhakate and Joshi's (2023) study found that the most significant dimensions of online reviews that evaluate online healthcare consultancy are medical treatment; doctors' behavior, knowledge, and experience; service; and patients' needs. AlNasser and AlMuhaideb (2024) additionally identified five main dimensions of patients' experiences and concluded that positive comments mainly refer to medical staff, while negative reactions are associated with pricing, appointments, and emergency services. Comments about customer service appear in both positive and negative reviews. Analyzing online word-of-mouth enables firms to systematically capture real-time and diverse customer feedback, providing a dynamic understanding of evolving perceptions that can be leveraged through text mining techniques to continuously improve service quality (Lu et al., 2023).

Studies of China's Healthcare Industry

Previous studies of healthcare service quality have covered different regions (see Fatima et al. (2018) for a review) around the world. Lam (1997), Li et al. (2015), Hu et al. (2016), Zhang et al. (2018), Tam (2019), Hu et al. (2020), and Wu et al. (2020) specifically focused on the Chinese healthcare system. Lam (1997) and Li et al. (2015) used the SERVQUAL scale and its five dimensions. Fan et al. (2017) also employed SERVQUAL to assess service quality in Chinese hospitals but added a new economic dimension. The latter cited authors concluded that, in general, patients' service quality expectations are lower than their corresponding perceptions of services. Tam (2019) in turn, developed a conceptual model of the relationships between perceived encounter quality, patient participation, self-efficacy, satisfaction, and loyalty intentions.

Hu et al. (2016) used the Chinese primary care assessment tool (PCAT) to compare patients' perceptions of primary care service quality in tertiary, secondary, and primary health facilities. The Chinese PCAT measures patients' experiences in 10 dimensions. These are first contact (i.e., utilization and access), continuity of care, coordination (i.e., referrals and information systems), comprehensiveness (i.e., services available and used), family centeredness, community orientation, and cultural competence.

Zhang et al. (2018) additionally analyzed negative comments about physicians shared on a Chinese health community website called "Ping An Good Doctor." The cited authors concluded that patients complain about problems throughout the entire process of medical consultations. The most frequent complaints are related to perceptions of insufficient consultation duration, impatient physicians, and inadequate therapeutic effects.

Wu et al. (2020) also gathered data from the Ping An Good Doctor website to study patients' comments shared online regarding three different stages: before, during, and after sales. The cited authors concluded that healthcare service quality at each stage shapes patients' experiences on both the physical and psychological level.

Tam's study (2019) targeted Hong Kong hospitals. According to the cited researcher's final model, customers' perceptions of service encounter quality comprise patient participation (i.e., the degree to which patients are involved in services' production) and physical environment (i.e., physical surroundings and tangibles' appearance). Other factors are technical quality (i.e., physicians' perceived technical abilities), empathy (i.e., interpersonal interaction quality), and communication (i.e., interaction between patients and physicians).

Finally, Hu et al. (2016) analyzed data from the China National Patient Survey, which includes questions organized according to five dimensions: process management, hospital environment, nursing care, physician care, and overall satisfaction. The cited study's results reveal that patients are more satisfied with healthcare in large hospitals with higher nurse-to-bed ratios.

Underpinning Theories

Three theoretical strands - signaling, information integration, and social support - operate within a broader service science framework and, taken together, help make sense of how patients articulate healthcare service quality in their online comments. Spence's (1973) seminal work on signaling theory posits that individuals (e.g., job candidates) use signals (e.g., education credentials) to convey their quality to employers. This theoretical approach is highly relevant to healthcare service quality as patients post their experiences on online platforms and potential patients interpret these narratives as signals of healthcare providers' quality (Dhakate & Joshi, 2023). Thus, signaling theory helps explain why online narratives act as indicators of service quality.

Information integration theory (Anderson, 1971), in turn, clarifies how individuals process and integrate multiple pieces of information to form judgments, attitudes, and decisions. Patients seeking healthcare services are exposed to various information sources (e.g., past experiences, hospital reputation, online reviews, and word of mouth) that are combined and weighted to form a final judgment of providers. This opinion influences whether patients will choose a particular hospital or doctor. Patients have both positive and negative experiences (Dhakate & Joshi, 2023, AlNasser & AlMuhaideb, 2024) so they might attribute different weights to information during their decision-making process. Information integration theory, therefore, elucidates how people treat and interpret signals—including patients' reviews—when making healthcare decisions.

Finally, social support theory explains how social interactions provide emotional, informational, and practical assistance and influence individuals' well-being, decision-making, and health outcomes (Cohen & Wills, 1985). When patients post reviews, narratives, and feedback about healthcare services on digital platforms, these people are engaging in social support behavior that affects other individuals' perceptions and decisions.

METHODOLOGY

Research Context

The empirical setting for this research was Meinian Onehealth, a company that ranks as China's leading private provider of health check-up and related services. This professional health management corporation was founded in 2004. Its main business is providing physical examinations (e.g., routine physical examinations and early tumor screening). These services represent more than 80% of the corporation's net revenues and integrated health consultations (i.e., medical messenger, telephone, and expert face-to-face consultations, as well as health lectures and salons), assessments, and interventions.

Meinian Onehealth's management model is built around prevention, pairing preventative care with treatment within a fully integrated examination–treatment–insurance loop. Physical examinations as part of disease prevention play an important role in the national health system, which focuses on preventive medicine and healthcare reform. It hosts what is currently the country's largest personal health information big data platform and maintains a national footprint of more than 600 medical and physical examination centres, reaching over 30 provinces and 100 key cities.

Data Collection

Online feedback on the corporation's physical examination services is generated by patients across all the Chinese regions where the company operates. Data for this study were gathered from two of the country's most prominent e-commerce platforms — Taobao and Jingdong — both of which allow users to rate their overall satisfaction from one to five stars, with the scale running from 1 (terrible) and 2 (poor) through 3 (average) to 4 (very good) and 5 (excellent).

After selecting a star rating, the patients post comments (i.e., Web reviews) about their healthcare experiences. The star ratings and comments were gathered and entered into an Excel spreadsheet. The final dataset included 954 and 1,363 reviews on Taobao and Jingdong, respectively, of the company's physical examination services. The patients' average rating was 4.7 stars on Taobao and 4.5 on Jingdong. To strengthen the robustness of the content analysis, the dataset was restricted to reviews exceeding a single line in length. In all, 500 positive reviews (star ratings of 4 and 5) and 300 negative reviews (star ratings of 1 and 2), all posted in 2018, were collected.

Data Analysis

The analysis of online reviews of the company's health management products was conducted with the Chinese software, Regional Operations Support Team Content Mining (ROST CM), which was developed by Wuhan University (Liu, 2013) [REMOVED REF FIELD]. The tool handles a wide range of Chinese-language text — from scholarly papers and microblog posts to chat logs and e-mails — and has been successfully deployed in a number of prior analyses (Zeng et al., 2015; Mei et al., 2024; Zheng et al., 2024). An example of this software's interface is shown in Figure 1.

Figure 1. ROST Content Mining software interface

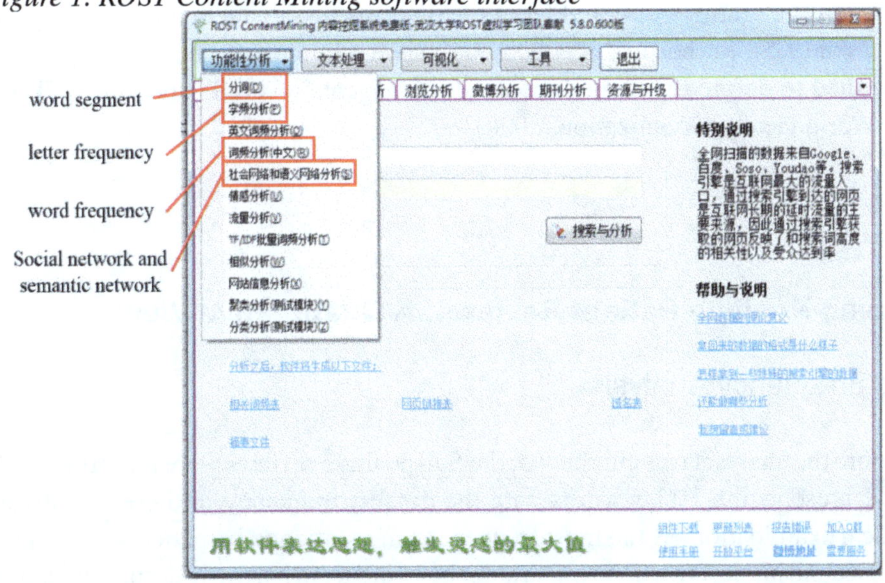

Many of the comments retrieved for this study were written in non-standard grammar - a feature that is largely inherent to online reviews, which typically combine direct opinions, brevity, conversational style, and a high degree of expressive freedom. To prepare the corpus for analysis, the texts were curated manually: irrelevant or filler items (for instance, "ok," "well," "often") were removed, while semantically close terms were collapsed into common labels (e.g., "clean" and "tidy"; "cheap" and "inexpensive"; "bargain" and "cost effective"). Three main techniques were then applied to the cleaned data — word frequency counts, social network analysis, and co-occurrence matrix construction.

The results were validated and the main themes shared online by both satisfied and dissatisfied patients were identified with the help of Leximancer tools. This software converts data extracted from natural language texts into semantic patterns, thereby enabling an automated, systematic analysis of qualitative information (Borges et al., 2025). One key advantage of Leximancer is its ability to detect themes with minimal researcher intervention, which enables a more objective, data-driven approach.

In addition, this software visually represents the main ideas within the texts as a concept map that offers valuable insights into how these ideas are interrelated. Leximancer analyses also facilitate comparisons of concepts, which permit the identification of divergences and similarities between groups within the dataset defined by tags. In the present study, satisfaction ratings were incorporated into the concept map as tags, thereby categorizing the themes highlighted into two groups: satisfaction (i.e., ratings of 4 and 5 out of 5) versus dissatisfaction (i.e., ratings of 1 and 2 out of 5). In the final phase, a qualitative method (i.e., narrative analysis) was applied to define the main dimensions of patients' overall experiences (Tam, 2019, World Health Organization, 2006).

RESULTS

Mapping Positive Patient Reviews: A Quantitative View

Word Frequency Analysis

Before the analysis was conducted, the 500 positive reviews were pre-processed. Table 1 presents the 30 keywords with the highest frequency in these narratives. "Physical examination" is the most frequent term mentioned by patients. "Service" has the second highest frequency. The latter keyword has a narrowly defined meaning in the online reviews, referring to the help and conveniences provided by staff in physical examinations, which is different from the meaning of service as it is used in health management services.

Table 1. Keywords with highest frequency of use in positive reviews

Number	Keywords	Frequency	Number	Keywords	Frequency
1	service	128	16	time	28
2	check	74	17	breakfast	27
3	attitude	57	18	hospital	25
4	report	51	19	queue	25

continued on following page

Table 1. Continued

Number	Keywords	Frequency	Number	Keywords	Frequency
5	customers	45	20	experience	24
6	doctor	41	21	suggest	23
7	staff	39	22	nurse	23
8	efficient	38	23	smoothly	22
9	convenient	35	24	reception	22
10	environment	33	25	online	21
11	items	32	26	enthusiastic	21
12	appointment	31	27	comprehensive	21
13	satisfied	31	28	clean	21
14	inexpensive	29	29	problem	20
15	patient	28	30	Helpful	18

Note. Based on data from Yufeng (2018)

Within positive reviews, customers frequently issue overall verdicts on service quality — phrases such as “good service,” “satisfactory service,” or “excellent service” recur throughout the corpus. Comments often zoom in on particular staff groups too: “the doctor and nurse services are good” or “the staff service is good” are illustrative. The word “check,” in this favourable context, is typically paired with appraisals like “everything was checked very comprehensively,” “the doctors checked me very closely,” and “the check-up results were satisfying.” “Attitude” emerges as a recurring secondary dimension, underscoring how the conduct of clinicians and front-line staff can tip an evaluation toward the positive end. A similar pattern surrounds the term “report.” For most patients, the most tangible aspect of their examination report is how quickly it is printed and made available - and the perceived quality of the report itself is something they gauge with relative ease.

Usually, the faster physical reports are printed, the more satisfied patients are. Other words used with high frequency are “doctor,” “staff,” “nurse,” and “customer,” confirming the co-creation nature of health services. Three further drivers consistently shape favourable patient feedback: the cleanliness and tidiness of the “environment,” the breadth and comprehensiveness of the examination “items” on offer, and the smooth running of the “appointment” process.

Semantic Network Analysis

The ROST CM software’s functional analysis features facilitate the plotting of semantic network maps that illustrate figuratively keywords’ relevance and assess each term’s importance. Two indicators jointly signal a keyword's relevance: the number of bivariate links it establishes with other terms and its overall frequency of occurrence. Although "physical examination" emerged as the most frequent word in the corpus, it proved semantically peripheral once the network structure was examined more closely; for that reason, it was dropped from the final map to keep the visualisation interpretable. This procedure also meant the semantic network only included the keywords found to be significant when each term's importance was analyzed. After removing any nonsignificant correlations, the final semantic network map for positive reviews was generated (see Figure 2). The most significant correlations are between service and attitude (43%), service and check (37%), service and staff (32%), and service and doctor (30%).

Figure 2. Semantic network of positive reviews

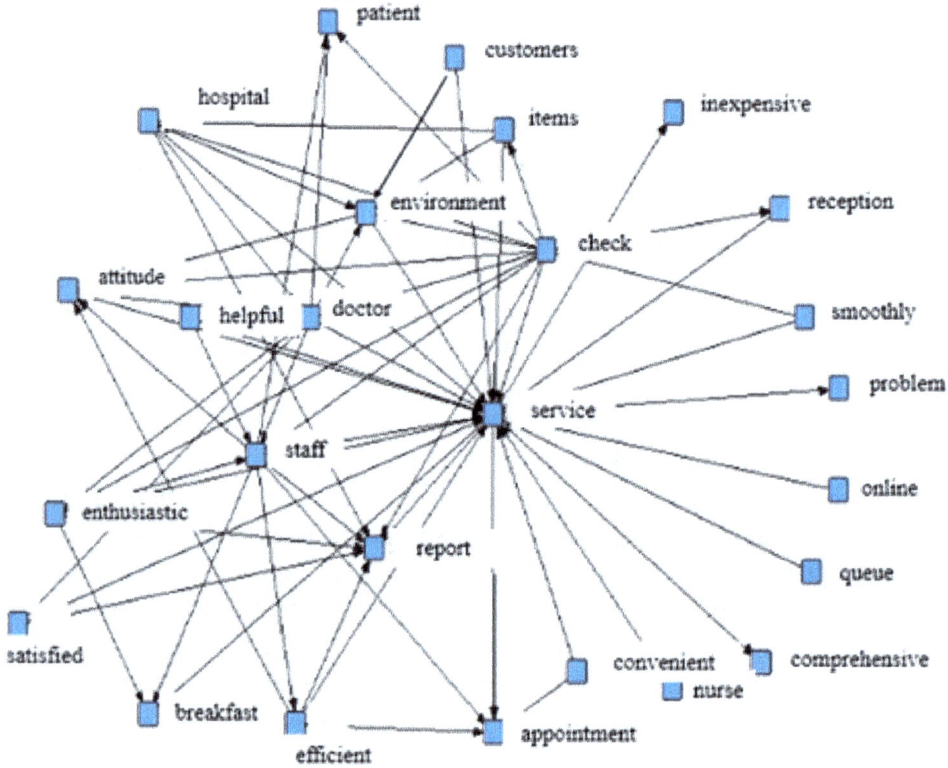

Note. Based on data from Yufeng (2018)

At the heart of the semantic network lies the term "service," which forms more links to surrounding keywords than any other node. This means that the main factor behind positive ratings is the good service patients experience during the physical examination process, including consultations before examinations, appointments, services, and consultations after examinations. Several other keywords also branch out widely across the network - among them "check," "doctor," "environment," "consultation," "time," and "report." Their prominence reflects what patients value most in practice: efficient examinations, professionally competent physicians, well-presented examination centres, and swift turnaround on reports. Moreover, the terms "items," "attitude," and "appointment" also have relatively high associations with some other keywords, indicating that consumers are quite concerned about examination items, the staff's attitude, and the appointment process. Recurring descriptors such as "patience," "convenience," and "efficiency" also populate the map, functioning across reviews as familiar markers of client satisfaction.

Mapping Negative Patient Reviews: A Quantitative View

Word Frequency Analysis

The negative subset comprised 300 reviews, which were pre-processed and then merged into a single corpus for ROST CM analysis. Following word segmentation, frequency statistics were generated to identify the dominant keywords; the top 30 are listed in Table 2.

Table 2. Keywords with highest frequency of use in negative reviews

Number	Keywords	Frequency	Number	Keywords	Frequency
1	attitude	89	16	nurse	29
2	service	84	17	breakfast	28
3	item	75	18	guidance	27
4	staff	67	19	terrible	27
5	check	64	20	environment	25
6	doctor	59	21	problem	23
7	appointment	39	22	parking	22
8	report	37	23	noisy	22
9	hospital	35	24	comprehensive	22
10	reception	34	25	online	22
11	experience	34	26	unprofessional	19
12	customer	33	27	perfunctory	18
13	expensive	32	28	consultation	18
14	time	30	29	queue	17
15	inconvenient	30	30	worth	15

Note. Based on data from Yufeng (2018)

The keyword "physical examination" is once again the most frequently used term. The keyword with the next highest frequency is "items." Reviews featuring this keyword surface repeated grievances about an examination offer perceived as too limited or poorly structured. "Check" comes in third by frequency - the same position it occupies in the positive corpus - yet the surrounding context inverts its meaning entirely: here, the word signals check-ups that patients judged perfunctory, incomplete, or unprofessional. Used in tandem, "items" and "check" map onto perceptions of the firm's technical and professional standing, pointing to substandard technical performance as a leading reason behind negative posts. In addition, the terms "staff," "attitude," "doctor," and "appointment" appear quite frequently.

Semantic Network Analysis

A functional analysis was carried out in ROST CM to map the correlations among keywords found in the selected negative reviews. After trimming away weak and uninformative associations, the final semantic network emerged (see Figure 3). The negative network proved noticeably denser than the positive one. Rather than a single anchoring node, four prominent hubs - service, attitude, queue, and items - sit at the centre, accompanied by a number of other influential terms. The structure most likely reflects how dissatisfied patients write: their reviews tend to be more granular, naming the specific factors that frustrated them and, as a result, generating tighter interconnections across the network. The strongest pairwise correlations involve service and attitude (49%), service and staff (42%), service and check (37%), service and item (36%), and attitude and problem (33%).

Figure 3. Semantic network map of negative reviews

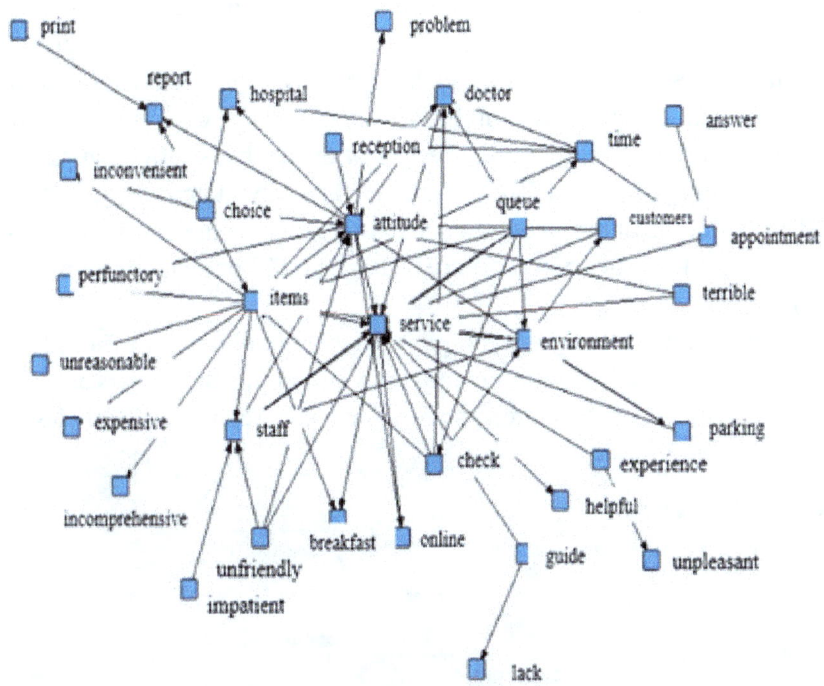

Note. Based on data from Yufeng (2018)

Three keywords dominate this semantic network: "service," "attitude," and "items." Service shortcomings are the single most common reason patients turn to negative reviews, and dissatisfaction with staff is typically channelled through descriptors like "terrible," "unfriendly," and "impatient." "Items" carries noticeably more weight here than in the positive map - both in frequency and in connectivity - pointing to its capacity to spark patient dissatisfaction. Nearby in the network sit phrases such as "not comprehensive" and "perfunctory" check-ups, together with grievances over "unreasonable" items. Other terms that are relatively highly connected are "time," "appointment," "experience," and "report." Related complaints mainly mention long waiting time for examinations, bad appointment services, and delays in printing reports, among other problems, all of which are unpleasant experiences that cause customers to write negative online reviews.

Concept Map

The Leximancer content analyses revealed 11 themes in patients' online descriptions of physical examination services. These topics were then grouped into eight main themes to facilitate further interpretation: physical examination, staff attention, medical check-up, hospital environment, price, consultation, procedure, and recommendation (Figure 4). The results of the analysis show that patients who give positive ratings are more likely to post reviews about core services and procedures. The themes most frequently linked to this group's narratives are examination (64 percent likelihood of co-occurrence), check-up (63 percent) and procedure (59 percent).

In contrast, patients that give their physical examinations low ratings (i.e., 1 or 2 out of 5 points) share narratives more frequently containing the themes of staff service and price. The most common themes are price (65 percent) and staff (58 percent).

Figure 4. Concept map

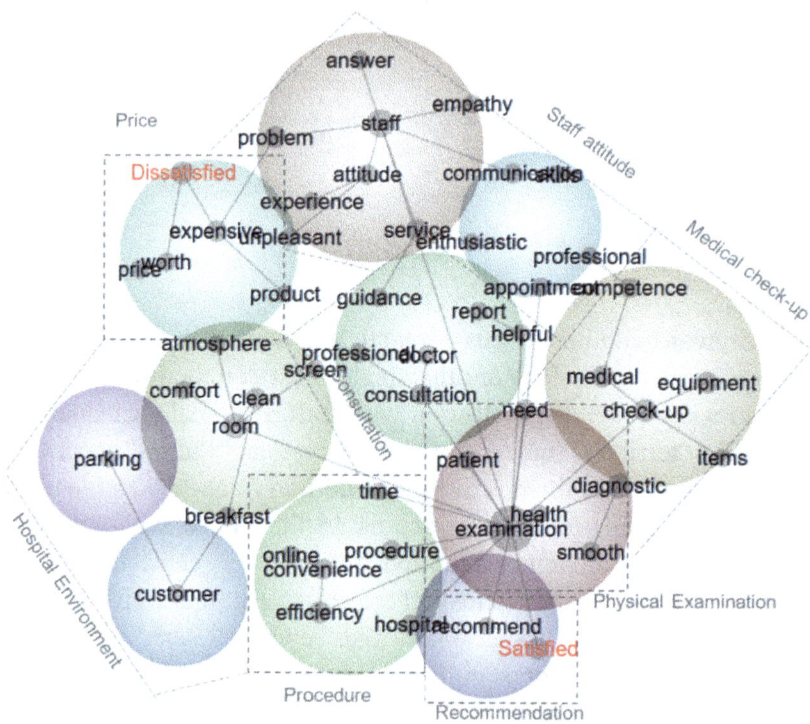

Qualitative Analysis

After considering the keywords' frequency and connections, an analysis was conducted of the main factors patients focus on when evaluating health management products that are part of physical examinations. Closely linked high-frequency keywords were subsequently consolidated into six overarching themes: staff attitude, medical check-up, hospital environment, price, procedure, and consultation. A handful of keywords fit naturally under more than one theme. The term "doctor," for instance, surfaces both when patients comment on attitude-related dimensions (service manner, friendliness) and when they assess clinical competence - placing it simultaneously within the staff attitude and medical check-up themes. The same applies to "hospital," since reviewers routinely compare the private health management firm at the centre of this study with public hospitals across multiple fronts: service, technology, environment, and pricing. Once the keywords were interpreted in light of their meaning and analytical weight, each of the six themes was populated with a corresponding set of terms. Illustrative excerpts from patient narratives - showing how customers make sense of their physical examination experiences - are presented under each theme that follows.

Staff Attitude

The staff attitude theme is linked with terms such as "attitude," "appointment," "convenience," "staff," "nurse," "customers," "online (service)," and "reception." Patients usually evaluate health management companies' services in the post-purchase phase, after physical examinations have been completed. However, the narratives are also related to service aspects before (e.g., online purchase consulting and reception) and during physical examinations.

A clear pattern across the reviews is the strong psychological dependence patients show on medical staff, whose presence and support they appear to value highly. Three terms encapsulate this: "doctor," "staff," and "attitude." Their prominence underscores the weight of the human dimension in shaping the patient experience and points to staff demeanor - that of doctors and other personnel alike — as one of the most decisive elements in customer evaluations. For instance, one patient shared, "[t]he customer service is quite good. Although the appointment roster was full, my appointment was adjusted to Saturday since that was when I was free." Another patient wrote, "[t]he staff [member] responsible for this sent a short message to remind me in advance about the physical examination." The staff attitude theme is also illustrated by a third review, which reads, "[a]ll the staff in the examination center are very good, and doctors are very enthusiastic about answering each question in detail to patients." Positive reviews highlighted kindness in healthcare roles and the comprehensiveness of care, while negative reviews pointed to poor communication, lack of empathy, and staff indifference.

Medical Check-Up

The theme of medical check-up is associated with the quality of diagnoses and treatments. The main concepts associated with this theme are "report," "doctor," "smooth (procedure)," "comprehensive(ness)," "experience," "items," "equipment," and "hospital." Patients frequently report such things as whether the check-up was quite efficient and/or detailed and whether it went smoothly. Other popular topics are whether physical examination items are comprehensive, the medical equipment is up-to-date, and the report is printed quickly. Items and efficiency stand out more sharply than other influential factors, and the gap widens noticeably on the negative side of the corpus. Lacking the technical know-how to assess the clinical merit of their examinations, patients tend to fall back on functional service quality cues when forming an overall judgement of their experience. Up-to-date, technologically advanced equipment used in physical examinations is also easily perceived by patients. One patient wrote, "[t]he doctors and nurses are very professional, the examination is thorough and detailed, and the items included in the check-up are comprehensive." Another patient shared, "[t]here are only a few items [included in the examination], which seem to be merely simple and routine checks."

Hospital Environment

The environment theme is dominated by questions of hygiene: whether corridors, toilets, and facilities come across as clean and well-kept tops the list of recurring concerns. The terms associated with this theme are "clean(liness)," customers, "parking (lot)," "satisfaction," "comfort," "noise," "breakfast," and "convenience." Parking availability emerges as a point of concern for some patients, who note whether the examination centre offers a lot on the premises. Breakfast is another recurring topic: since most centres serve it routinely to examination customers, food quality - readily judged at first hand - finds its way into the reviews. Patients also recall noise levels and other tangibles that affect their experiences. For example, one review reads, "[t]he screen on the door of the room conveniently calls out customers' numbers as a reminder."

Price

The price theme's most often mentioned terms are "inexpensive (service)," "expensive (product)," and "worth," indicating that patients pay attention to the value for money of health management service products. Pricing is rarely discussed in absolute terms: reviewers typically set the company's fees against what public hospitals charge, using the comparison to articulate their own subjective read on value for money. To ensure patients are satisfied, their overall experience should make them feel that the physical examination is worth the fees charged. A patient wrote, "[t]he service is not worth the price, so I think I will not go there again, and [I] do not recommend this service." Another patient shared, "[t]he service is just so-so, and [it's] definitely not worth 2,000 yuan."

Procedure

The procedure theme is led by three high-frequency terms: "efficiency," "time," and "queue." Their prominence makes clear how much importance patients place on the length of the wait they have to endure. Crowded waiting areas are a frequent target of negative feedback, with reviewers describing the volume of customers queuing for physical examinations as distinctly unpleasant.The optimization of physical examination procedures and a short queue and waiting time are thus important drivers of patient satisfaction.

A patient reported, "[i]f you are going to have a physical examination, you should go to the center at a time when there are not too many people waiting and when doctors have more time available." Another customer wrote, "[t]here are a lot of people waiting for check-ups, so each item is done relatively hastily." A further client commented that "[o]nline booking and reservation is simple and convenient."

Consultation

The consultation theme is anchored by five high-profile terms – "consultation," "helpful (staff)," "report," "doctor," and "hospital" — whose prominence reveals that patients view health education and the interpretation of examination reports as critically important parts of their experience. Negative reviews often mention that insufficient medical guidance is given to the centers' customers. Clearly, health education counseling always needs to be included throughout the examination process. Providers need to deliver comprehensive health education at every stage of the customer journey — before, during, and after the examination itself. For example, a patient shared, "the [d]octors gave helpful advice in response to my questions." Another patient wrote, "after the examination, they call [the patients in] to receive informative feedback."

DISCUSSION

This study sought to answer two research questions, the first of which was as follows: What are the main dimensions of narratives about physical examination services shared by Chinese private hospitals' patients online? A close reading of the online review corpus brought to the surface the main dimensions that define the physical examination experience.

Regarding the top 30 most frequent keywords, around 73% were shared in both positive and negative reviews. Although the reviews under study were posted in the post-purchase phase of experiences, the most common terms used by both satisfied and dissatisfied patients are related to all stages of physical examination experiences. Keywords that are specific to negative reviews are "consultation," "expensive services," "insufficient guidance," "noise," "parking lots," "perfunctory check-ups," and "terrible and unprofessional staff." The terms associated with positive reviews are "cleanliness," "convenience," "efficiency," "enthusiasm," "inexpensive services," "satisfaction," "smooth procedures," and "suggestions." The price for services adds a new dimension to research on public primary care services (Hu et al., 2016).

As in Zhang et al.'s study (Zhang et al., 2018), the present study's reviews included not only content about experiences (e.g., services, checks, environments, reports, and breakfast) but also emotional responses to experiences (e.g., satisfaction and unfriendly, terrible, unpleasant, and enthusiastic staff). According to signaling theory (Spence, 1973), such mentions serve as quality signals that reduce uncertainty and guide patients' trust in providers.

Given the diversity of comments posted by different patients, their perceptions clearly vary. For example, some customers consider the services expensive, while other clients report that services are inexpensive. Moreover, 22 of the top keywords, including "report," "environment," "doctor," "staff," and "nurse," appear in the narratives shared by both satisfied and dissatisfied patients.

Taken together, the correlation and semantic network analyses pointed to six themes that capture the main forces behind customer satisfaction and dissatisfaction - service attitude, medical check-up, hospital environment, procedure, consultation, and price. These findings confirm that perceived healthcare quality is related not only to outcomes but also to the entire process (Um & Lau, 2018).

The service theme is mainly related to healthcare providers' attitudes and the personalized attention offered by different personnel (i.e., doctors, nurses, and other staff). This theme fits well with the concept of quality interactions with medical staff (Swain & Kar, 2018, Um & Lau, 2018) including staff attitude, doctors' behavior (Dhakate & Joshi, 2023) personalized attention, and information availability, which all contribute to a customer-friendly environment (Fatima et al., 2018). The hospital staff's attitude and communication can be understood as a supplemental value dimension in healthcare service provision (Miao et al., 2020).

The medical check-up theme highlights the importance of using advanced technology and up-to-date equipment in physical examinations and the perceived benefits of highly professional medical staff, which significantly influence consumers' evaluations. This theme is linked to medical examinations' technical quality (Swain & Kar, 2018, Fu et al., 2011, Eleuch, 2011) and, in turn, to clinical procedure outcomes' quality. The latter factor is related to the provision of adequate diagnoses, use of up-to-date equipment, the way the staff carries out examinations, and medical reports' quality.

The environment theme is in line with the concept of environmental quality (Um & Lau, 2018) and the dimensions of physical environment (Fatima et al., 2018, Trivedi & Jagani, 2018) and physical maintenance (Shabbir et al., 2016). These factors include tangible (Shafei et al., 2019) and intangible characteristics of hospital facilities, such as cleanliness, comfort Giovanis et al., 2018), ambience, accessibility, food, resources (Swain & Kar, 2018), a noise-free environment (Trivedi & Jagani, 2018), and parking areas.

The price theme is associated with value for money, which corresponds to the economic dimension added by Fan et al. (2017) to the SERVQUAL model and the service cost dimension identified by Zarei (2015). Notably, Fan et al. (2017) concluded that economic factors create the largest gap between patients' expectations and perceptions in Chinese hospitals. Miao et al. (2020) further established that healthcare services' monetary costs are an important driver of patient satisfaction.

The procedure theme frames efficiency in concrete terms: a smooth physical examination process is one that consolidates everything into a single, one-stop experience for the customer. This theme is connected to the dimensions of operational efficiency (Miranda et al., 2012), administrative quality (Um & Lau, 2018), and procedural quality (Swain & Kar, 2018) which include admission, discharge, waiting time, patient safety and/or privacy, billing, and follow-up. The procedure theme is thus associated with the concept of healthcare facilitators who provide core health services while adding value to patients' experiences by making them easier. This factor includes optimizing different aspects of the physical examination process, such as admission, waiting time in queues, and consistent quality over time (Giovanis et al., 2018). The procedure theme can be said to correspond to Wu et al.'s (2020) transaction cycle perspective on service quality. The consultation theme highlights two further satisfaction levers: stronger health education on the provider side and ongoing follow-up of customers' health status over time. This theme addresses the concept of primary care, which facilitates providing healthcare from facilities closer to target populations (Li et al., 2020, Liu et al., 2018).

The present study also answered a second research question: Do the main dimensions shared online vary by satisfied and dissatisfied patients? The dimension analysis was facilitated by Leximancer tools. The results reveal that the most frequent themes shared by satisfied patients are related to core services, examination, check-up and procedures, while dissatisfied patients are more likely to write about prices and staff attitudes. Price is a variable highlighted in negative reviews by AlNaseer and AlMuhaideb (2024). The current empirical research confirmed the asymmetric nature of satisfaction determinants in this context.

CONCLUSION

This study sought to answer the first research question: What are the main dimensions of narratives about physical examination services shared by Chinese private hospitals' patients online? The analysis focused on data from a large private health management corporation operating in China, whose most prominent type of service is physical examinations. By gathering relevant health data, such examinations enable providers to identify potential conditions at an early stage and intervene - preventively or curatively - before they progress.

The research included identifying the main factors affecting consumers' experiences and satisfaction with this company's services by conducting content analyses of patients' online reviews. Six themes emerge from the results as the principal drivers of both customer satisfaction and dissatisfaction — service attitude, medical check-up, hospital environment, procedure, consultation, and price.This study's findings provide further evidence of social media data and content analysis's usefulness in terms of healthcare service quality assessments. It concludes that the growing integration of digital health tools will play a pivotal role in reshaping patient experiences and service quality perceptions. This study addressed the second research question: Do the main dimensions shared online vary by satisfied and dissatisfied patients? Both groups are likely to comment on staff attitudes. Dissatisfied customers also tend to mention the pricing of services. In contrast, satisfied patients concentrate more often on core services.

Theoretical Contributions

This study's results make a number of contributions to the theoretical advancement of the field. First, in contrast to previous research on healthcare service quality in China (e.g., Hu et al., 2016, Zhang et al., 2018, Li et al., 2015, Lam, 1997), the current study targeted a specific research context: a private health management services company's provision of physical examinations. These examinations and health condition diagnoses are two of the pillars of primary healthcare management (Li et al., 2020). Private institutions must provide service quality (Wagstaff et al., 2009) especially because of Chinese patients' preference for state-owned facilities (Yip & Hsiao, 2015).

Second, this study's significant findings confirm the advantages of using content analysis of reviews shared on e-commerce websites in healthcare service quality research (Aljafari et al., 2023, Um & Lau, 2018, Zhang et al., 2018, and Zhang et al., 2019). Consistent with social support theory (Cohen & Wills, 1985) shared reviews offer emotional relief to reviewers and useful guidance to other patients.

Third, the present study employed mixed method content analyses using software that facilitated the processing of Chinese-language texts. The design paired two complementary strands: a quantitative analysis run through ROST CM - covering word frequency, correlation, and semantic network techniques - and a qualitative, narrative reading of the web reviews themselves.

Fourth, this study identified dimensions of patients' narratives in all phases, in contrast to Zhang et al.'s research,20 which separately analyzed online complaints about different aspects. The phases analyzed in the present study included the pre-consultation (i.e., registration and waiting), consultation (i.e., examination, physician attitudes, and consultation), and post-consultation (i.e., perceptions of treatments' effects) phases, as well as core services and other services. This study also applied the information integration and signaling theories, which facilitated an overview of the main themes shared online by both satisfied and dissatisfied patients.

Managerial Implications

Because this research focused on a private health management company in China, the findings also have a practical value. Healthcare managers can use online reviews to understand the drivers of satisfaction and dissatisfaction in order to improve their companies' perceived service quality and patients' wellbeing. Company managers can specifically focus on the six dimensions identified to enhance their clients' experiences, increase these individuals' satisfaction, generate more positive reviews, and improve their hospitals' image.

The most essential dimension proved to be health providers' service attitudes. This result highlights the role of "soft" aspects of healthcare service delivery (Zhang et al., 2018). Managers could introduce empathy and communication training to strengthen patient–staff interactions. For example, specific programs on patient communication and emotional support could be implemented to improve staff responsiveness. Medical check-ups and consultations are the core medical services linked with technical quality, which includes physical examinations and the outcomes that motivate customers to visit private hospitals, including primary healthcare concerns.

Optimizing patient flow through digital scheduling can reduce waiting times and improve perceived efficiency. Hospitals' environments and procedures add further value to core products. Finally, the value for money perceived by patients when evaluating costs is an important dimension. Implementing clear and flexible pricing options can strengthen patients' sense of fairness and confidence in the service.

Limitations and Future Research

Not unexpectedly, the present research also has some limitations that should be highlighted. First, the findings on consumers' experiences and satisfaction with private health management service enterprises in China were based on an analysis of one company's reviews. Regardless of how representative this corporation may be, the conclusions cannot be generalized without confirmation from additional research. To ensure a deeper and more comprehensive exploration of this topic, multiple specific companies need to be studied. E-commerce reviews may reflect the perspectives of more digitally active and urban users, which can influence representativeness. Future research could compare the dimensions of patient experiences present in public versus private hospitals and examine whether similar patterns arise in other emerging markets.

Second, social media data provide clear benefits to researchers, but the current results were based solely on reviews posted by patients who decided to share their experience online. These individuals' opinions will most likely only affect the decision-making processes of frequent users of social media.

Last, patients from different demographic profiles (e.g., gender and age group) and underlying health conditions require different types of physical examination, and these clients might have different needs. Thus, the six dimensions identified need to be tested further using different methods, such as in-depth interviews with healthcare stakeholders and patient surveys that collect demographic data.

Overall, additional research is needed on how health managers respond to positive and negative online reviews and how this reaction affects patients' decision-making processes. The present study confirmed that patients share narratives about all steps of the physical examination experience, including online and offline components, so future research should construct a customer journey map to highlight physical touchpoints.

REFERENCES

Akdere, M., Top, M., & Tekingündüz, S. (2020). Examining patient perceptions of service quality in Turkish hospitals: The SERVPERF model. *Total Quality Management & Business Excellence, 31*(3–4), 342–352. DOI: 10.1080/14783363.2018.1427501

Alborie, H. M., & Damanhouri, A. M. S. (2013). Patients' satisfaction of service quality in Saudi hospitals: A SERVQUAL analysis. *International Journal of Health Care Quality Assurance, 26*(1), 20–30. DOI: 10.1108/09526861311288613

Aljafari, R., Soh, F., Setia, P., & Agarwal, R. (2023). The local environment matters: Evidence from digital healthcare services for patient engagement. *Journal of the Academy of Marketing Science, 52*(5), 1343–1365. DOI: 10.1007/s11747-023-00972-0

AlNasser, S., & AlMuhaideb, S. (2024). Listening to patients: Advanced Arabic aspect-based sentiment analysis using transformer models towards better healthcare. *Big Data and Cognitive Computing, 8*(11), 156. DOI: 10.3390/bdcc8110156

Altuntas, S., Dereli, T., & Kaya, I. (2020). Monitoring patient dissatisfaction: A methodology based on SERVQUAL scale and statistical process control charts. *Total Quality Management & Business Excellence, 31*(9–10), 978–1008. DOI: 10.1080/14783363.2018.1457434

Anderson, N. H. (1971). Integration theory and attitude change. *Psychological Review, 78*(3), 171–206. DOI: 10.1037/h0030834

Borges, A. P., Rodrigues, P., Brochado, A., & Sousa, A. (2025). Mindfulness as a mediating mechanism between health importance and positive mental well-being. *International Journal of Pharmaceutical and Healthcare Marketing, 19*(3), 773–793. Advance online publication. DOI: 10.1108/IJPHM-07-2024-0069

Bowers, M. R., Swan, J. E., & Koehler, W. F. (1994). What attributes determine quality and satisfaction with health care delivery? *Health Care Management Review, 19*(4), 49–55. DOI: 10.1097/00004010-199401940-00006

Cao, X., Rajagopalan, S., & Tong, C. (2024). Impact of vertical integration in a referral-based healthcare system. *Omega, 12*, 102998. DOI: 10.1016/j.omega.2023.102998

Chao, J., Lu, B., Zhang, H., Zhu, L., Jin, H., & Liu, P. (2017). Healthcare system responsiveness in Jiangsu Province, China. *BMC Health Services Research, 17*(1), 31. DOI: 10.1186/s12913-017-1980-2

Chen, A., Li, L. J., & Wang, J. S. (2016). The experiential elements of patient satisfaction using the phenomenological qualitative study. *Zhongguo Weisheng Zhiliang Guanli*, *9*(5), 1–4.

Chen, Z. (2009). Launch of the health-care reform plan in China. *Lancet*, *373*(9672), 1322–1324. DOI: 10.1016/S0140-6736(09)60753-4

Cohen, S., & Wills, T. A. (1985). Stress, social support, and the buffering hypothesis. *Psychological Bulletin*, *98*(2), 310–357. DOI: 10.1037/0033-2909.98.2.310

Cronin, J. J.Jr, & Taylor, S. A. (1994). SERVPERF versus SERVQUAL: Reconciling performance-based and perceptions-minus-expectations measurement of service quality. *Journal of Marketing*, *58*(2), 125–131. DOI: 10.1177/002224299405800110

Dhakate, N., & Joshi, R. (2023). Classification of reviews of e-healthcare services to improve patient satisfaction: Insights from an emerging economy. *Journal of Business Research*, *164*, 114015. DOI: 10.1016/j.jbusres.2023.114015

Eleuch, A. K. (2011). Healthcare service quality perception in Japan. *International Journal of Health Care Quality Assurance*, *24*(6), 417–429. DOI: 10.1108/09526861111150680

Fan, L.-H., Gao, L., Liu, X., Zhao, S. H., Mu, H., Li, Z., Shi, L., Wang, L., Jia, X., Ha, M., & Lou, F. (2017). Patients' perceptions of service quality in China: An investigation using the SERVQUAL model. *PLoS One*, *2*(12), e0190123. DOI: 10.1371/journal.pone.0190123

Fatima, T., Malik, S. A., & Shabbir, A. (2018). Hospital healthcare service quality, patient satisfaction and loyalty: An investigation in context of private healthcare systems. *International Journal of Quality & Reliability Management*, *35*(6), 1195–1214. https://doi.org/ https://doi.org/10.1108/IJQRM-02-2017-0031. DOI: 10.1108/IJQRM-02-2017-0031

Feng, J., & Zhang, T. (2009). Comparison of models of ownership structure in the health care and its Chinese choice. *Jianghai Journal*, *6*, 74–79.

Frampton, S. B., & Guastellos, S. (2008). Honoring the life of a pioneer in patient-centered care: Harvey Picker (1915–2008). *The Patient*, *1*(2), 73–75. DOI: 10.2165/01312067-200801020-00001

Fu, M. L., Feng, Z. Y., & Chen, S. C. (2011). The enlightenment from health management experience in developed countries. *Chinese Health Service Management*, *3*(2), 233–236.

Giovanis, A., Pierrakos, G., Rizomyliotis, I., & Binioris, S. (2018). Assessing service quality and customer behavioral responses in hospital outpatient services: A formative measurement approach. *International Journal of Quality and Service Sciences*, *10*(2), 98–116. DOI: 10.1108/IJQSS-03-2017-0023

Hu, L., Ding, H., Liu, S., Wang, Z., Hu, G., & Liu, Y. (2020). Influence of patient and hospital characteristics on inpatient satisfaction in China's tertiary hospitals: A cross-sectional study. *Health Expectations : An International Journal of Public Participation in Health Care and Health Policy*, *23*(1), 115–124. DOI: 10.1111/hex.12974

Hu, R., Liao, Y., Du, Z., Hao, Y., Liang, H. and Sh,i L. (2016). Types of health care facilities and the quality of primary care: A study of characteristics and experiences of Chinese patients in Guangdong Province, China. *BMC Health Services Research*, 16(a):335. DOI: 10.1186/s12913-016-1604-2

Lam, S. S. (1997). SERVQUAL: A tool for measuring patients' opinions of hospital service quality in Hong Kong. *Total Quality Management*, *8*(4), 145–152. DOI: 10.1080/0954412979587

Li, M., Lowrie, D. B., Huang, C.-Y., Lu, X.-C., Zhu, Y.-C., Wu, X.-H., Shayiti, M., Tan, Q.-Z., Yang, H.-L., Chen, S.-Y., Zhao, P., He, S.-H., Wang, X.-R., & Lu, H.-Z. (2015). Evaluating patients' perception of service quality at hospitals in nine Chinese cities by use of the SERVQUAL scale. *Asian Pacific Journal of Tropical Biomedicine*, *5*(6), 497–504. DOI: 10.1016/j.apjtb.2015.02.003

Li, X., Krumholz, H. M., Yip, W., Cheng, K. K., De Maeseneer, J., Meng, Q., Mossialos, E., Li, C., Lu, J., Su, M., Zhang, Q., Xu, D. R., Li, L., Normand, S. T., Peto, R., Li, J., Wang, Z., Yan, H., Gao, R., & Hu, S. (2020). Quality of primary health care in China: Challenges and recommendations. *Lancet*, *395*(10239), 1802–1812. DOI: 10.1016/S0140-6736(20)30122-7

Li, X., Lu, J., Hu, S., Cheng, K. K., De Maeseneer, J., Meng, Q., Mossialos, E., Xu, D. R., Yip, W., Zhang, H., Krumholz, H. M., Jiang, L., & Hu, S. (2017). The primary health-care system in China. *Lancet*, *390*(10112), 2584–2594. DOI: 10.1016/S0140-6736(17)33109-4

Liu, Q. Q. (2013). Discrimination of forest tourism concept based on ROST-CM analysis. [Social Sciences]. *Journal of Central South University of Forestry and Technology*, *7*(1), 20–23. DOI: 10.1007/s11771-000-0006-z

Liu, Y., Kong, Q., Yuan, S., & Klundert, J. (2018). Factors influencing choice of health system access level in China: A systematic review. *PLoS One*, *13*(8), e0201887. https://doi.org//. DOI: 10.1371/journal.pone.0201887

Liu, Y. F., & Wang, Z. (2016). The development model and its enlightenment of health management service industry in the United States. *Journal of the Asia Pacific Economy*, *3*, 75–81.

Lu, L., Xu, P., Wang, Y.-Y., & Wang, Y. (2023). Measuring service quality with text analytics: Considering both importance and performance of consumer opinions on social and non-social online platforms. *Journal of Business Research*, *169*, 114298. DOI: 10.1016/j.jbusres.2023.114298

Luo, H. (2016). The released program of 'Healthy China 2030'. *Science and Technology Daily*, *1*, 10–26.

Meesala, A., & Paul, J. (2018). Service quality, consumer satisfaction and loyalty in hospitals: Thinking for the future. *Journal of Retailing and Consumer Services*, *40*, 261–269. DOI: 10.1016/j.jretconser.2016.10.011

Mei, Z., Li, W., Chen, J., Yin, H., Song, Y., Tu, W., Ding, Z., Bai, Y., Jin, S., & Xu, G. (2024). The transformation of 20-year social participation policies of older people in China: Network analysis and text analysis. *PLoS One*, *19*(8), e0308401. DOI: 10.1371/journal.pone.0308401

Miao, R., Zhang, H., Wu, Q., Zhang, J., & Jiang, Z. (2019). Using structural equation modeling to analyze patient value, satisfaction, and loyalty: A case study of healthcare in China. *International Journal of Production Research*, *58*(2), 577–596. DOI: 10.1080/00207543.2019.1598595

Miranda, F. J., Chamorro, A., Murillo, L. R., & Vega, J. (2012). Primary health care services quality in Spain: A formative measurement approach using PLS path modeling. *International Journal of Quality and Service Sciences*, *4*(4), 387–398. DOI: 10.1108/17566691211288368

Moghadam, M. N., & Amiresmaili, M. (2009). Hospital services quality assessment—Hospitals of Kerman University of Medical Sciences as a tangible example of a developing country. *International Journal of Health Care Quality Assurance*, *24*(1), 57–66. DOI: 10.1108/09526861111098247

National Health and Family Planning Commission of the People's Republic of China. (2015). *Further improving the action plan for medical services*. http://www.nhfpc.gov.cn/yzygj/ylfwjh/gxyg_index.shtml

Parasuraman, A., Berry, L. L., & Zeithaml, V. A. (1988). SERVQUAL: A multiple-item scale for measuring consumer perceptions of service quality. *Journal of Retailing*, *64*(1), 12–40.

Peng, J. M., & Lin, Y. (2009). The blend of Confucianism, Taoism and Buddhism in Sun Simiao medical ethics thought. *Medical Philosophy, 30*(17), 23–24.

Rao, K. Q., Yin, L., & Liu, Y. L. (2000). The effect on the development of social economy from the health transition of Chinese residents and the change of the demand for health services. *Zhongguo Weisheng Jingji, 9*, 5–11.

Raposo, M. L., Alves, H. M., & Duarte, P. A. (2009). Dimensions of service quality and satisfaction in healthcare: A patient's satisfaction index. *Service Business, 3*(1), 85–100. DOI: 10.1007/s11628-008-0055-1

Rashid, W. E. W., & Jusoff, H. K. (2009). Service quality in health care setting. *International Journal of Health Care Quality Assurance, 22*(5), 471–482. DOI: 10.1108/09526860910975580

Shabbir, A., Malik, S. A., & Malik, S. A. (2016). Measuring patients' healthcare service quality perceptions, satisfaction, and loyalty in public and private sector hospitals in Pakistan. *International Journal of Quality & Reliability Management, 33*(5), 538–557. DOI: 10.1108/IJQRM-06-2014-0074

Shafei, I., Walburg, J., & Taher, A. (2019). Verifying alternative measures of healthcare service quality. *International Journal of Health Care Quality Assurance, 32*(2), 516–533. DOI: 10.1108/IJHCQA-05-2016-0069

Spence, M. (1973). Job market signaling. *The Quarterly Journal of Economics, 87*(3), 355–374. DOI: 10.2307/1882010

Swain, S., & Kar, N. C. (2018). Hospital service quality as antecedent of patient satisfaction—A conceptual framework. *International Journal of Pharmaceutical and Healthcare Marketing, 12*(3), 251–269. DOI: 10.1108/IJPHM-06-2016-0028

Tam, J. L. M. (2019). Examining the role of customer self-efficacy in service encounters. *Services Marketing Quarterly, 40*(4), 269–284. DOI: 10.1080/15332969.2019.1666534

The General Office of the State Council of the People's Republic of China. (2015). *Notice of the General Office of the State Council on issuing several policies and measures for promoting the accelerated development of private medical institutions.* https://www.gov.cn/zhengce/content/2015-06/15/content_9845.htm

Trivedi, R., & Jagani, K. (2018). Perceived service quality, repeat use of healthcare services and inpatient satisfaction in emerging economy: Empirical evidences from India. *International Journal of Pharmaceutical and Healthcare Marketing, 12*(3), 288–306. DOI: 10.1108/IJPHM-11-2017-0065

Um, K. H., & Lau, A. K. W. (2018). Healthcare service failure: How dissatisfied patients respond to poor service quality. *International Journal of Operations & Production Management*, *38*(5), 1245–1270. DOI: 10.1108/IJOPM-11-2016-0669

Valencia-Arias, A., Piedrahita, L. B., Zapata, A. B., & Arias, M. L. B. (2018). Mapping the healthcare service quality domain: A bibliometric analysis. *Journal of Clinical and Diagnostic Research : JCDR*, *12*(8), IC01–IC05. DOI: 10.7860/JCDR/2018/30361.11863

Vogus, T. J., & McClelland, L. C. (2016). When the customer is the patient: Lessons from healthcare research on patient satisfaction and service quality ratings. *Human Resource Management Review*, *26*(1), 37–49. DOI: 10.1016/j.hrmr.2015.09.005

Wagstaff, A., Yip, W., Lindelow, M., & Hsiao, W. C. (2009). China's health system and its reform: A review of recent studies. *Health Economics*, *18*(S2), S7–S23. DOI: 10.1002/hec.1518

Wang, X., Geng, N., Jiang, S., Zhou, L., & Jiang, Z. (2021). Optimal design of healthcare services after the separation of prescribing and dispensing. *International Journal of Production Research*, *60*(9), 2918–2941. DOI: 10.1080/00207543.2021.1906459

World Health Organization. (2006). *Quality of care: A process for making strategic choices in health systems*. WHO Press.

Wu, H., Deng, Z., Wang, B., & Wu, T. (2020). Online service qualities in the multistage process and patients' compliments: A transaction cycle perspective. *Information & Management*, *57*(5), 103230. DOI: 10.1016/j.im.2019.103230

Xu, X. P., Ke, D. G., Deng, D. N., Houser, S. H., Li, X. N., Wang, Q., & Shan, N. C. (2019). An innovative medical consultation model in mainland China: Acceptance and perceptions. *International Journal of Health Care Quality Assurance*, *32*(7), 1057. DOI: 10.1108/IJHCQA-02-2017-0033

Yip, W., & Hsiao, W. C. (2015). What drove the cycles of Chinese health system reforms? *Health Systems and Reform*, *1*(1), 52–61. DOI: 10.4161/23288604.2014.995005

Yufeng, X. (2018). *Consumer experience and satisfaction of private health management service enterprises in China* [Doctoral dissertation, Iscte – Instituto Universitário de Lisboa]. Iscte Repository. http://hdl.handle.net/10071/17314

Zarei, E. (2015). Service Quality of Hospital Outpatient Departments: Patients' Perspective. *International Journal of Health Care Quality Assurance*, *28*(8), 778–790. DOI: 10.1108/IJHCQA-09-2014-0097

Zeng, X. H., Zheng, Y. X., & Zhang, Q. (2015). Study on definition of smart tourism based on content analysis. *Resources Development & Market, 10*, 1246–1249.

Zhang, M., Guo, X., & Wu, T. (2019). Impact of free contributions on private benefits in online healthcare communities. *International Journal of Electronic Commerce, 23*(4), 492–523. DOI: 10.1080/10864415.2019.1655208

Zhang, W., Deng, Z., Hong, Z., Evans, R., Ma, J., & Zhang, H. (2018). Unhappy patients are not alike: Content analysis of the negative comments from China's Good Doctor Website. *Journal of Medical Internet Research, 20*(1), e35. DOI: 10.2196/jmir.8223

Zhang, Y., Zhang, L., Zhang, X., Yang, M. M., Zhang, S., Li, S.-J., & Huang, Y.-Y. (2018). Hospital service quality and patient loyalty: The mediation effect of empathy. *Journal of Business and Industrial Marketing, 33*(8), 1176–1186. DOI: 10.1108/JBIM-02-2018-0072

Zheng, Y., Zeng, M., Deng, B., Bin, H., Liu, F., & Lin, X. (2024). Topic mining and sentiment analysis based on the online review from MOOC platform's logistics course. *SAGE Open, 14*(4), 21582440241303486. Advance online publication. DOI: 10.1177/21582440241303486

Chapter 8
Analysis of Ethical Issues in Medical Decision-Making Driven by Artificial Intelligence and Governance Strategies:
Focusing on the Diversified Governance Network With Multi-Stakeholder Collaboration

Poshan Yu
http://orcid.org/0000-0003-1069-3675
Soochow University, China & European Business Institute, Luxembourg & Australian Studies Centre, Shanghai University, China

Yiheng Chen
http://orcid.org/0009-0008-5047-2811
Independent Researcher, China

Chandra Lukita
http://orcid.org/0009-0006-6035-8241
Universitas Catur Insan Cendekia, Indonesia

ABSTRACT

With the growing complexity of global health challenges, the demand for efficient medical services is rising. AI in medical decision-making brings new opportunities but also ethical concerns. This study analyzes research trends in AI-medicine, ex-

DOI: 10.4018/979-8-2600-2238-2.ch008

plores ethical issues in AI-driven medical decision-making, and proposes solutions. Based on stakeholder theory, it shows patients face privacy risks, hospitals have liability issues, and the government struggles with regulation. A multi-stakeholder collaborative governance model is suggested to address these. Using Citespace, the research pinpoints key areas to guide future studies.

INTRODUCTION

In today's medical field, the application of artificial intelligence is developing at an unprecedented pace. With its powerful data processing and analysis capabilities, artificial intelligence has brought new ideas to medical decision - making. It shows great potential in aspects such as disease diagnosis and treatment plan selection, and is expected to improve medical efficiency and quality, and address current global health challenges. However, this application has also given rise to many complex ethical issues that urgently need to be resolved(Reddy et al., 2020). It is of great significance to conduct research on these issues. On the one hand, medical decisions are directly related to patients' lives, health, and rights. If ethical disputes arise in the application of artificial intelligence in this area, it may lead to serious consequences such as misdiagnosis and mistreatment. On the other hand, with the deep integration of artificial intelligence in the medical field, if these ethical issues are not properly addressed, it will hinder the sustainable development of artificial intelligence in the medical industry and also affect the public's trust in medical technology.

This study focuses on " Analysis of Ethical Issues in AI - Driven Medical Decision - Making and Governance Strategies ". The core research questions are: what specific ethical problems do artificial intelligence and medical decision-making face, and how can we achieve their long-term development starting from the present situation?To explore this important topic, this study conducts a visual analysis of existing literature with the help of CiteSpace software, sorts out the current application status and progress of artificial intelligence in medicine, and excavates relevant research hotspots and trends. Secondly, from the perspective of the stakeholder theory, we will delve deeply into the ethical issues and dilemmas of artificial intelligence in medical applications. By identifying various stakeholders involved, such as patients, hospitals, and the government, we can better understand their interests, concerns, and the ethical challenges they face. Finally, based on our analysis results, we will explore a multi-dimensional collaborative governance model for artificial intelligence in the medical field. This research is of great significance for promoting the ethical application of artificial intelligence in the medical field and safeguarding the well-being of patients worldwide.

LITERATURE REVIEW

The integration of artificial intelligence and medical decision-making is profoundly transforming the landscape of the healthcare industry. While striving to enhance the efficiency and precision of medical care, a multitude of ethical issues have emerged concomitantly. A thorough exploration of these issues holds significant importance for promoting the robust, compliant, and sustainable development of AI in medical decision-making, safeguarding the rights and interests of patients, and upholding the ethical principles of the healthcare sector. Consequently, systematically reviewing high-quality academic literature and summarizing the existing achievements and deficiencies constitute an essential prerequisite for deepening research in this field.

In the realm of artificial intelligence, the paper titled "Artificial Intelligence in Medicine" has conducted an in-depth study on it. The author delved profoundly into the core technologies of AI, such as the application principles of machine learning and deep learning in the medical field. It was pointed out that AI is capable of providing support for medical decision-making by mining massive amounts of medical data. However, the formidable challenge of the interpretability of complex algorithms urgently requires a solution(Hamet & Tremblay, 2017). In terms of medical technology, the paper "The Role of AI in Hospitals and Clinics: Transforming Healthcare in the 21st Century" explores the application of artificial intelligence in healthcare technology. Through a critical assessment of the transformative potential of AI, it encourages interdisciplinary dialogue among researchers, clinicians, and technical experts, thereby promoting the development of AI-driven solutions that prioritize ethical standards, fairness, and a patient-centered approach(Varnosfaderani & Forouzanfar, 2024). In terms of ethical issues, the paper "Ethical considerations for the use of artificial intelligence in medical decision-making capacity assessments" delves deeply into the ethical considerations involved when artificial intelligence is used for decision-making capacity assessments. It points out that artificial intelligence is highly vulnerable to biased input data, which can lead to biased decisions. This gives rise to issues of autonomy and brings about uncertainty regarding who should be held responsible for the final decision-making outcomes(MacIntyre et al., 2023). In the aspect of medical decision-making, the paper "Revolutionizing healthcare: the role of artificial intelligence in clinical practice" comprehensively analyzes the potential applications of artificial intelligence in disease diagnosis, treatment recommendations and other aspects. It also mentions that artificial intelligence can enhance accuracy, reduce costs, save time, and minimize human errors, thus thoroughly revolutionizing personalized medicine(Alowais et al., 2023). In terms of transparency, the paper "Towards Transparent Healthcare: Advancing Local Explanation Methods in Explainable Artificial Intelligence" emphasizes that the key to user trust lies in the transparency and reliability of artificial intelligence by exploring the application of explainable artificial intelligence in healthcare(Metta et al., 2024). The paper "Unbox the black-box for the medical explainable AI via multi-modal and multi-centre data fusion: A mini-review, two showcases and beyond" also points out that the lack of interpretability of the artificial intelligence black-box model may undermine our confidence in it. The deficiency of interpretability and transparency in most existing artificial intelligence systems may also be one of the reasons why it is difficult for AI tools to be successfully applied and integrated into daily clinical practice(G. Yang et al., 2022). In terms of data privacy, the paper titled "The ethical, legal and social implications of using artificial intelligence systems in breast cancer care" points out that the application of artificial intelligence in medical decision-making involves the collection, storage, and use of a large amount of patients' sensitive data, which poses severe challenges to data privacy. For instance, during the data collection stage, patients often find it difficult to know the specific purposes and destinations of the data(Carter et al., 2020). In terms of the definition of responsibility, the paper "AI in Radiology: Navigating Medical Responsibility" studies and investigates the legal challenges faced by artificial intelligence in medical applications within the field of radiology. It analyzes relevant case law and literature, with a particular focus on the issue of the attribution of professional responsibility, highlighting the urgency of establishing a sound responsibility framework(Contaldo et al., 2024). In terms of multi-agent collaboration, the paper "Multi-stakeholder preferences for the use of artificial intelligence in healthcare: A systematic review and thematic analysis" states that to strengthen multi-agent collaboration, clinicians will need to adapt to their evolving roles. There should be further cooperation between healthcare professionals and AI developers. By introducing new AI applications in the clinical environment, they should prioritize and develop applications that meet key clinical needs and streamline clinical workflows(Vo et al., 2023).

Although certain achievements have been made in existing research, there are still numerous deficiencies. Firstly, with the rapid development of technology, new ethical risks keep emerging, and the existing research lags behind in keeping up with these changes. The current research hotspots are constantly evolving. Secondly, there is a shortage of research on strategies for addressing the ethical issues of AI in healthcare.

This paper aims to fill this gap by conducting a CiteSpace analysis of Artificial Intelligence and Medical Ethics and answering the following research questions: What specific ethical problems do artificial intelligence and medical decision - making face, and how can we achieve their long - term development starting from the present?

Sub - questions:

1. With the development of artificial intelligence in the medical field, what are the current research hotspots?
2. Why does artificial intelligence lead to ethical issues in medical decision-making?
3. How can we provide solution models for these ethical issues?

METHODOLOGY

Based on previous research, we conducted a literature search in the Web of Science using the keywords "AI" and "ethics in medical". In order to conduct a more rigorous analysis, we focused our target solely on the Web of Science Core Collection. Eventually, a total of 1,414 pieces of literature were obtained. Then, we set the retrieval period between 2015 and 2025, and a total of 1,320 pieces of literature were sorted out. We carried out a meticulous screening of these articles, deleting Meeting Abstracts, Letters, and the like. Finally, 1,226 articles were selected for a systematic analysis. We imported these pieces of literature into Citespace. After the deduplication and screening functions provided by the system itself, a total of 616 pieces of available literature were ultimately obtained. Citespace is a tool used for the visual analysis and research of academic literature in research fields, research domains, or disciplines (Chen, 2004). It constructs a network of a series of underlying entities and their relationships, which are derived from representative datasets in the corresponding knowledge fields. The structural patterns and trends, combined with the temporal patterns and indicators, provide analysts with information about the significant developments in the research field(Chen, 2020). We conducted a visual research through keyword co-occurrence analysis and keyword clustering analysis, and scientifically examined the connection between AI and medical ethics. According to the analysis of CiteSpace, we have identified the research hotspots and development directions in aspects such as AI and medical ethics in recent years. At the same time, it also demonstrates the close connections among different fields.

Figure 1. The screening of articles from Web of Science

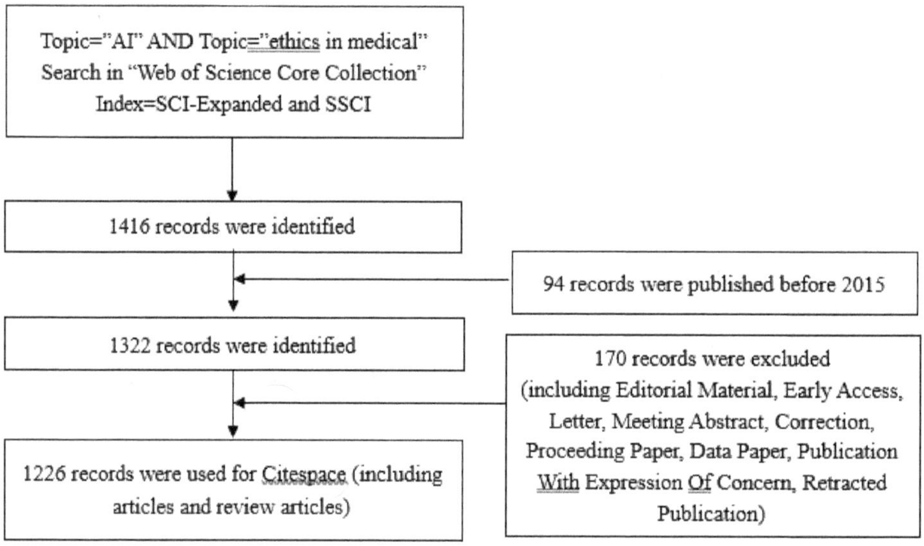

Source: Web of Science

DISCUSSION

The Analysis of CiteSpace

We imported 1,226 pieces of literature into CiteSpace. By utilizing the software's automatic deduplication function, we finally obtained 616 pieces of available literature. We set the node type as keywords, adjusted the scale factor k to 18, and selected the options of pruning sliced networks and pruning the merged network. Eventually, we created a CiteSpace knowledge graph.

Figure 2. the results of the keyword co-occurrence network analysis of the research on artificial intelligence in the field of medical ethics.

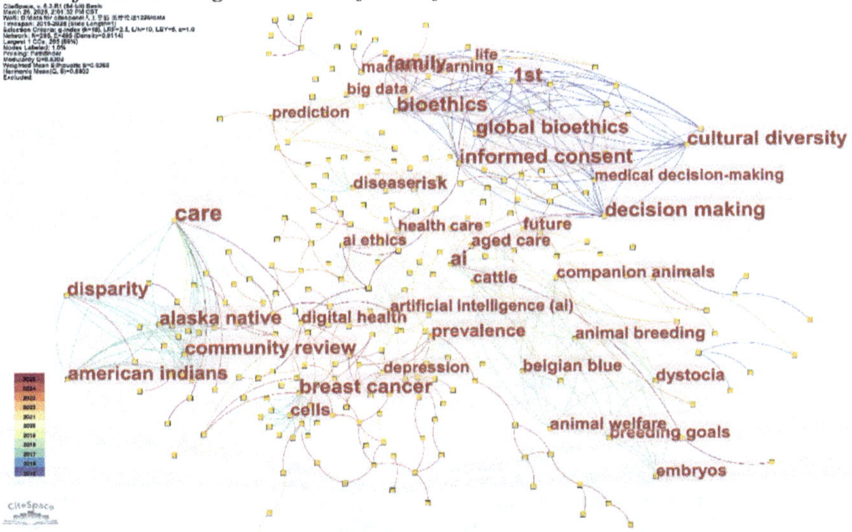

Figure 1 shows the results of the keyword co-occurrence network analysis of the research on artificial intelligence in the field of medical ethics. As can be seen from the figure, the keywords in the main research areas are "artificial intelligence (ai)", "bioethics", "medical decision-making", etc. While the relevant keywords in the medical field are "health care", "aged care", "breast cancer", etc., which reflect the applied research of artificial intelligence in different medical scenarios, including disease diagnosis and treatment, and the care of specific groups of people. The keywords related to ethics include "informed consent", "global bioethics", etc., which reflect the ethical issues involved in the medical application of artificial intelligence, such as the protection of patients' rights and interests and global ethical norms.

The color bar at the lower left corner of the figure also represents different years. The connections between various keywords are of corresponding colors, indicating the time when they first appeared or became active. For example, some keywords that are closely related to the development of artificial intelligence technology are mostly surrounded by red, which shows that the integration of artificial intelligence and medicine is currently a research hotspot. In particular, the research on the application of artificial intelligence in medical decision-making is an issue that people are paying increasing attention to.

The connections between the nodes in the figure indicate the co-occurrence relationships between the keywords. The thicker the connection, the more times the two keywords appear together in the same piece of literature, and the stronger the research correlation between them. Through the distribution of the connections, we can see the connections and intersections between different research topics. For example, there is a close correlation among artificial intelligence, medical decision-making, and ethics.

Figure 3. the results of the Clustering Distribution Diagram of the research on artificial intelligence in the field of medical ethics.

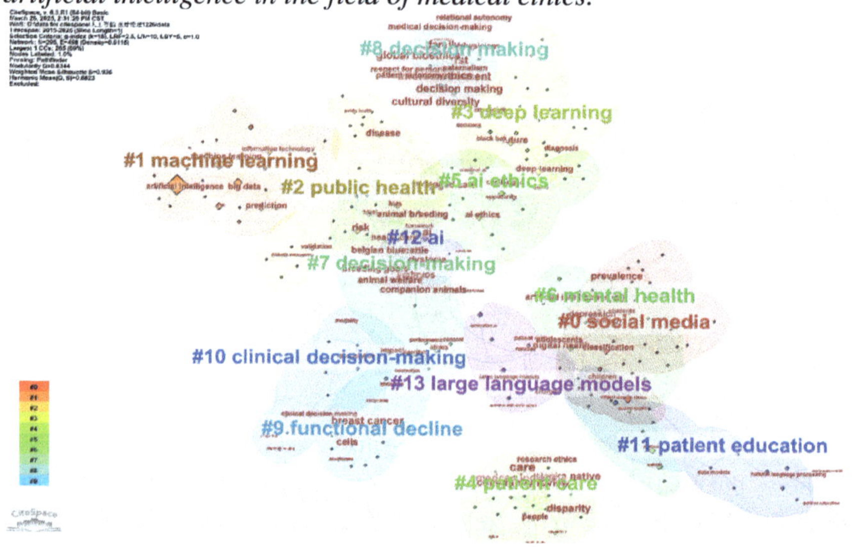

In the clustering analysis Figure 2, the clustering modularity value Q = 0.8344 > 0.3, which means that the clustering structure is significant; the clustering average silhouette value S = 0.936 > 0.7, indicating that the results are convincing. The average silhouette value S = 0.936, which is close to 1, implies that the homogeneity of the clustering is relatively good. In the figure, the colored areas with numbers represent different clusters, and each cluster is composed of a group of related keywords, reflecting specific research topics. For example, machine learning, ai ethics, artificial intelligence, deep learning, decision making, clinical decision-making, etc., are all current research hotspots. Keywords such as "artificial intelligence", "big data", and "prediction" appear around "machine learning", indicating the application of machine learning technology in artificial intelligence and medical prediction in recent years, as well as its combination with big data. The keyword "ai ethics" is the core of the cluster, reflecting the discussion of ethical issues in the application of artificial intelligence in the medical field. At the same time, the cluster of the keyword "ai" has a large overlapping area with the clusters of "decision-making" and "ai ethics", indicating that there is a lot of interdisciplinary research in the aspect of artificial intelligence assisting medical decision-making.

Examining the Ethical Issues and Dilemmas of Medical Artificial Intelligence Based on the Stakeholder Theory

With the rapid development of artificial intelligence, its technology is transforming the development of the medical field. Scholars and practitioners have debated the philosophical, ethical, legal, and regulatory impacts of medical AI, and empirical studies on stakeholders' knowledge and attitudes have begun to emerge(Tang et al., 2023). The stakeholder theory is an enterprise management theory that gradually developed in countries such as the United States and the United Kingdom, which have long adhered to the external control-oriented corporate governance model, around the 1960s. The stakeholder theory was initially developed as a theory of strategic management, or more precisely, as a perspective of strategic management(Bridoux & Stoelhorst, 2022). This theory encourages organizations to recognize and consider the stakeholders existing within or outside the organization, promoting the understanding and management of stakeholders' needs, desires, and requirements. In turn, it enables organizations to formulate strategies to maximize the creation of their value and maintain their long-term success and sustainability(Mahajan et al., 2023). Nowadays, this theory is also applied to other fields, such as healthcare and education, to analyze and solve complex problems involving multiple interest subjects in these fields(Dlugatch et al., 2023).

The application of AI in the medical scenario involves numerous stakeholders. Patients are the direct users, and their health, privacy, and right to autonomous decision-making are affected(Richardson et al., 2021); hospitals are the places where the technology is applied, which are related to the quality of medical services, the definition of responsibility, professional development, etc.; the government undertakes the regulatory responsibility and needs to protect public interests and regulate the development of the industry(Roski et al., 2021). The stakeholder theory focuses on all groups affected by an organization's decisions and actions, which can comprehensively cover these subjects and analyze the interests and ethical dilemmas of all parties. For example, in terms of data privacy, decision-making in the medical field often intersects with high-risk scenarios and highly sensitive data(Ossa, Milford, et al., 2024). Hospitals need to use data rationally to provide services and conduct data governance, which includes establishing data - sharing practices to promote trust and protect patients' privacy(Saw & Ng, 2022). Although artificial intelligence has brought many positive benefits to healthcare, the ethical issues surrounding it are diverse and complex, involving privacy, data protection, transparency, interpretability, data bias, the definition of responsibility, etc(McLennan et al., 2022). Compared with medicine, the development of artificial intelligence lacks sound legal and professional accountability mechanisms(Mittelstadt, 2019). The autonomous and opaque learning and decision - making of artificial intelligence in a dynamic environment can lead to some unique technical, ethical, and legal consequences(Corfmat et al., 2025). Therefore, it is crucial to develop relevant laws and regulations, which is conducive to countries leveraging the potential advantages of artificial intelligence while minimizing any attendant risks(Da Silva et al., 2022). At present, stakeholders do not trust the independent diagnosis of AI and do not believe that it can completely replace doctors(L. Yang et al., 2022). For example, if medical chatbots provide incorrect advice, diagnoses, or prescriptions, they may cause harm. The harm of misdiagnosis is exacerbated when chatbots can instill so much trust in patients that they become overconfident in the diagnosis(Fournier-Tombs & McHardy, 2023). These issues are interrelated, and one issue may affect the interests of multiple parties. For example, algorithmic bias may have potential impacts on issues such as patient discrimination, safety, and privacy in healthcare(Katznelson & Gerke, 2021). The use of biased algorithms by hospitals can affect diagnosis and treatment, and the government also needs to regulate the fairness of algorithms(Corfmat et al., 2025). These biases include technical and social biases, which often reflect a compromise in the quality of care provided to marginalized groups(Sankar et al., 2024). The stakeholder theory emphasizes considering the interest relationships and interactions among different subjects from an overall perspective, which helps to analyze the complexity and internal connections of ethical issues and find the root causes and solutions(Nora et al., 2023).

For patients, the application of medical artificial intelligence poses potential risks in terms of privacy protection and data security(Richardson et al., 2021). Patient data is a valuable resource in healthcare and lies at the core of AI systems. By analyzing patterns in health data, AI can predict diseases, suggest treatment methods, and improve patient outcomes(Moulaei et al., 2025). However, if this large amount of sensitive personal health data is leaked or misused, it will seriously violate patients' privacy(Corfmat et al., 2025). The Privacy Protection Study Commission (PPSC), established under the Privacy Act of 1974, noted that as of 1977, medical researchers often used patients' clinical health records in research without consent(Evans, 2023). At the same time, since AI algorithms often exhibit the characteristic of a "black box" in medical decision-making, to a certain extent, it affects the transparency of the application of artificial intelligence in medical decision-making(Durán & Jongsma, 2021). AI transparency refers to ensuring that humans understand how an AI system operates and the clarity of its accuracy, including informing patients of the errors made by the AI system to improve user trust and usability(Kunar et al., 2024). As AI systems are integrated into various decision-making processes, there is an increasing debate in the scientific and policy communities about the extent to which those who develop AI or are subject to AI decisions can understand how the resulting decision-making mechanisms operate and why specific decisions are made(G. Yang et al., 2022). Patients may find it difficult to fully participate in medical decision-making due to a lack of understanding, and it is difficult for them to fully express their autonomous will and preferences(Sand et al., 2022). To reduce patients' fears of such impersonal care, doctors should pay more attention to the transformation of their relational roles, handle uncertain areas, balance competitive risks, and finally provide emotional support to patients(Amann et al., 2023). In addition, the fairness and accessibility of medical artificial intelligence are also worthy of attention. Advanced technologies may be concentrated in developed regions or large medical institutions, and the cost of use may discourage some patients, affecting the fair access to medical services(Kempt et al., 2022). At the same time, if artificial intelligence is used without restrictions in the medical field, it may exacerbate racial and gender inequalities and endanger patient safety(Chauhan & Gullapalli, 2021).

As the direct application subject of medical artificial intelligence, hospitals face the dilemma of ambiguous liability definition(Herrmann et al., 2024). Liability and accountability are sometimes used interchangeably and are rarely defined, and there is a controversy over whether an AI system can be held accountable or whether the ultimate responsibility is always borne by humans(Christoforaki & Beyan, 2022). When artificial intelligence is integrated into clinical practice, allocating liability in the case of negative outcomes becomes both complex and crucial(Contaldo et al., 2024). However, under the current legal status, in the event of a medical malpractice, it is difficult to determine the liable party when artificial intelligence is used. Due to these controversial aspects, it is difficult to provide clear criteria in court, thus further complicating the allocation of liability(Ungureanu et al., 2025). This unclear liability not only undermines patients' rights and interests but also puts hospitals in a passive position in medical disputes. The excessive dependence of hospitals on medical artificial intelligence may hinder the professional skill development of medical staff. Long-term reliance on machine diagnosis will weaken their ability to think independently and make clinical judgments. There are also deficiencies in the ethical review and regulatory implementation of hospitals. The ethical review mechanism is not yet perfect, and there is a lack of a standardized process for the ethical evaluation of medical artificial intelligence. In practical operations, there may be situations of lax review and ineffective supervision.

The government plays a crucial regulatory and guiding role in the development of medical artificial intelligence, but it also faces many challenges at present. Firstly, research involving the use of artificial intelligence to promote health is also being conducted in large companies and smaller start - ups, which may fall outside the scope of research ethics regulation in some jurisdictions(Shaw et al., 2024). Secondly, policies and regulations lag behind technological development. A complete legal and regulatory system has not been established to regulate the research, development, application, and management of artificial intelligence in healthcare, leaving legal gaps in key areas(Roski et al., 2021). Finally, regulatory authorities have mostly been reactive as they attempt to keep up with the rapid development of artificial intelligence(Polevikov, 2023). At the regulatory level, it is necessary to strengthen data quality management and improve algorithm transparency and traceability to reduce algorithmic bias(Zhang & Zhang, 2023). These long - standing discussions on AI ethics and social issues have led to recent research surrounding the EU AI Act(Willem et al., 2024). The government also needs to optimize resource allocation. Currently, there is a phenomenon of uneven resource distribution, which is not conducive to the widespread popularization of the technology. In addition, the supervision of medical artificial intelligence involves multiple departments, and cross-departmental coordination is difficult. The division of responsibilities is not clear, and problems such as multiple management and policy conflicts are likely to occur, affecting the efficiency of supervision.

The following table centers around the core theme of medical AI ethics. Based on demonstrating the particularity of medical AI ethics issues, it analyzes the challenges and difficulties of medical AI ethics governance and places the governance of ethical risks within the social - technical system of medical AI. This table is organized from multiple dimensions, covering not only technical challenges but also factors in social, legal, ethical, and many other aspects. It provides a clear and systematic framework for understanding medical AI ethics topics, clearly presenting the full picture of medical AI ethics issues. This helps researchers and relevant practitioners to deeply understand the key issues and coping strategies in this field, thus promoting the sound development of medical AI in line with ethical norms.

Table 1.

Category	Details
Particularities of Ethical Issues	**Unique Application Context:** In the medical field, the uniqueness of the application context is extremely prominent. It places higher demands on the ethical values of medical artificial intelligence than other fields. Once homogeneous ethical issues arise, they not only attract high attention but also lead to serious consequences. This requires that decisions must be patient - centered and comprehensively consider multiple factors. **Failure to Meet Closed - loop Conditions:** Patients' conditions vary widely, medical activities are complex, and there are unknown variables in application scenarios. Most scenarios can hardly meet the requirements of strong closure. Relying solely on specific ethical norms cannot properly address these issues, so the participation of multiple stakeholders in ethical governance is urgently needed. **Need for a Stronger Trust Bond:** Trust is a fundamental value in the doctor - patient relationship and significantly influences the application of medical artificial intelligence devices. General artificial intelligence gains trust through technology and other means. However, due to its close connection with life and health, medical artificial intelligence may face trust crises both in terms of technological stability and in the relationship between doctors and patients.
Main Problems in Ethical Governance	**Inadequate Governance Basis:** Although all parties have reached a certain consensus on the ethical governance of medical artificial intelligence, there is still a lack of a unified basis for ethical principles. After the integration of bioethics and artificial intelligence ethical principles, there are still problems in terms of applicability and sufficiency in practical applications. Moreover, the update speed of ethical principles often lags behind technological development, thus leading to chaos in governance. **Unclear Governance Objects:** The technology of medical artificial intelligence has not formed a stable model, and ethical issues are difficult to fully anticipate. Ethical governance needs to focus on the social - technical system. At present, governance is still in the exploration stage, with the objects, scopes, and boundaries of governance being ambiguous. It is urgent to determine the objects and subjects of governance to achieve precise governance and thus effectively address complex ethical challenges. **Incomplete Governance Mechanisms:** The ethical governance system in the field of biomedicine is mature, and medical artificial intelligence is subject to strict review. However, the current medical ethical governance mechanism cannot be directly applied. There is not only a lack of standardized regulations and accountability mechanisms, but also a need for more stakeholders to participate. At present, there is also a lack of effective strategies to collect and feedback ethical demands. **Urgent Need to Enhance Governance Awareness:** Medical artificial intelligence is currently in the niche incubation stage. The public has not yet differentiated its ethical issues from quality issues and has a serious lack of understanding of governance concepts and other aspects. The awareness of ethical governance among directly affected groups such as physicians is weak, and their enthusiasm for participating in governance is low. At the same time, stakeholders may "stand by," which not only affects the protection of their own rights and interests but also hinders their in - depth understanding of ethical governance.

continued on following page

Table 1. Continued

Category	Details
Analysis of the Difficulties in Ethical Governance	**Technological Continuous Innovation and "Unpredictable" Application Scenarios:** The digital and intelligent transformation of healthcare provides innovative resources for medical artificial intelligence, and the scenario - driven approach makes its development diversified. However, the rapid development of technology has increased the types of ethical risks, such as algorithmic bias and data privacy risks. This requires a high - speed response ability from the ethical governance mechanism, thus increasing the difficulty of governance. **Diverse Ethical Demands of Stakeholders are "Difficult to Reconcile":** Medical artificial intelligence needs to balance the ethical demands of different stakeholders. However, the evaluation framework of ethical guidelines has its limitations. There are continuous conflicts among the moral concerns and values of different subjects, and factors such as regional culture lead to significant differences in ethical standards, making it difficult to reconcile these ethical demands. **Confusion in the Attribution of Responsibility and Liability for Technology:** The complexity of technology leads to the generalization and blurring of the responsible subjects. When there are mistakes in diagnosis and treatment, the distribution of responsibilities is uncertain, and it is difficult to identify the responsible subjects in the path of legalization. Moreover, in practical applications, the frequent interaction among multiple subjects in the technological process further increases the difficulty of liability determination. The technical decision-making is opaque and has poor interpretability, and there is no endogenous human-like intentionality, which plunges ethical governance into the dilemma of blurred responsibilities. **Difficulty in Obtaining Scientific Evidence for Governance Decisions:** How to improve the transparency and interpretability of technical decision-making is a key issue that urgently needs to be solved in the development of medical artificial intelligence. The ethical governance of medical artificial intelligence requires scientific and quantifiable evidence. Currently, the understanding of its ethical issues mostly remains at the level of theoretical speculation, and there is a lack of systematic arguments. There are many difficulties in obtaining scientific evidence, including the need for researchers to possess knowledge in multiple fields, the influence of the subjectivity of stakeholders and researchers, the lack of standards for questionnaire design, and the possible triggering of scientific research ethical issues, etc. These have greatly hindered the scientific promotion of ethical governance.

Exploration of the Governance Model for the Ethics of Artificial Intelligence in Healthcare — Based on Multi - Dimensional Collaboration

In the current era of rapid technological development, medical artificial intelligence (AI) is integrating into the healthcare industry at an unprecedented speed, profoundly transforming the traditional medical model. At this moment, exploring a scientific and reasonable governance model for medical AI is of utmost importance.

It plays an irreplaceable role in balancing the relationship between technological innovation and ethical norms.

However, at the present stage, there are some problems in the governance of medical AI, and it should not merely become a measure for post-hoc remediation. The formation of an AI regulatory framework requires the integration of considerations from moral, regulatory, technical, social, and practical aspects. These multiple perspectives contribute to all aspects of the evolving regulatory paradigm(Zhou & Gattinger, 2024). Currently, ensuring the ethical value system and behavior of AI systems is a major concern worldwide(Thurzo, 2025). Therefore, we should actively construct internationally universal ethical guidelines for medical AI, making the adherence to ethical norms an inherent value pursuit in the development of medical AI. Such values should not merely stay on the surface but should be shaped into a deeply ingrained quality and culture, permeating every aspect of the collaborative governance among diverse stakeholders in medical AI.

Based on the above background and needs, this paper constructs an institutional framework aimed at addressing the ethical issues of medical AI. This framework comprehensively takes into account various factors such as technology, ethics, and law. Through a series of measures, including clarifying the responsibilities of all parties, standardizing technical processes, and establishing a supervision mechanism, it safeguards the healthy development of medical AI and helps to promote the sustainable development of this industry.

Figure 4. an institutional framework aimed at addressing the ethical issues of medical AI

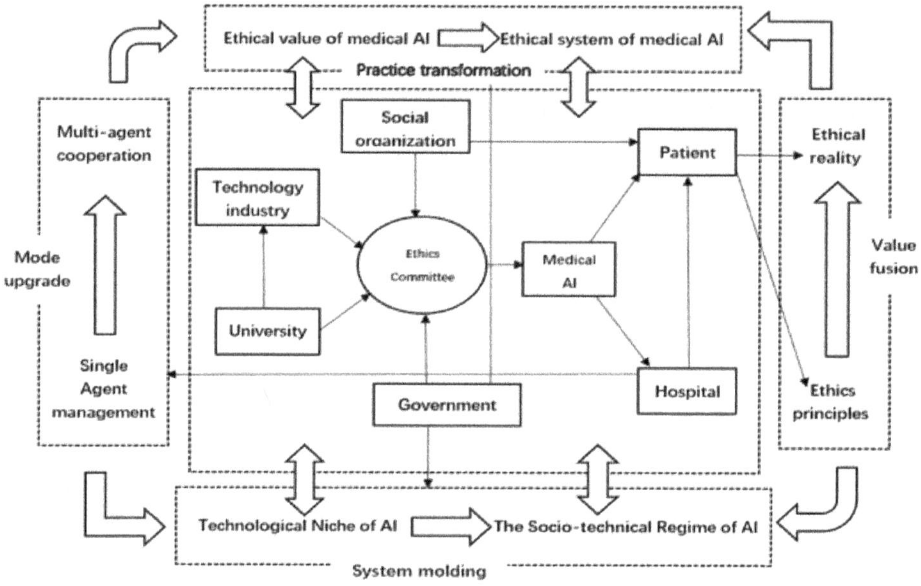

Source: Modified by Authors based on (2024)

Multi - Stakeholder Collaboration: Building a Diverse Governance Network

The resolution of ethical issues in artificial intelligence (AI) in healthcare cannot rely on a single entity. Instead, it should promote an upgrade from single - entity management to a multi - stakeholder collaborative model. According to the stakeholder theory, the survival and development of the industry depend on the support and cooperation of these stakeholders. To achieve "fairness, trustworthiness, respect, loyalty, care, and cooperation" as the inherent attributes of stakeholder relationships, stakeholders need to act sincerely(Valentinov & Roth, 2024). Therefore, when formulating strategies and making decisions, it is necessary to comprehensively consider the interests of all parties and balance the relationships among different stakeholders(Nora et al., 2023). In the development process of medical artificial intelligence, the role played by government departments is of vital importance. Their primary responsibility is to formulate scientific and reasonable macro policies and a sound regulatory system. At the same time, government departments also need to shoulder the heavy responsibility of supervising and managing the entire industry. They must carry out comprehensive tests and necessary approval processes to ensure that all ethical guidelines and regulations are effectively implemented(Wang et al., 2024). Take the field of data protection as an example. It is urgent for the government to introduce strict data protection regulations. These regulations can strictly restrict the behavior of medical artificial intelligence systems in the collection, use, and storage of patient data, fundamentally preventing issues such as illegal collection of patients' sensitive information, arbitrary abuse of data, and data breaches caused by improper storage, thus comprehensively protecting patients' privacy security. At present, various management and consulting institutions have developed a wide range of ethical principles, encouraging institutional decision-makers to apply these principles to specific practical decisions(Palmer & Schwan, 2024). At the same time, governments, advocacy groups, and other national and international organizations are formulating AI governance guidelines and ethical standards in an attempt to enhance public confidence(Kerasidou et al., 2022).

At the same time, universities and relevant professional institutions, with their rich scientific research resources and talent reserves, should become important forces in technological research and development and ethical research. Modern AI technology poses more challenges to ensuring moral compliance (Ossa, Lorenzini, et al., 2024). On the one hand, they should devote a great deal of effort to continuously optimizing artificial intelligence technology and actively promoting the in-depth development of its algorithms. Through continuous technological breakthroughs, artificial intelligence can play a greater role in medical diagnosis, significantly improving the accuracy and reliability of diagnosis, and providing strong support for precise treatment of patients. For example, in the field of medical imaging diagnosis, optimized algorithms can more keenly capture the characteristics of lesions, enabling professionals to improve the early diagnosis of different diseases and reduce diagnostic errors(Al Kuwaiti et al., 2023). On the other hand, it is equally urgent to conduct in-depth ethical research. This can provide solid theoretical support for the rational application of technology and ensure that medical artificial intelligence develops on the right track. However, building an artificial intelligence system that meets ethical and safety standards is no easy task, and it is a formidable challenge. It requires substantial investment in aspects such as data governance, algorithm management, and a thorough assessment of the social and environmental impacts of artificial intelligence. It also requires interdisciplinary and cross-departmental cooperation among data scientists, healthcare providers, and policymakers(Siala & Wang, 2022).

The technology industry plays an irreplaceable and crucial role in the process of transforming scientific research achievements from theoretical concepts into practical applications. In the field of medical artificial intelligence, as a significant force in technological innovation, enterprises must not overlook the constraints of ethics while pursuing technological breakthroughs and commercial interests. Enterprises need to deeply integrate ethical considerations into the design, development, and subsequent iterative processes of their products. From data collection and algorithm optimization to the realization of product functions, every link should adhere to ethical standards. In this way, it can be ensured that the medical artificial intelligence products and services provided to the market not only possess advanced technical performance but also stand up to ethical scrutiny.

At the same time, social organizations also have unique value in the development process of medical artificial intelligence. Social organizations should actively engage in it and give full play to their social influence. For example, by carrying out a variety of popular science and publicity activities, using multiple online and offline channels to popularize knowledge about the principles, application scenarios, and potential risks of medical artificial intelligence to the public, so as to enhance the public's level of awareness and understanding of related issues. Meanwhile, social media platforms can be used to provide real-time, diverse, and dynamic data, reflecting the ideas and feelings of a wide range of social strata, and gaining an in-depth understanding of the public's concerns about AI, making it an important tool for understanding and solving problems(Maghsoudi et al., 2024).

Medical institutions, as the direct users of AI, need to implement ethical principles in daily medical practices. Rather than simply focusing on the technical and design aspects of these systems, we should pay more attention to the forward-looking responsibilities of doctors who use such systems(Sand et al., 2022). Medical staff should use AI - based healthcare technology correctly as an auxiliary tool for diagnosis and treatment rather than relying on it completely. At the same time, medical institutions should establish internal ethical review mechanisms to strictly evaluate and supervise the introduced AI - based healthcare technology. In clinical practice, doctors should not only apply moral principles but also regard patients as unique individuals and establish a genuine rapport with them(Okamoto et al., 2025).

Patients, as the ultimate users of AI in healthcare, should have their rights fully protected. Patients have the right to understand the working principles of AI, data usage, and potential risks, and should have full informed consent and the right to choose in medical decision - making.

Transparency and communication are central ideas proposed by professionals to make AI tools acceptable to clinical and non - clinical medical staff and patients(Fazakarley et al., 2023). With the integration of artificial intelligence-based decision-making tools, the bilateral doctor-patient relationship may transform into a trilateral relationship(Cartolovni et al., 2022). Given the potential limitations and biases in AI - generated recommendations, it is crucial to establish feedback and collaboration channels between medical professionals and patients(Ueda et al., 2024). By constructing an effective communication mechanism, patients can fully express their needs and concerns, thereby increasing trust in the technology.

Ethical Values: The Transformation From Concept to Practice

Artificial intelligences themselves embody values, as they require actions and choices, but their practical applications are modeled or programmed by the engineers who build the systems(Keskinbora, 2019). The ethical value of medical artificial intelligence is rich in connotation and far-reaching in significance, covering many key aspects. Upholding the values of non-maleficence, respect for human autonomy, and the maintenance of fairness and quality are of paramount importance in any medical setting(Petersson et al., 2023). First and foremost, the protection of patients' rights and interests is of utmost importance, which means fully respecting patients' rights to privacy, informed consent, and autonomous choice. Patients' personal health data is extremely sensitive information and should be properly protected throughout the entire life cycle of medical artificial intelligence. Secondly, the connection between artificial intelligence technology and health equity in terms of accessibility is considered crucial for healthcare(Rubeis et al., 2022). Therefore, the pursuit of medical fairness is also one of the core ethical values. Moreover, the requirements for technical safety cannot be ignored. Medical artificial intelligence systems must possess a high degree of stability and reliability to prevent harm to patients caused by technical failures.

These important values should not merely remain at the theoretical level but should be effectively integrated into the entire research and development process of medical artificial intelligence. During the design phase, full consideration should be given to patient privacy protection, and advanced encryption technologies and access control mechanisms should be adopted to ensure the security of patient data from the source. For example, multi-layer encryption algorithms can be used to encrypt patients' medical record data, and only authorized personnel can access and use this data. During the application phase, it is necessary to ensure the fairness of algorithms. Through extensive data testing and verification, unequal distribution of medical resources caused by algorithmic bias can be avoided.

The practical transformation of these abstract ethical values into operable ethical systems is the key to the standardized development of medical artificial intelligence. Ethical systems should comprehensively and meticulously specify the ethical guidelines and norms for medical artificial intelligence at every stage, such as data management specifications, algorithm review processes, and liability - tracing mechanisms. At the same time, corresponding supervision and enforcement mechanisms should be established. AI software is often proprietary, and external researchers usually have little or no access to training data or performance evaluations. Therefore, ensuring that developers fulfill their obligations in terms of performance transparency and fairness may require the support of independent auditors, researchers, or government agencies to ensure the healthy development of medical artificial intelligence in line with ethical norms(Herington et al., 2023).

Institutional Shaping: The Integrated Development of Technology and Society

The robust development of medical artificial intelligence cannot be achieved without a sound social-technical system as solid support. However, the construction of such a system is by no means an overnight task, but a gradual process. When starting from the technological niche stage, ethical considerations should be placed in a crucial position, with an emphasis on the forward-looking prediction and prevention of ethical issues. R&D teams, regulatory authorities, and industry experts need to maintain a keen sense of insight, carefully analyze the technical architecture, data processing models, and application scenarios, and anticipate possible ethical risks such as algorithmic bias, data privacy leakage, and ambiguous liability definition. In the market niche stage, further expand the application scope of the technology while strengthening the supervision of the technology to ensure its ethical compliance in commercial applications. Eventually, through continuous development and improvement, a stable socio - technical system will be formed.

Value Integration: The Organic Unity of Ethics and Technology

Value integration is the ultimate goal of solving the ethical problems of artificial intelligence in healthcare, that is, to achieve the organic integration of ethical principles and ethical practice. Ethical principles are the basic norms for the development of artificial intelligence in healthcare, including respecting patients' autonomy, protecting patient privacy, and ensuring medical fairness. In practical application scenarios, deeply integrating ethical principles into the technical design, operation processes, and service models of medical artificial intelligence is the key to ensuring its healthy development. This requires us to transform ethical norms from external constraints into the inherent attributes of technology and run them through every link of research, development, and application.

The ethical governance of medical artificial intelligence is by no means a one-time project, and a dynamic adjustment mechanism needs to be established. In practical application scenarios, with the iterative development of technology and changes in social needs, new ethical issues will continue to emerge. This requires us to promptly adjust and improve ethical principles based on practical feedback. For example, when the algorithm shows diagnostic biases in a specific population, it is necessary to re-examine the data collection standards and model training rules; when patients have concerns about data sharing, the privacy protection agreement should be optimized. Through continuous iterative optimization, ethical principles can not only conform to the characteristics of the medical industry but also have clear implementation standards, truly becoming the navigation instrument for technological development.

Value integration is the core path to the sustainable development of medical artificial intelligence. Technological innovation should not come at the cost of sacrificing ethical values. Instead, ethical requirements such as the protection of patients' rights and interests and medical fairness should be internalized as the core indicators of technological research and development. Only when technological innovation and ethical norms resonate in harmony can the social value of medical artificial intelligence be maximized.

Facing complex ethical challenges, the governance of medical artificial intelligence requires the construction of an all-round and multi-level collaborative system. Government departments should play a guiding role in formulating policies and establish unified industry standards and regulatory frameworks; scientific research institutions should strengthen interdisciplinary research and cooperation to form transparent regulatory guidelines, which is an important step in winning trust and ensuring the safety, reliability, and fairness of AI systems(Khan et al., 2025); enterprises need to embed ethical requirements into the whole life cycle management of their products; social organizations should build platforms for public participation to promote multi-party dialogue; finally, patients and the public should also be involved, as patients and the public are important voices in formulating effective and ethical AI governance(Frost et al., 2022). At the same time, a complete chain should be established, from the extraction of ethical values to institutional design, from standard formulation to supervision and implementation, to ensure that ethical governance covers all aspects such as technological research and development, clinical application, and market promotion. Only by pooling the strength of all parties and forming a joint governance force can we promote the steady and long-term development of medical artificial intelligence on the track of compliance with ethical norms and truly achieve its ultimate goal of serving human health.

CONCLUSION

This study undertakes a comprehensive exploration of the ethical issues in artificial intelligence (AI) within the medical decision - making scenario and proposes a multi - dimensional collaborative governance model. The research findings offer significant insights into the current state of AI in healthcare and provide a solid foundation for future development.

By leveraging CiteSpace analysis, we have successfully identified the research hotspots and development trends in the field of AI and medical ethics. This not only helps us understand the current research landscape but also provides directions for future research. It is evident that the integration of AI and medical decision - making is a rapidly evolving area, with continuous emergence of new topics and challenges.

Based on the stakeholder theory, we have deeply analyzed the ethical issues and dilemmas faced by patients, hospitals, and the government. Patients are confronted with privacy and data security risks, as well as limitations in their participation in medical decision - making. Hospitals struggle with ambiguous liability definitions and insufficient ethical review and supervision. The government faces challenges such as lagging policies and regulations, resource allocation issues, and cross - departmental coordination difficulties. These findings highlight the complexity of ethical issues in medical AI and the need for a comprehensive and systematic approach to address them.

In response to these issues, the proposed multi - dimensional collaborative governance model offers a practical solution. Multi - stakeholder collaboration can effectively balance the interests of different parties and build a diversified governance network. The transformation of ethical values from concept to practice can ensure that ethical considerations are integrated into every aspect of AI development and application. The integrated development of technology and society can shape a sound institutional system, providing a favorable environment for the sustainable development of medical AI. Value integration can achieve the organic unity of ethics and technology, enabling AI to innovate while adhering to ethical principles.

However, it should be noted that the implementation of this governance model still faces some challenges. For example, in multi - stakeholder collaboration, there may be conflicts of interest and differences in values among different parties, which require effective communication and coordination mechanisms. The transformation of ethical values into practice needs to overcome the obstacles of technological complexity and cost. The shaping of the institutional system requires long - term efforts and continuous improvement. Value integration also needs to adapt to the continuous development of technology and the changing social environment.

In conclusion, although the application of AI in medical decision - making brings many opportunities, it also poses significant ethical challenges. By addressing these challenges through the proposed multi - dimensional collaborative governance model, we can promote the healthy and sustainable development of AI in healthcare. Future research should focus on further improving the governance model, strengthening empirical research, and enhancing international cooperation to ensure that AI in healthcare can truly benefit human health while adhering to ethical principles. This study not only contributes to the academic understanding of medical AI ethics but also provides practical guidance for the development and application of AI in the medical field.

REFERENCES

Al Kuwaiti, A., Nazer, K., Al-Reedy, A., Al-Shehri, S., Al-Muhanna, A., Subbarayalu, A. V., Al Muhanna, D., & Al-Muhanna, F. A. (2023). A Review of the Role of Artificial Intelligence in Healthcare. *Journal of Personalized Medicine*, *13*(6), 951. Advance online publication. DOI: 10.3390/jpm13060951 PMID: 37373940

Alowais, S. A., Alghamdi, S. S., Alsuhebany, N., Alqahtani, T., Alshaya, A. I., Almohareb, S. N., Aldairem, A., Alrashed, M., Bin Saleh, K., Badreldin, H. A., Al Yami, M. S., Al Harbi, S., & Albekairy, A. M. (2023). Revolutionizing healthcare: The role of artificial intelligence in clinical practice. *BMC Medical Education*, *23*(1), 689. Advance online publication. DOI: 10.1186/s12909-023-04698-z PMID: 37740191

Amann, J., Vayena, E., Ormond, K. E., Frey, D., Madai, V. I., & Blasimme, A. (2023). Expectations and attitudes towards medical artificial intelligence: A qualitative study in the field of stroke. *PLoS One*, *18*(1), e0279088. Advance online publication. DOI: 10.1371/journal.pone.0279088 PMID: 36630325

Bridoux, F., & Stoelhorst, J. W. (2022). Stakeholder theory, strategy, and organization: Past, present, and future. *Strategic Organization*, *20*(4), 797–809. DOI: 10.1177/14761270221127628

Carter, S. M., Rogers, W., Win, K. T., Frazer, H., Richards, B., & Houssami, N. (2020). The ethical, legal and social implications of using artificial intelligence systems in breast cancer care. *The Breast : Official Journal of the European Society of Mastology*, *49*, 25–32. DOI: 10.1016/j.breast.2019.10.001 PMID: 31677530

Cartolovni, A., Tomicic, A., & Mosler, E. L. (2022). Ethical, legal, and social considerations of AI-based medical decision-support tools: A scoping review. *International Journal of Medical Informatics*, *161*, 104738. Advance online publication. DOI: 10.1016/j.ijmedinf.2022.104738 PMID: 35299098

Chauhan, C., & Gullapalli, R. R. (2021). Ethics of AI in Pathology <i>Current Paradigms and Emerging Issues</i>. *The American Journal of Pathology*, *191*(10), 1673–1683. DOI: 10.1016/j.ajpath.2021.06.011 PMID: 34252382

Chen, C. (2004). Searching for intellectual turning points: Progressive knowledge domain visualization. *Proceedings of the National Academy of Sciences of the United States of America*, *101*(suppl_1), 5303–5310. https://doi.org/doi:10.1073/pnas.0307513100. DOI: 10.1073/pnas.0307513100 PMID: 14724295

Chen, C. (2020). A Glimpse of the First Eight Months of the COVID-19 Literature on Microsoft Academic Graph: Themes, Citation Contexts, and Uncertainties [Methods]. *Frontiers in Research Metrics and Analytics*, *5*, 607286. Advance online publication. DOI: 10.3389/frma.2020.607286 PMID: 33870064

Christoforaki, M., & Beyan, O. (2022). AI Ethics-A Bird's Eye View. *Applied Sciences (Basel, Switzerland)*, *12*(9), 4130. Advance online publication. DOI: 10.3390/app12094130

Contaldo, M. T., Pasceri, G., Vignati, G., Bracchi, L., Triggiani, S., & Carrafiello, G. (2024). AI in Radiology: Navigating Medical Responsibility. *Diagnostics (Basel)*, *14*(14), 1506. Advance online publication. DOI: 10.3390/diagnostics14141506 PMID: 39061643

Corfmat, M., Martineau, J. T., & Régis, C. (2025). High-reward, high-risk technologies? An ethical and legal account of AI development in healthcare. *BMC Medical Ethics*, *26*(1), 4. Advance online publication. DOI: 10.1186/s12910-024-01158-1 PMID: 39815254

Da Silva, M., Horsley, T., Singh, D., Da Silva, E., Ly, V., Thomas, B., Daniel, R. C., Chagal-Feferkorn, K. A., Iantomasi, S., White, K., Kent, A., & Flood, C. M. (2022). Legal concerns in health-related artificial intelligence: A scoping review protocol. *Systematic Reviews*, *11*(1), 123. Advance online publication. DOI: 10.1186/s13643-022-01939-y PMID: 35715812

Dlugatch, R., Georgieva, A., & Kerasidou, A. (2023). Trustworthy artificial intelligence and ethical design: Public perceptions of trustworthiness of an AI-based decision-support tool in the context of intrapartum care. *BMC Medical Ethics*, *24*(1), 42. Advance online publication. DOI: 10.1186/s12910-023-00917-w PMID: 37340408

Durán, J. M., & Jongsma, K. R. (2021). Who is afraid of black box algorithms? On the epistemological and ethical basis of trust in medical AI. *Journal of Medical Ethics*, *47*(5), 329–335. DOI: 10.1136/medethics-2020-106820 PMID: 33737318

Evans, B. J. (2023). Rules for robots, and why medical AI breaks them. *Journal of Law and the Biosciences*, *10*(1), lsad001. Advance online publication. DOI: 10.1093/jlb/lsad001 PMID: 36815975

Fazakarley, C. A., Breen, M., Leeson, P., Thompson, B., & Williamson, V. (2023). Experiences of using artificial intelligence in healthcare: A qualitative study of UK clinician and key stakeholder perspectives. *BMJ Open*, *13*(12), e076950. Advance online publication. DOI: 10.1136/bmjopen-2023-076950 PMID: 38081671

Fournier-Tombs, E., & McHardy, J. (2023). A Medical Ethics Framework for Conversational Artificial Intelligence. *Journal of Medical Internet Research*, *25*, e43068. Advance online publication. DOI: 10.2196/43068 PMID: 37224277

Frost, E. K., Bosward, R., Aquino, Y. S., Braunack-Mayer, A., & Carter, S. M. (2022). Public views on ethical issues in healthcare artificial intelligence: Protocol for a scoping review. *Systematic Reviews*, *11*(1), 142. Advance online publication. DOI: 10.1186/s13643-022-02012-4 PMID: 35841073

Hamet, P., & Tremblay, J. (2017). Artificial intelligence in medicine. *Metabolism: Clinical and Experimental*, *69*, S36–S40. DOI: 10.1016/j.metabol.2017.01.011 PMID: 28126242

Herington, J., McCradden, M. D., Creel, K., Boellaard, R., Jones, E. C., Jha, A. K., Rahmim, A., Scott, P. J. H., Sunderland, J. J., Wahl, R. L., Zuehlsdorff, S., & Saboury, B. (2023). Ethical Considerations for Artificial Intelligence in Medical Imaging: Deployment and Governance. *Journal of Nuclear Medicine*, *64*(10), 1509–1515. DOI: 10.2967/jnumed.123.266110 PMID: 37620051

Herrmann, M., Wabro, A., & Winkler, E. (2024). Percentages and reasons: AI explainability and ultimate human responsibility within the medical field. *Ethics and Information Technology*, *26*(2), 26. Advance online publication. DOI: 10.1007/s10676-024-09764-8

Katznelson, G., & Gerke, S. (2021). The need for health AI ethics in medical school education. *Advances in Health Sciences Education : Theory and Practice*, *26*(4), 1447–1458. DOI: 10.1007/s10459-021-10040-3 PMID: 33655433

Kempt, H., Heilinger, J. C., & Nagel, S. K. (2022). Relative explainability and double standards in medical decision-making Should medical AI be subjected to higher standards in medical decision-making than doctors? *Ethics and Information Technology*, *24*(2), 20. Advance online publication. DOI: 10.1007/s10676-022-09646-x

Kerasidou, C., Kerasidou, A., Buscher, M., & Wilkinson, S. (2022). Before and beyond trust: Reliance in medical AI. *Journal of Medical Ethics*, *48*(11), 852–856. DOI: 10.1136/medethics-2020-107095 PMID: 34426519

Keskinbora, K. H. (2019). Medical ethics considerations on artificial intelligence. *Journal of Clinical Neuroscience : Official Journal of the Neurosurgical Society of Australasia*, *64*, 277–282. DOI: 10.1016/j.jocn.2019.03.001 PMID: 30878282

Khan, M. M., Shah, N., Shaikh, N., Thabet, A., Alrabayah, T., & Belkhair, S. (2025). Towards secure and trusted AI in healthcare: A systematic review of emerging innovations and ethical challenges. *International Journal of Medical Informatics*, *195*, 105780. Advance online publication. DOI: 10.1016/j.ijmedinf.2024.105780 PMID: 39753062

Kunar, M. A., Montana, G., & Watson, D. G. (2024). Increasing transparency of computer-aided detection impairs decision-making in visual search. *Psychonomic Bulletin & Review*. Advance online publication. DOI: 10.3758/s13423-024-02601-5 PMID: 39448515

MacIntyre, M. R., Cockerill, R. G., Mirza, O. F., & Appel, J. M. (2023). Ethical considerations for the use of artificial intelligence in medical decision-making capacity assessments. *Psychiatry Research*, *328*, 115466. Advance online publication. DOI: 10.1016/j.psychres.2023.115466 PMID: 37717548

Maghsoudi, M., Mohammadi, A., & Habibipour, S. (2024). Navigating and Addressing Public Concerns in AI: Insights From Social Media Analytics and Delphi. *IEEE Access : Practical Innovations, Open Solutions*, *12*, 126043–126062. DOI: 10.1109/ACCESS.2024.3440660

Mahajan, R., Lim, W. M., Sareen, M., Kumar, S., & Panwar, R. (2023). Stakeholder theory. *Journal of Business Research*, *166*, 114104. Advance online publication. DOI: 10.1016/j.jbusres.2023.114104

McLennan, S., Fiske, A., Tigard, D., Müller, R., Haddadin, S., & Buyx, A. (2022). Embedded ethics: A proposal for integrating ethics into the development of medical AI. *BMC Medical Ethics*, *23*(1), 6. Advance online publication. DOI: 10.1186/s12910-022-00746-3 PMID: 35081955

Metta, C., Beretta, A., Pellungrini, R., Rinzivillo, S., & Giannotti, F. (2024). Towards Transparent Healthcare: Advancing Local Explanation Methods in Explainable Artificial Intelligence. *Bioengineering (Basel, Switzerland)*, *11*(4), 369. Advance online publication. DOI: 10.3390/bioengineering11040369 PMID: 38671790

Mittelstadt, B. (2019). Principles alone cannot guarantee ethical AI. *Nature Machine Intelligence*, *1*(11), 501–507. DOI: 10.1038/s42256-019-0114-4

Moulaei, K., Akhlaghpour, S., & Fatehi, F. (2025). Patient consent for the secondary use of health data in artificial intelligence (AI) models: A scoping review. *International Journal of Medical Informatics*, *198*, 105872. Advance online publication. DOI: 10.1016/j.ijmedinf.2025.105872 PMID: 40107041

Nora, G. A. M., Alberton, A., & Ayala, D. H. F. (2023). Stakeholder theory and actor-network theory: The stakeholder engagement in energy transitions. *Business Strategy and the Environment*, *32*(1), 673–685. DOI: 10.1002/bse.3168

Okamoto, S., Kataoka, M., Itano, M., & Sawai, T. (2025). AI-based medical ethics education: Examining the potential of large language models as a tool for virtue cultivation. *BMC Medical Education*, *25*(1), 185. Advance online publication. DOI: 10.1186/s12909-025-06801-y PMID: 39910559

Ossa, L. A., Lorenzini, G., Milford, S. R., Shaw, D., Elger, B. S., & Rost, M. (2024). Integrating ethics in AI development: A qualitative study. *BMC Medical Ethics*, *25*(1), 10. Advance online publication. DOI: 10.1186/s12910-023-01000-0 PMID: 38262986

Ossa, L. A., Milford, S. R., Rost, M., Leist, A. K., Shaw, D. M., & Elger, B. S. (2024). AI Through Ethical Lenses: A Discourse Analysis of Guidelines for AI in Healthcare. *Science and Engineering Ethics*, *30*(3), 24. Advance online publication. DOI: 10.1007/s11948-024-00486-0 PMID: 38833207

Palmer, A., & Schwan, D. (2024). More Process, Less Principles: The Ethics of Deploying AI and Robotics in Medicine. *Cambridge Quarterly of Healthcare Ethics, 33*(1), 121-134, Article Pii s0963180123000087. https://doi.org/DOI: 10.1017/S0963180123000087

Petersson, L., Vincent, K., Svedberg, P., Nygren, J. M., & Larsson, I. (2023). Ethical considerations in implementing AI for mortality prediction in the emergency department: Linking theory and practice. *Digital Health*, *9*, 20552076231206588. Advance online publication. DOI: 10.1177/20552076231206588 PMID: 37829612

Polevikov, S. (2023). Advancing AI in healthcare: A comprehensive review of best practices. *Clinica Chimica Acta; International Journal of Clinical Chemistry*, *548*, 117519. Advance online publication. DOI: 10.1016/j.cca.2023.117519 PMID: 37595864

Reddy, S., Allan, S., Coghlan, S., & Cooper, P. (2020). A governance model for the application of AI in health care. *Journal of the American Medical Informatics Association : JAMIA*, *27*(3), 491–497. DOI: 10.1093/jamia/ocz192 PMID: 31682262

Richardson, J. P., Smith, C., Curtis, S., Watson, S., Zhu, X., Barry, B., & Sharp, R. R. (2021). Patient apprehensions about the use of artificial intelligence in healthcare. *NPJ Digital Medicine*, *4*(1), 140. Advance online publication. DOI: 10.1038/s41746-021-00509-1 PMID: 34548621

Roski, J., Maier, E. J., Vigilante, K., Kane, E. A., & Matheny, M. E. (2021). Enhancing trust in AI through industry self-governance. *Journal of the American Medical Informatics Association : JAMIA, 28*(7), 1582–1590. DOI: 10.1093/jamia/ocab065 PMID: 33895824

Rubeis, G., Dubbala, K., & Metzler, I. (2022). "Democratizing" artificial intelligence in medicine and healthcare: Mapping the uses of an elusive term. *Frontiers in Genetics, 13*, 902542. Advance online publication. DOI: 10.3389/fgene.2022.902542 PMID: 36046243

Sand, M., Durán, J. M., & Jongsma, K. R. (2022). Responsibility beyond design: Physicians' requirements for ethical medical AI. *Bioethics, 36*(2), 162–169. DOI: 10.1111/bioe.12887 PMID: 34089625

Sankar, B. S., Gilliland, D., Rincon, J., Hermjakob, H., Yan, Y., Adam, I., Lemaster, G., Wang, D., Watson, K., Bui, A., Wang, W., & Ping, P. P. (2024). Building an Ethical and Trustworthy Biomedical AI Ecosystem for the Translational and Clinical Integration of Foundation Models. *Bioengineering (Basel, Switzerland), 11*(10), 984. Advance online publication. DOI: 10.3390/bioengineering11100984 PMID: 39451360

Saw, S. N., & Ng, K. H. (2022). Current challenges of implementing artificial intelligence in medical imaging. *Physica Medica : PM : An International Journal Devoted to the Applications of Physics to Medicine and Biology : Official Journal of the Italian Association of Biomedical Physics (AIFB), 100*, 12–17. DOI: 10.1016/j.ejmp.2022.06.003 PMID: 35714523

Shaw, J., Ali, J., Atuire, C. A., Cheah, P. Y., Español, A. G., Gichoya, J. W., Hunt, A., Jjingo, D., Littler, K., Paolotti, D., & Vayena, E. (2024). Research ethics and artificial intelligence for global health: Perspectives from the global forum on bioethics in research. *BMC Medical Ethics, 25*(1), 46. Advance online publication. DOI: 10.1186/s12910-024-01044-w PMID: 38637857

Siala, H., & Wang, Y. C. (2022). SHIFTing artificial intelligence to be responsible in healthcare: A systematic review. *Social Science & Medicine, 296*, 114782. Advance online publication. DOI: 10.1016/j.socscimed.2022.114782 PMID: 35152047

Tang, L., Li, J. X., & Fantus, S. (2023). Medical artificial intelligence ethics: A systematic review of empirical studies. *Digital Health, 9*, 20552076231186064. Advance online publication. DOI: 10.1177/20552076231186064 PMID: 37434728

Thurzo, A. (2025). Provable AI Ethics and Explainability in Medical and Educational AI Agents: Trustworthy Ethical Firewall. *Electronics (Basel), 14*(7), 1294. Advance online publication. DOI: 10.3390/electronics14071294

Ueda, D., Kakinuma, T., Fujita, S., Kamagata, K., Fushimi, Y., Ito, R., Matsui, Y., Nozaki, T., Nakaura, T., Fujima, N., Tatsugami, F., Yanagawa, M., Hirata, K., Yamada, A., Tsuboyama, T., Kawamura, M., Fujioka, T., & Naganawa, S. (2024). Fairness of artificial intelligence in healthcare: Review and recommendations. *Japanese Journal of Radiology*, *42*(1), 3–15. DOI: 10.1007/s11604-023-01474-3 PMID: 37540463

Ungureanu, A. M., Matei, S. C., & Malita, D. (2025). Controversies in the Application of AI in Radiology-Is There Medico-Legal Support? Aspects from Romanian Practice. *Diagnostics (Basel)*, *15*(2), 230. Advance online publication. DOI: 10.3390/diagnostics15020230 PMID: 39857113

Valentinov, V., & Roth, S. (2024). Relationality in transaction cost economics and stakeholder theory: A new conceptual framework. *Business Ethics, the Environment & Responsibility*, *33*(3), 535–546. DOI: 10.1111/beer.12652

Varnosfaderani, S. M., & Forouzanfar, M. (2024). The Role of AI in Hospitals and Clinics: Transforming Healthcare in the 21st Century. *Bioengineering (Basel, Switzerland)*, *11*(4), 337. Advance online publication. DOI: 10.3390/bioengineering11040337 PMID: 38671759

Vo, V., Chen, G., Aquino, Y. S., Carter, S. M., Do, Q. N., & Woode, M. E. (2023). Multi-stakeholder preferences for the use of artificial intelligence in healthcare: A systematic review and thematic analysis. *Social Science & Medicine*, *338*, 116357. Advance online publication. DOI: 10.1016/j.socscimed.2023.116357 PMID: 37949020

Wang, B. J., Asan, O., & Zhang, Y. Q. (2024). Shaping the future of chronic disease management: Insights into patient needs for AI-based homecare systems. *International Journal of Medical Informatics*, *181*, 105301. Advance online publication. DOI: 10.1016/j.ijmedinf.2023.105301 PMID: 38029700

Willem, T., Fritzsche, M. C., Zimmermann, B. M., Sierawska, A., Breuer, S., Braun, M., Ruess, A. K., Bak, M., Schönweitz, F. B., Meier, L. J., Fiske, A., Tigard, D., Müller, R., McLennan, S., & Buyx, A. (2024). Embedded Ethics in Practice: A Toolbox for Integrating the Analysis of Ethical and Social Issues into Healthcare AI Research. *Science and Engineering Ethics*, *31*(1), 3. Advance online publication. DOI: 10.1007/s11948-024-00523-y PMID: 39718728

Yang, G., Ye, Q. H., & Xia, J. (2022). Unbox the black-box for the medical explainable AI via multi-modal and multi-centre data fusion: A mini-review, two showcases and beyond. *Information Fusion*, *77*, 29–52. DOI: 10.1016/j.inffus.2021.07.016 PMID: 34980946

Yang, L., Ene, I. C., Belaghi, R. A., Koff, D., Stein, N., & Santaguida, P. (2022). Stakeholders' perspectives on the future of artificial intelligence in radiology: A scoping review. *European Radiology*, *32*(3), 1477–1495. DOI: 10.1007/s00330-021-08214-z PMID: 34545445

Zhang, J., & Zhang, Z. M. (2023). Ethics and governance of trustworthy medical artificial intelligence. *BMC Medical Informatics and Decision Making*, *23*(1), 7. Advance online publication. DOI: 10.1186/s12911-023-02103-9 PMID: 36639799

Zhou, K. R., & Gattinger, G. (2024). The Evolving Regulatory Paradigm of AI in MedTech: A Review of Perspectives and Where We Are Today. *Therapeutic Innovation & Regulatory Science*, *58*(3), 456–464. DOI: 10.1007/s43441-024-00628-3 PMID: 38528278

Chapter 9
Ethical Frameworks for AI-Driven Medical Innovations:
Balancing Progress and Patient Welfare

Poshan Yu
http://orcid.org/0000-0003-1069-3675
Soochow University, China & European Business Institute, Luxembourg & Australian Studies Centre, Shanghai University, China

Xinyuan Jiang
http://orcid.org/0009-0003-1998-1195
Independent Researcher, China

Chandra Lukita
http://orcid.org/0009-0006-6035-8241
Universitas Catur Insan Cendekia, Indonesia

ABSTRACT

The integration of AI in healthcare brings innovation but also ethical challenges. Using Citespace for bibliometric analysis of 2010 - 2025 literature from WoS and CNKI, the study identifies thematic hotspots and knowledge gaps in tech-related ethics for medicine. Western research emphasizes algorithmic fairness, while Eastern work focuses on ethical governance. Seven key gaps exist, including lack of cross-cultural harmonization. The study proposes ethical guidelines like participatory validation

DOI: 10.4018/979-8-2600-2238-2.ch009

and culturally adaptive governance. Comparing regional policies shows the need to embed ethics in AI design. A triadic framework integrating technical, ethical, and clinical aspects offers strategies to balance AI's potential with patient well-being.

INTRODUCTION

In recent years, artificial intelligence (AI) has emerged as a revolutionary force in the health technology field, driving a new wave of medical innovations (Saheb et al., 2021). From diagnostic tools that can detect diseases at early stages with remarkable accuracy to personalized treatment plans tailored to an individual's genetic makeup, AI holds the promise of transforming healthcare (Varnosfaderani & Forouzanfar, 2024). These advancements are particularly critical in addressing persistent global health challenges, and improving medical outcomes, making healthcare more accessible and effective. For instance, AI-powered telemedicine platforms have enabled remote diagnosis in rural Sub-Saharan Africa, where physician shortages leave millions without timely care (Manyazewal et al., 2021). Similarly, predictive algorithms for disease outbreaks—such as those deployed during the COVID-19 pandemic—demonstrate AI's capacity to mitigate large-scale public health crises by optimizing resource allocation and containment strategies (Drew et al., 2020). This aligns with recent case studies from China, which highlight how emerging technologies like AI-driven diagnostics and blockchain-secured health records can modernize healthcare systems while navigating localized infrastructural and ethical constraints (Wang et al., 2024).

However, as AI-driven medical innovations continue to proliferate, they bring with them a host of complex ethical challenges (Federico & Trotsyuk, 2024). The fundamental need to protect patient welfare often comes into conflict with the pursuit of technological progress. Recent studies on China's digital healthcare transformation reveal that rapid AI adoption in clinical settings—such as centralized diagnostic platforms and blockchain-based health records—has not only improved operational efficiency but also exposed tensions between technological scalability and localized ethical governance (Yu et al., 2022). This tension is magnified in global health contexts, where technological solutions must navigate cultural heterogeneity, infrastructural limitations, and entrenched socioeconomic disparities. For example, while AI-enabled diagnostic tools may enhance efficiency in high-income settings, their deployment in low- and middle-income countries (LMICs) risks exacerbating inequities and false diagnosis rate if not paired with investments in digital literacy and infrastructure (Adhikari et al., 2025). Additionally, AI algorithms may be vulnerable to biases, which could lead to unfair treatment of certain patient groups (Chin et al., 2023). There are also concerns regarding data privacy

(Wang et al., 2023), as AI systems rely on vast amounts of patient data. Moreover, the use of AI in medical decision-making may raise questions about accountability and transparency (Bouderhem, 2024). Therefore, there is a need to consider how AI developers can be practically assisted to anticipate, identify and address ethical issues regarding AI technologies (McLennan et al., 2022).

The integration of AI into global health systems demands more than technical prowess—it requires a commitment to equity-centered design. Technologies such as mobile health applications, wearable biosensors, and blockchain-secured electronic health records have shown potential to democratize healthcare access (Barragan-Montero et al., 2021). China's public-private partnership (PPP) model in regional healthcare networks—where state-led infrastructure investments are combined with private-sector technological innovations—demonstrates how collaborative governance can accelerate AI deployment while addressing systemic barriers like resource disparities and ethical oversight gaps (Yu & Xu, 2022). Yet, their success hinges on addressing systemic barriers. For example, AI models trained on datasets from high-income populations often fail to generalize to LMIC contexts, perpetuating diagnostic inaccuracies for marginalized groups (Adhikari et al., 2025). Research has shown that "A number of Artificial Intelligence (AI) ethics frameworks have been published in the last 6 years in response to the growing concerns posed by the adoption of AI in different sectors, including healthcare" (Goirand et al., 2021). Understanding these gaps is crucial for developing comprehensive ethical frameworks. To truly address these global health challenges, ethical frameworks must prioritize not only technical robustness but also cultural adaptability and participatory governance (Reddy et al., 2020). To this end, we used a Citespace-based bibliometric analysis to examine research trends in AI ethics in medicine from 2010 to 2025. This analysis allowed us to identify the dominant thematic hotspots in the existing literature, highlighting areas of focus as well as areas that require further investigation.

This study adopts a multidisciplinary approach, integrating insights from various fields such as computer science, medical ethics, and healthcare policy. By doing so, we aim to develop a more holistic understanding of the global ethical challenges surrounding AI-driven medical innovations, echoing recent scholarship that emphasizes the critical role of cross-disciplinary frameworks in addressing ethical complexities of generative AI systems (Yu et al., 2024). Our analysis extends beyond Western-centric paradigms to explore how hybrid ethical models—combining global standards with region-specific adaptations—can foster equitable health technology deployment. Our findings will not only contribute to the academic literature but also provide practical guidance for policymakers, healthcare providers, and AI developers, enabling them to make more informed decisions and ensure that AI is used in a manner that promotes both technological progress and patient welfare.

LITERATURE REVIEW

Identify Research Gap

Despite extensive research on Artificial Intelligence (AI) in medicine and its ethical implications, a critical gap persists in systematically examining the triadic interplay among AI, ethics, and medical innovation with a focus on patient welfare and healthcare equity (Dalton-Brown, 2020). While existing studies have explored pairwise relationships—such as AI and efficiency (Topol, 2019) or AI and ethical governance (Goirand et al., 2021)—few have integrated these dimensions into a cohesive framework that balances technological progress with societal impact. Critically, as Mittelstadt (2019) argues, ethical principles alone cannot guarantee responsible AI deployment and their practical implementation requires complementary mechanisms such as participatory governance and adaptive accountability structures, which remain underexplored in current frameworks. Key unresolved challenges include:

1. Epistemological tensions between AI-driven decisions and physician-patient relationships (Obermeyer et al., 2019) (Ploug & Holm, 2020)
2. Regional disparities in ethical frameworks, with Western policies emphasizing algorithmic accountability (e.g. EU AI Act) and Eastern approaches prioritizing institutional governance (e.g. China's ethical review systems) (Cath, 2018)
3. Lack of empirical metrics to evaluate ethical compliance in AI-medicine integration (Char et al., 2018) (McLennan et al., 2022)

This gap is further underscored by bibliometric analysis using CiteSpace, which reveals fragmented scholarly trajectories: Web of Science (WoS) literature focuses on bias mitigation (Rajkomar et al., 2018), while China National Knowledge Infrastructure (CNKI) emphasizes stakeholder education (Tuzov & Lin, 2024). Neither adequately addresses cross-cultural harmonization or longitudinal societal impacts—a void this study fills by mapping latent connections and proposing a patient-centric, multidisciplinary framework, which was supported by Gerke (2020).

By mapping these disparities, this study fills the gap through a unified framework that bridges AI-driven efficiency, healthcare equity, and participatory ethics—informed by CiteSpace's latent linkage detection and critique of existing regional policies (e.g. EU AI Act's risk-based mandates vs. China's systemic governance).

Research Questions

This study proposes one main research question, which is further broken into three specific sub-questions, to fill the research gaps identified before:

- Main research question: How can ethical frameworks be systematically designed and implemented to balance technological progress in AI-driven medical innovations with the protection of patient welfare?
- Sub-question 1: What are the dominant hotspots, knowledge gaps in existing research on AI ethics in medicine (2010–2025), as revealed by a Citespace-based bibliometric analysis?
- Sub-question 2: Given the CiteSpace analysis, how can we translate these hotspots into actionable ethical guidelines that are specifically tailored to AI-driven medical innovations, while also filling the identified knowledge gaps?
- Sub-question 3: How do the ethical instructions derived from the CiteSpace-informed analysis compare with the existing regional policies (such as those in the EU, USA, UK, and Canada) in terms of their comprehensiveness, enforceability, and adaptability to different healthcare systems, and what lessons can be learned from these comparisons to improve the overall ethical framework?

METHODOLOGY

Method

This study adopted a Citespace-based bibliometric method to conduct a scientific research collaboration analysis on the collected documents. We utilized CiteSpace, a bibliometric tool crafted by Prof. Chaomei Chen. Employing this instrument, a bibliometric analysis of the relevant literature was conducted, and the findings were presented in a visual format.

CiteSpace 5.2.R2 is a citation visual analysis software, developed from the background of scientometrics and knowledge visualization, which is specifically used to identify potential knowledge contained in scientific literature. This software can help researchers understand the basic knowledge of the discipline, find classical literature in the field, discover research frontiers, and clarify the context of research evolution (Chen, 2016).

CiteSpace converts the concepts within a research domain into mapping functions that link research frontiers and intellectual bases (Ding & Yang, 2022). The three concepts formulated within the framework of this mapping function concept play a crucial role in addressing the following three issues: (a) determining the essence of the research frontier, (b) labeling the research area, and (c) detecting new trends and abrupt changes over time. CiteSpace has been used by users in more than 100 countries, and more than 15,000 papers have been published using the CiteSpace tool (Su et al., 2019).

The CiteSpace software works as Fig. 1 based on previous studies. From a time-series perspective, it has the capacity to uncover newly emerging topics and evolving research trends (Chen, 2006). Moreover, CiteSpace generates graphs composed of nodes and lines. Depending on diverse research requirements, node types can represent authors, institutions, countries, terms, keywords, categories, cited authors, cited references, or cited journals. The magnitude of each node corresponds to the frequency of references or occurrences; specifically, larger nodes signify higher frequencies. Lines in the graph depict relationships between nodes. A greater thickness of the line indicates a stronger connection between the relevant nodes (Zhuang et al., 2022).

Figure 1. The conceptual model of CiteSpace

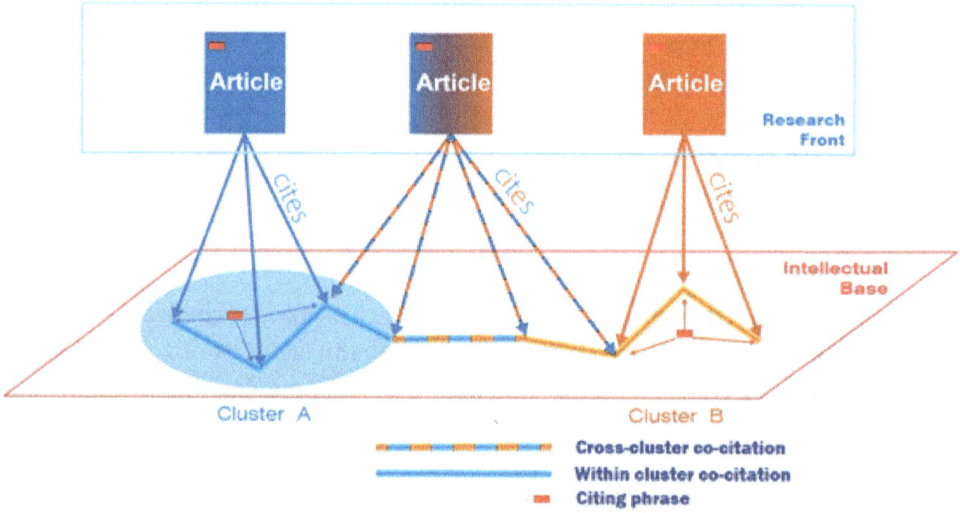

(Chen, 2006)
Source: WoS

Clustering refers to segregating a collection of physical or intangible objects into distinct groups. The group that emerges from this clustering process is known as a cluster, essentially an aggregation of objects. Elements within the same cluster exhibit significant similarity. In contrast, there's a notable degree of dissimilarity between elements belonging to different clusters. In CiteSpace, the clustering label is derived from the citation document and can be extracted from the title or index or summary of the cited document (Chen, 2020).

Data Selection

Our study employs data sourced from the Web of Science (WoS) Core Collection, specifically drawing on the Science Citation Index Expanded (SCIE) and Social Sciences Citation Index (SSCI). The rationale for selecting this database is threefold: (1) The WoS covers a wide range of publications from different fields, which includes over 15,000 journals and 50,000,000 classified publications in 251 categories and 150 research areas (Merigó & Yang, 2017); (2) WoS is a proper database because it contains a set of data, such as titles, authors, institutions, countries, abstracts, keywords, references, citation counts, impact factors and others (Gaviria-Marin et al., 2019); (3) WoS is widely used and recognized worldwide, and have been considered authoritative indices, thus ensuring that research results are more representative and convincing .

To ensure the accuracy and precise analysis results, we follow strict guidelines during the search and selection phase, as showed in Fig. 2. We set three search strategies for literature retrieval:

1) Search with the criteria 'Topic = AI AND Topic = Ethics'.
2) Use 'Topic = AI AND Topic = Medical' as the search terms.
3) Employ 'Topic = AI AND Topic = Ethics AND Topic = Medical'.

The indexing is set for SCI-EXPANDED and SSCI within the Web of Science Core Collection (WOSCC). The time span for the literature search ranges from January 1, 2010, to March 28, 2025. Subsequently, we will conduct a comparative analysis of the number of documents corresponding to these three retrieval strategies. By meticulously examining the quantity and content of the retrieved literature, we aim to pinpoint the research gaps, which will serve as valuable guides for our research endeavors in this field.

Figure 2. Qualitative Description of the Research Methodology

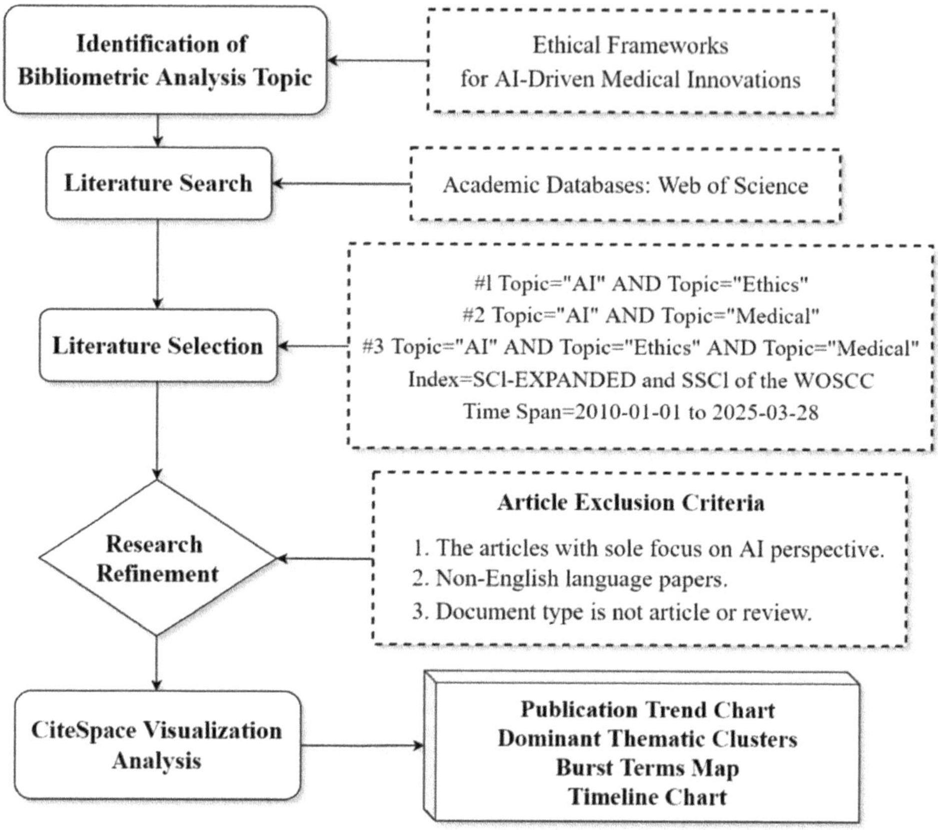

CITESPACE ANALYSIS

Publication Trends Overtime

The annual number of publications represents the field's quantity evolution and can assist scholars in predicting the field's future development (Geng et al., 2024). Through searching and screening, we finally obtained 315 articles and 117 reviews focused on AI-ethics in medicine on Web of Science. Meanwhile, we also obtained 418 documents focused on this field from China National Knowledge Infrastructure.

Fig. 3 shows the chronological distribution of publications in the platform research field.

The first discernible publications in this dataset emerged in 2017. Since then, the number of publications has been steadily climbing. This growth trajectory can be segmented into three distinct phases. The initial phase, spanning from 2017 to 2019, witnessed a minimal number of publications, with only a handful of papers released each year, signaling an embryonic stage of research activity. In the intermediate stage, from 2020 to 2022, the number of papers published on both WOS and CNKI increased notably, with the total number of publications more than doubling compared to the previous phase, indicating a period of rapid expansion and maturation, much like a seed-time timeline. The final stage, from 2023 to 2024, has seen an exponential surge in the total number of publications, with a dramatic increase in both WOS-published papers and CNKI-published articles. This substantial uptick represents a blossoming era, suggesting that research in this area has reached a highly active and productive phase.

Figure 3. Publication trends, 2012-2025

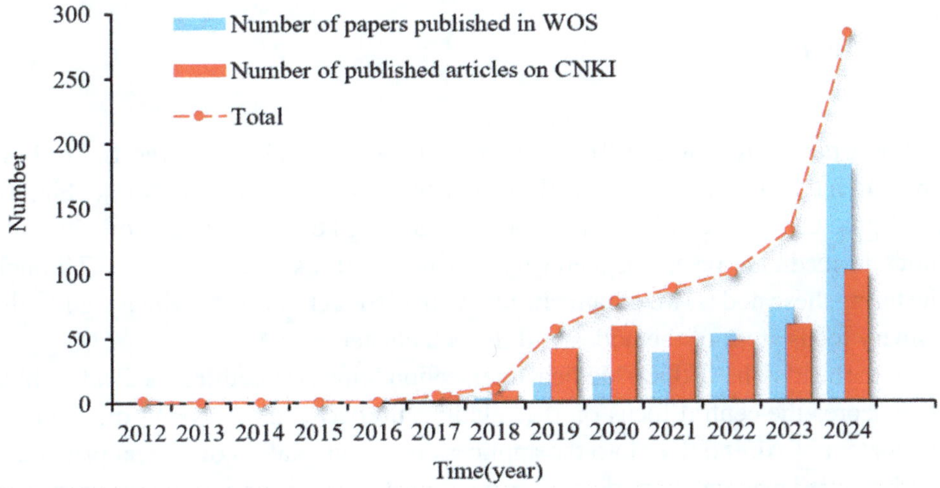

Source: WoS and CNKI

Dominant Thematic Clusters Analysis

Figure 4. Clustering keyword network in the field of AI ethics in medicine from WoS

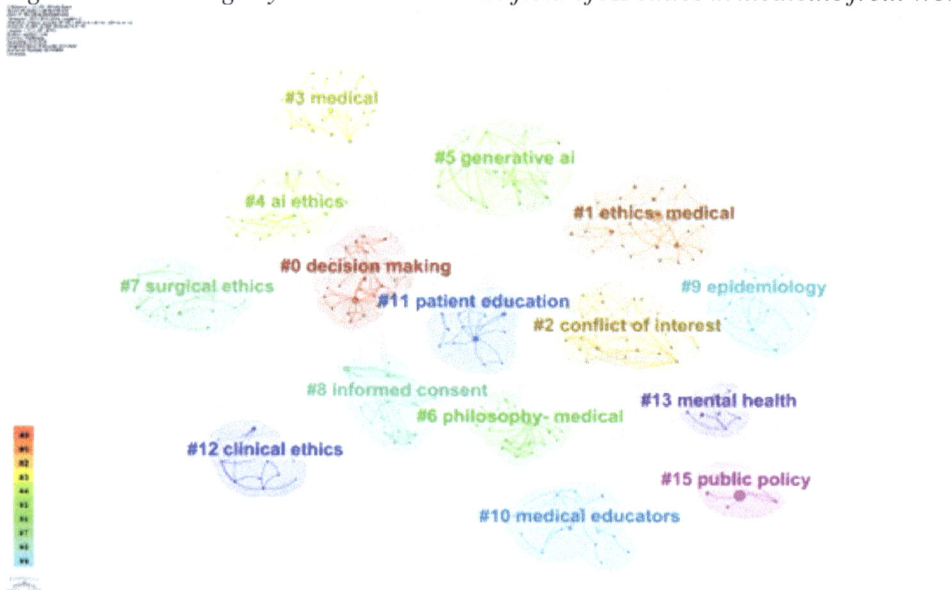

Source: WoS

We arrange all articles (2010–2025) from Web of Science in the field of AI ethics in medicine in a hierarchical manner through a clustering network (Fig. 4). The figure depicts the collaboration network among keywords in the domain of AI ethics in medicine research, featuring 297 nodes and 487 connections. Through clustering these nodes, we obtain clusters with distinct keywords, which signify the primary focus areas of the nodes within each cluster.

At the heart is the "Ethics-Medical Intersection" cluster (#1 ethics-medical), which underscores the central focus on the relationship between ethics and medicine in the context of AI. It delves into the application and adaptation of ethical principles in AI-enabled medical scenarios, covering aspects like fairness, accountability, and transparency in medical decision-making.

Closely related are the "AI-Specific Ethical Concerns" clusters (#4 ai ethics, #5 generative ai), highlighting the increasing attention given to the unique ethical challenges posed by AI. For generative AI, issues such as the authenticity of generated medical information and output bias are in focus, while the broader 'ai ethics' cluster encompasses fundamental concerns like data privacy and algorithmic bias in medical diagnosis and treatment.

The "Clinical and Surgical Ethics" clusters (#12 clinical ethics, #7 surgical ethics) concentrate on the practical implications of medical ethics when AI is introduced. In clinical settings, this involves examining the impact on patient-doctor relationships and informed consent, while in surgical contexts, it explores the use of AI-assisted tools and the ethical implications of AI-based surgical decision-making.

Finally, the "Patient-related Considerations" clusters (#11 patient education, #8 informed consent) emphasize the significance of the patient's role. Patient education is essential for patients to understand AI-based healthcare, and informed consent becomes more intricate with AI-driven technologies, prompting questions about necessary patient knowledge and effective consent-obtaining methods.

Figure 5. Clustering keyword network in the field of AI ethics in medicine from CNKI

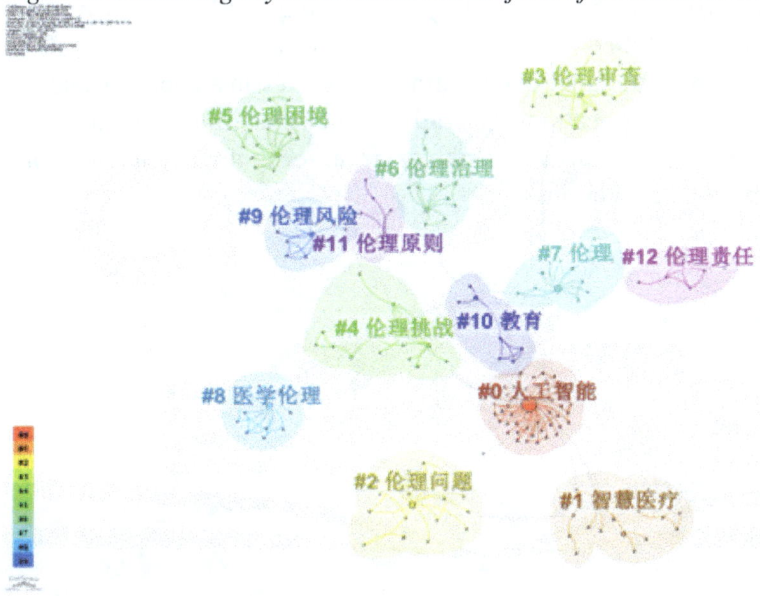

Source: CNKI

At the same time, we also organize all relevant articles from China National Knowledge Infrastructure through a clustering network (Fig. 5), with 240 nodes and 285 connections. At the core is the "Core AI and Medical Application Cluster," where #0 人工智能 (Artificial Intelligence) acts as the foundational overarching technology, around which all related concepts orbit. Adjacent to it, #1 智慧医疗 (Smart Healthcare) focuses on leveraging AI to enhance healthcare delivery in areas like diagnosis and treatment planning.

The "Ethical Issues and Challenges Cluster" encompasses #2 伦理问题 (Ethical Issues), which covers a wide array of moral concerns at the AI-medicine intersection; #4 伦理挑战 (Ethical Challenges), highlighting the hurdles in making AI-based medical practices ethical; and #5 伦理困境 (Ethical Dilemmas), dealing with complex scenarios of competing ethical considerations.

The "Ethical Governance and Review Cluster" features #3 伦理审查 (Ethical Review), underscoring the importance of review mechanisms for AI-driven medical tech, and #6 伦理治理 (Ethical Governance), concerning the systems and policies for regulating ethical AI use in medicine.

The "Ethical Fundamentals Cluster" includes #7 伦理 (Ethics), providing the theoretical base; #9 伦理风险 (Ethical Risks), analyzing risks of unethical AI use like threats to patient autonomy; #11 伦理原则 (Ethical Principles), emphasizing the need for key ethical tenets; and #12 伦理责任 (Ethical Responsibilities), determining stakeholder responsibilities for ethical AI use.

Lastly, the "Specialized and Supplementary Cluster" has #8 医学伦理 (Medical Ethics) bridging traditional medical ethics with AI-specific issues, and #10 教育 (Education) stressing the importance of educating all involved in AI-related medical activities about its ethical implications. Overall, these clusters illuminate the multifaceted nature of research in AI medical ethics, from technological applications to ethical governance and education.

Burst Terms Map Analysis

Figure 6. Burst terms map of articles on WoS

Top 24 Keywords with the Strongest Citation Bursts

Keywords	Year	Strength	Begin	End
ethics medical	2010	1.88	**2010**	2016
care	2011	3	**2011**	2018
education	2011	1.31	**2011**	2012
disorders	2012	1.31	**2012**	2015
conflict of interest	2013	1.35	**2013**	2014
clinical trials	2014	1.64	**2014**	2022
impact	2014	1.24	**2014**	2015
children	2015	2.03	**2015**	2019
life	2015	1.32	**2015**	2016
big data	2018	2.19	**2018**	2021
machine learning	2019	7.92	**2019**	2021
classification	2019	1.45	**2019**	2020
bias	2020	3.8	**2020**	2022
medical ethics	2011	2.21	**2020**	2021
performance	2021	2.54	**2021**	2022
technology	2021	2.15	**2021**	2022
risk assessment	2021	2.05	**2021**	2022
segmentation	2021	1.55	**2021**	2023
clinical ethics	2021	1.24	**2021**	2023
medical imaging	2022	1.9	**2022**	2023
privacy	2022	1.9	**2022**	2023
implementation	2022	1.52	**2022**	2023
ai	2020	1.42	**2022**	2023
guidelines	2011	1.21	**2022**	2023

Source: WoS

Figure 7. Burst terms map of articles on CNKI

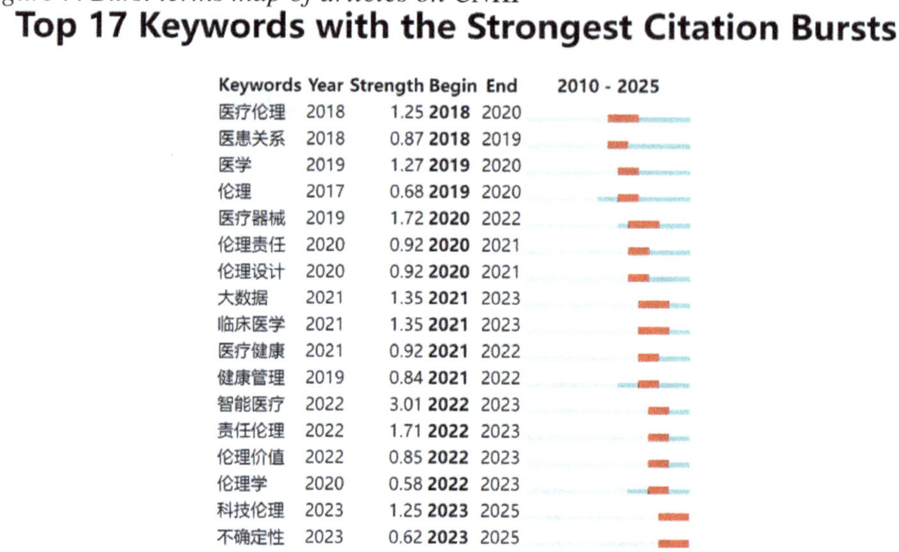

Source: CNKI

The two maps (Fig. 6, Fig. 7) of citation burst terms from Web of Science (WoS) and China National Knowledge Infrastructure (CNKI) reveals a dynamic interplay between global ethical concerns and region-specific priorities in the discourse surrounding AI-driven medical innovations. Over the past decade, both datasets underscore the transformative potential of technologies like big data and machine learning, while simultaneously highlighting the ethical complexities they introduce. Globally, WoS trends reflect a sustained emphasis on challenges such as algorithmic bias, privacy risks, and the ethical implications of clinical trials involving vulnerable populations like children. Terms like "bias" (2019–2021) and "AI guidelines" (2019–2021) signal a growing push for regulatory frameworks to address fairness and transparency in AI applications. Similarly, CNKI's focus on "大数据" (big data, 2021–2023) and "智能医疗" (intelligent healthcare, 2022–2023) aligns with these global themes but contextualizes them within China's unique socio-technical landscape, emphasizing systemic harmony and the integration of ethics into technological design.

Regional divergences, however, illuminate distinct cultural and institutional priorities. The WoS corpus prioritizes individual rights and institutional accountability, as seen in bursts like "conflict of interest" (2013–2014) and "clinical ethics" (2014–2022), reflecting Western debates around autonomy and regulatory rigor. In contrast, CNKI's emphasis on relational ethics—such as "医患关系" (doctor-patient relationship, 2018–2019) and "伦理责任" (ethical responsibility, 2020–2021)—

reveals a stronger focus on collective welfare and systemic trust, mirroring China's recent policy shifts toward "governance by design" and techno-ethical integration. Temporal trends further illustrate this evolution: early discourse in both regions centered on foundational principles like "medical ethics" (WoS) and "医学" (medicine, CNKI), while later phases shifted toward actionable frameworks, such as WoS's "risk assessment" (2021–2023) and CNKI's "科技伦理" (technology ethics, 2023–2025).

These insights collectively advocate for a hybrid ethical framework that harmonizes global standards with localized adaptations. For instance, integrating WoS-driven priorities like bias mitigation and privacy safeguards with CNKI's relational focus on doctor-patient trust could foster more culturally resonant AI systems. Additionally, addressing emerging challenges like "不确定性" (uncertainty, CNKI 2023–2025) requires adaptive governance models that anticipate unpredictable AI outcomes while maintaining patient welfare as a core imperative. By bridging Western regulatory rigor with Eastern systemic ethics, stakeholders can develop AI innovations that not only advance medical progress but also uphold the dignity, safety, and equitable treatment of patients worldwide. This synthesis underscores the necessity of interdisciplinary collaboration and cross-cultural dialogue to navigate the ethical labyrinth of AI in healthcare, ensuring that technological advancements remain anchored in universally shared values of justice and human flourishing.

Timeline Chart Analysis

Figure 8. Timeline chart of papers on WoS

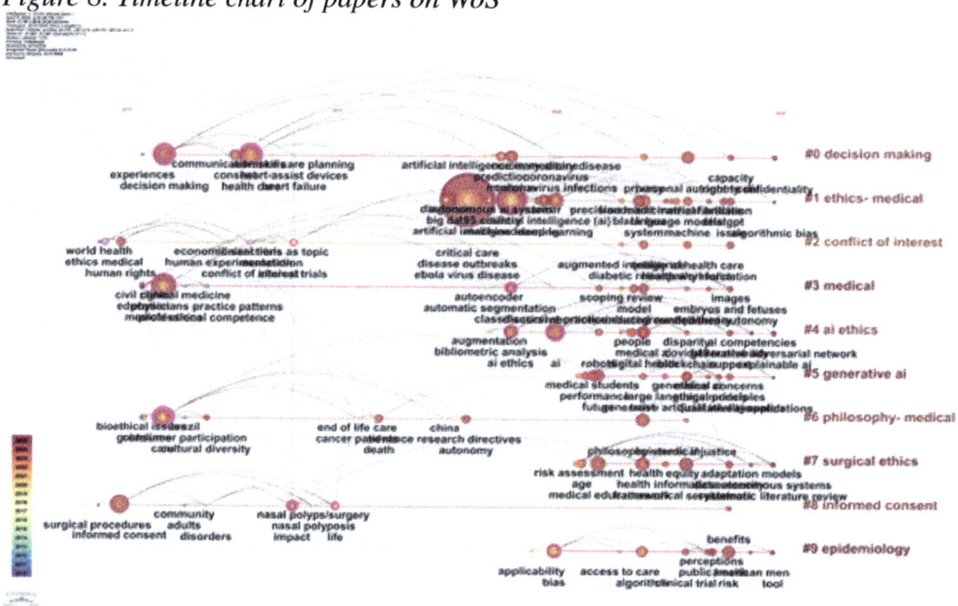

Source: WoS

Figure 9. Timeline chart of papers on CNKI

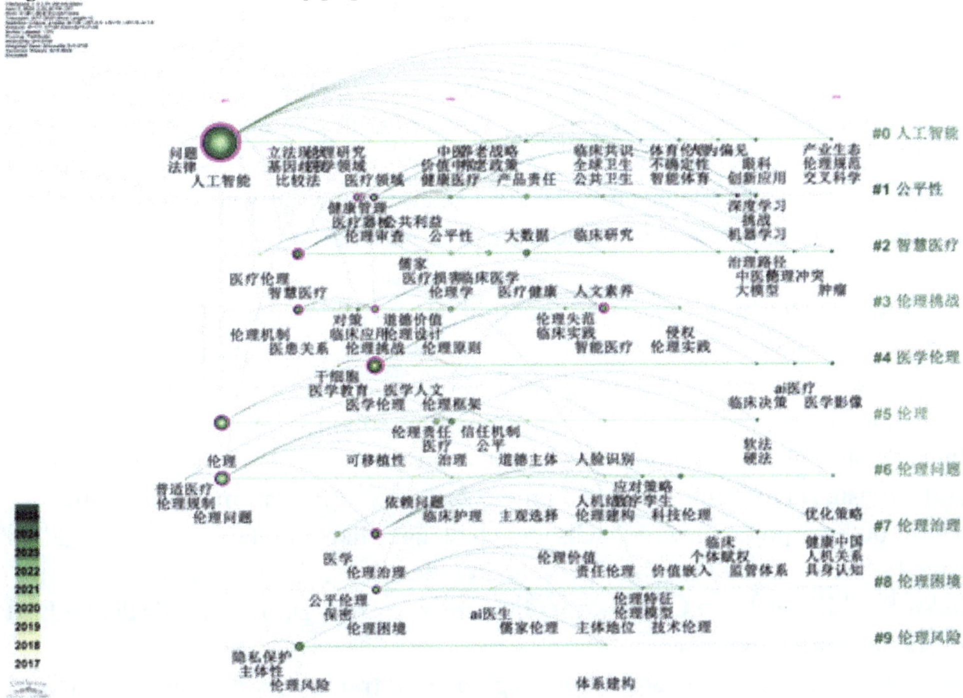

Source: CNKI

The timeline analyses of publications from Web of Science (WoS) and China National Knowledge Infrastructure (CNKI) reveal distinct yet complementary perspectives on the ethical challenges of AI-driven medical innovations. The WoS data presents a broad, interdisciplinary landscape where concerns like decision-making autonomy, algorithmic accountability, and clinical ethic intersect with technical themes such as predictor analytics and artificial intelligence in medical science. This corpus reflects Western scholarship's emphasis on individual rights, procedural transparency, and the tension between technological capabilities ("high-quality intelligence labs") and systemic risks ("dangerous systems"). Notably, the clustering of terms like "ethics-medical", "human experimentation" and "conflict of interest" underscores a sustained focus on research integrity and patient agency, while "cultural medicine" and "globalization" hint at nascent discussions about cross-cultural applicability.

In contrast, CNKI's timeline demonstrates China's structured approach to AI ethics, organized around explicit normative categories like "伦理规范" (ethical norms), "责任伦理" (responsibility ethics), and "公平性" (fairness). The prominence

continued on following page

Table 1. Continued

of Confucian-inspired concepts—such as "儒家伦理" (Confucian ethics) and "道德主体" (moral agency)—highlights a cultural grounding in collective welfare and hierarchical harmony. Technical domains are systematically paired with governance frameworks reflecting state-driven integration of ethics into AI development. Distinctively, CNKI publications emphasize design-stage ethics ("伦理设计" [ethical design], "价值嵌入" [value embedding]), suggesting proactive institutional efforts to preempt risks, unlike WoS's more reactive focus on mitigating existing harms (e.g. "algorithmic bias").

Three critical insights emerge. First, divergent ethical priorities shape implementation: WoS stresses individual consent and post-hoc accountability, while CNKI prioritizes systemic stability and pre-emptive value alignment. Second, cultural frameworks profoundly influence problem-solving—Western individualism fuels debates about autonomy ("directives autonomy" in WoS), whereas Chinese collectivism centers on relational duties ("人机关系" [human-machine relations]). Third, both corpora converge on urgent challenges like data fairness ("公平性" in CNKI; "biased algorithms" in WoS) and clinical integration ("clinical concerns" in WoS; "临床应用" in CNKI), signaling universal recognition of AI's dual-edged impact on patient welfare.

To balance innovation with ethics, a glocalized framework is essential: integrating Western procedural rigor (e.g. audit trails, transparent algorithms) with Eastern design-phase ethics (e.g. value-sensitive engineering). For instance, CNKI's "伦理模型" [ethical models] could inform WoS's "decision-making" paradigms to create AI systems that are both technically robust and culturally resonant. Similarly, WoS's emphasis on "cultural diversity" must expand beyond token inclusion to address CNKI's documented "伦理困境"(ethical dilemmas) in non-Western contexts. Policymakers should foster transnational dialogues—perhaps through WHO-sponsored guidelines—that harmonize these perspectives, ensuring AI advancements uphold contextualized justice without stifling progress.

Knowledge Gaps

Table 1. Knowledge gaps of AI ethics in medicine

Knowledge Gap	Description
Cross-Cultural and Global Ethical Frameworks	Limited integration of Western (individualist) and Eastern (collectivist) ethical paradigms into global AI ethics guidelines.
Long-Term Societal and Psychological Impacts	Absence of longitudinal studies on AI's societal effects (e.g. erosion of trust in healthcare) and psychological impacts on patients.
Technical-Social Interdisciplinary Solutions	Lack of concrete technical tools (e.g. bias mitigation) integrated with ethical governance models.
Under-Researched Medical Subfields	Mental health, geriatrics, and palliative care are underrepresented, especially for vulnerable populations (e.g. dementia patients).
Empirical Metrics for Ethical Compliance	Minimal research on measurable outcomes (e.g. audit frameworks, patient satisfaction) to evaluate ethical AI deployment.
Generative AI's Ethical Boundaries in Practice	Unresolved accountability for AI-generated clinical recommendations and legal liability frameworks.
Interdisciplinary Collaboration Models	Siloed approaches dominate; no robust models bridging AI developers, clinicians, and ethicists.

Key Trends in Existing Research

By conducting a comprehensive Citespace-based bibliometric analysis of the literature from the two aforementioned platforms, we can derive new insights into potential research directions.

Table 2. Key Trends in Existing Research

Key Trend	Description
Ethical Principles at the Core	Global emphasis on adapting classical bioethics (e.g. autonomy, fairness) to AI-driven medical contexts.
AI-Specific Challenges Gaining Traction	Rising focus on generative AI ethics (e.g. bias, misinformation) and algorithmic fairness in diagnosis.
Patient-Centric Frameworks	Growing emphasis on patient education, informed consent, and reshaping doctor-patient relationships.
Governance and Systemic Review Mechanisms	CNKI prioritizes policy frameworks (伦理治理), while WoS addresses governance via accountability.
Integration of Traditional and AI-Specific Ethics	Efforts to reconcile traditional medical ethics (e.g. surgical ethics) with AI's role in clinical decision-making.

Actionable Ethical Instructions Extracted From Bibliometric Analysis

1) For Ethics-Medical Intersection: When developing and implementing AI-based medical decision-making tools, ensure strict adherence to principles of fairness, accountability, and transparency. This involves clear documentation of how AI algorithms operate, regular audits to prevent discriminatory outcomes, and establishing channels for patients and medical professionals to question and understand AI-derived decisions.
2) Regarding AI-Specific Ethical Concerns: In the context of generative AI in medicine, establish verification mechanisms to authenticate the medical information it generates. For all AI applications, implement robust data privacy protocols, conduct regular checks for algorithmic bias, and ensure that the moral implications of AI-made decisions in diagnosis and treatment are thoroughly evaluated and justified.
3) Concerning Clinical and Surgical Ethics: In clinical settings, when using AI, enhance patient-doctor communication to clarify how AI impacts care. Streamline and clarify the informed consent process for AI-related medical procedures. In surgical applications, develop ethical guidelines for the use of AI-assisted tools, including provisions for human override in case of algorithmic failures and clear delineation of responsibility between human surgeons and AI systems.
4) For Patient-related Considerations: Prioritize the development of educational materials to inform patients about the role of AI in their medical care. These materials should be accessible, understandable, and cover aspects such as how AI algorithms work, potential benefits and risks, and patients' rights. When obtaining informed consent for AI-driven treatments, provide comprehensive and simplified information, and ensure patients have sufficient time and support to make an informed decision.
5) To Address Knowledge Gaps in Public Policy and Multidisciplinary Synergy: Encourage policymakers to actively engage with ethicists, medical professionals, and AI researchers to develop inclusive public policies for AI in medicine. At the academic and research level, foster more interdisciplinary collaborations, for example, between philosophy departments, medical schools, and computer science faculties. These collaborations should aim to integrate philosophical insights on ethics, educational strategies for medical professionals and patients, and technological expertise to create a more holistic approach to AI ethics in medicine.

EXISTING REGIONAL POLICIES DISCUSSION

Table 3. Existing regional policies of AI ethics in healthcare

Region	Policy Name	Authority	Year	Key AI Medical Ethics Provisions
EU	Ethics Guidelines for Trustworthy AI	EU High-Level Expert Group	2019	Proposes ethical principles for AI in healthcare: human oversight, safety, privacy, transparency, and fairness (non-binding guidelines).
	Medical Device Regulation (MDR)	European Commission	2021	Mandates clinical safety verification and data transparency disclosure for AI-driven medical devices.
	AI Act	European Commission	2024	Classifies medical AI as high-risk; mandates clinical validation, data quality audits, and real-time monitoring (passed in 2024).
USA	AI/ML-Based Software as a Medical Device Action Plan	FDA	2021	Requires dynamic algorithm monitoring, clinical validation, and user training for AI systems.
	NIH Guidelines for AI in Health Research	National Institutes of Health	2022	Emphasizes data privacy, algorithmic transparency, and patient involvement in research design (federal funding standards).
	Executive Order on Safe, Secure, and Trustworthy AI	White House	2023	Mandates fairness testing for medical AI and directs federal agencies to establish safety standards.
UK	NHS AI Lab Ethics Framework	NHSX	2020	Requires medical AI tools to undergo clinical efficacy and societal equity assessments.
	Health and Care Act 2022 (AI Provisions)	UK Parliament	2022	Establishes an AI regulatory framework, requiring dataset transparency and algorithmic audits.
	AI Safety Summit Outcomes	UK Government	2023	Publishes medical AI safety guidelines, emphasizing accountability and patient right to explanation.
Canada	Directive on Automated Decision-Making	Treasury Board of Canada	2019	Requires public healthcare AI systems to be transparent, appealable, and ethically reviewed.
	Artificial Intelligence and Data Act (AIDA)	Innovation, Science and Economic Development Canada	2022	Mandates real-time performance monitoring and safety certification for high-risk medical AI (under legislative process).
	CIHR Guidelines for AI in Health Research	Canadian Institutes of Health Research	2023	Highlights patient consent, data privacy, and algorithmic fairness in AI deployment.

Source: Compiled by the authors based on EU AI Act (2024), U.S. FDA AI/ML-Based Software as a Medical Device Action Plan (2021), UK Health and Care Act 2022, Canada's Artificial Intelligence and Data Act (2022), and related national AI policy documents from 2019-2024.

Comparing Ethical Instructions and Regional Policies

The integration of artificial intelligence (AI) into healthcare systems has prompted a global proliferation of ethical frameworks and regulatory policies, reflecting both the transformative potential and profound risks of these technologies. A comparative analysis of regional approaches reveals evolving attempts to balance innovation with patient safety and ethical accountability. The European Union's regulatory trajectory exemplifies this tension, progressing from non-binding ethical guidelines in 2019 to the legally enforceable AI Act of 2024, which categorizes medical AI as high-risk and mandates clinical validation, data quality audits, and real-time monitoring. This graduated approach mirrors broader international patterns where early ethical principles gradually crystallize into specific technical requirements, as seen in the U.S. FDA's 2021 action plan for algorithm monitoring and Canada's proposed Artificial Intelligence and Data Act (AIDA) with its safety certification mandates. However, these policies collectively underscore a critical gap between technical compliance and the philosophical underpinnings of medical ethics, necessitating deeper engagement with the moral dimensions of human-AI collaboration in care delivery.

The clustering of ethical recommendations exposes fundamental challenges that existing regulations inadequately address. While policies like the EU Medical Device Regulation (MDR) and UK Health and Care Act 2022 emphasize clinical safety and dataset transparency, they remain silent on the epistemological crisis emerging when AI diagnostic tools challenge physician judgment or when algorithmic predictions contradict patient lived experiences. This lacuna becomes particularly acute in surgical contexts, where proposed ethical guidelines for human override mechanisms must contend with the temporal realities of operating rooms – split-second decisions that defy post-hoc accountability frameworks. The NIH and CIHR guidelines' emphasis on patient involvement in research design points toward participatory ethics models, yet most current frameworks retain paternalistic structures that treat patients as data subjects rather than epistemic partners in AI development.

Multidisciplinary integration emerges as both a persistent challenge and potential solution. The UK AI Safety Summit's accountability guidelines and Canada's Directive on Automated Decision-Making implicitly recognize that algorithmic transparency alone cannot resolve value conflicts between efficiency-driven healthcare systems and patient autonomy imperatives. This necessitates the institutionalization of cross-disciplinary dialogue mechanisms that go beyond current academic collaborations, embedding ethicists and social scientists directly into regulatory bodies and clinical AI implementation teams. The NHS AI Lab Ethics Framework's requirement for societal equity assessments suggests a promising model, but its effectiveness hinges on operationalizing philosophical concepts like distributive justice into concrete audit parameters – a translation challenge that existing technical standards for bias detection inadequately address.

Ultimately, the evolving policy landscape reveals an uncomfortable truth: current ethical frameworks remain reactive adaptations to technological capabilities rather than proactive articulations of medicine's normative aspirations (Moodley, 2024). The White House's 2023 Executive Order on fairness testing and the EU's emphasis on human oversight gesture toward maintaining medicine's humanistic core, but they risk reducing ethical practice to compliance checklists. True integration requires reimagining medical education to cultivate "algorithmic literacy" among practitioners, redesigning informed consent processes as iterative dialogues about probabilistic AI outputs, and reconceptualizing patient autonomy in an era where treatment recommendations emerge from neural networks rather than solely human cognition. As international regulations converge on risk-based classification systems, the critical challenge lies in preserving medicine's moral dimensions while harnessing AI's analytical power—a balance demanding continuous negotiation between technological possibility, regulatory constraint, and the irreducible complexity of healing relationships.

Suggestions for ethical frameworks

The systematic design and implementation of ethical frameworks for AI-driven medical innovations necessitates a paradigm shift from fragmented regulatory compliance to culturally adaptive, epistemologically inclusive governance architectures. Current regional policies, while advancing critical safeguards—such as the EU AI Act's high-risk classification with clinical validation mandates (van Kolfschooten & van Oirschot, 2024) and Canada's proposed AIDA requirements for real-time monitoring—reveal a persistent disconnect between technical specifications and the lived ethical complexities of patient care. To bridge this gap, ethical frameworks must evolve into dynamic socio-technical ecosystems that harmonize three dimensions: context-sensitive policy integration, patient-centered epistemic justice, and embedded interdisciplinary praxis. These dimensions must address the knowledge gaps identified in cross-cultural ethical harmonization, long-term societal impacts, and global solution design while leveraging emerging trends in patient-centric governance and generative AI ethics.

A critical starting point lies in reconceptualizing regulatory interoperability. The EU's graduated approach—from non-binding guidelines (2019) to enforceable legislation (2024)—demonstrates the value of iterative policy maturation. However, its emphasis on risk classification risks oversimplifying ethical dilemmas inherent in AI's probabilistic outputs, particularly in underrepresented domains like geriatrics and palliative care. Integrating the UK Health and Care Act's algorithmic audit requirements with Canada's Directive on Automated Decision-Making could create a hybrid governance model where technical transparency (e.g. dataset disclosures) coexists with procedural justice mechanisms (e.g. patient appeal processes). For instance, the FDA's dynamic monitoring protocols could be augmented by the NHS AI Lab's societal equity assessments, operationalized through culturally calibrated bias detection algorithms that account for regional variations in healthcare access and ethical priorities. Such an approach would address the cross-cultural knowledge gap by embedding comparative ethical analyses—contrasting Western individualist autonomy with Eastern collectivist welfare principles—into algorithmic training datasets and regulatory review criteria.

At the heart of patient welfare protection lies the imperative to institutionalize epistemic pluralism in AI evaluation. Current policies like the NIH's patient involvement guidelines and the UK AI Safety Summit's emphasis on explanation rights remain constrained by paternalistic frameworks that treat patients as passive recipients rather than co-designers of AI systems. A transformative solution would involve participatory validation protocols, where AI diagnostic tools undergo dual validation: statistical accuracy testing and qualitative assessments by patient panels representing diverse illness experiences. For example, a diabetic patient's experiential knowledge of hypoglycemia symptoms could refine AI models trained solely on biochemical markers, addressing the under-researched psychological impacts of AI-driven diagnoses. This aligns with recommendations for patient education but extends them into co-creation mechanisms, such as AI interfaces that dynamically adjust explanations based on a patient's health literacy level, as suggested by CIHR's consent guidelines. Such interfaces could leverage generative AI to produce personalized educational content while incorporating verification mechanisms—akin to the EU MDR's transparency mandates—to prevent misinformation.

Operationalizing these principles demands embedded ethics infrastructure within healthcare institutions and AI development pipelines. The White House Executive Order's fairness testing requirements and Canada's AIDA safety certification processes could be reimagined through translational ethics units—permanent interdisciplinary teams comprising ethicists, clinicians, data scientists, and patient advocates. These units would serve dual functions: guiding real-time ethical adjustments during AI deployment (e.g. modifying surgical AI's error thresholds based on intraoperative human feedback) and conducting longitudinal studies on AI's societal impacts, such as trust erosion in marginalized communities. Drawing from the NHS's efficacy assessments, such units could develop ethic-technical benchmarks that quantify trade-offs between diagnostic speed and interpretability, informed by public deliberative forums as proposed in Canadian policies. For generative AI in mental health applications—a critically under-researched area—these units could establish accountability chains using blockchain-audited decision trails, ensuring clarity in liability distribution between developers, clinicians, and algorithms, as hinted at in the UK AI Safety Summit outcomes.

Ultimately, balancing innovation and welfare requires ethics as a generative design constraint rather than a post-hoc checkpoint. This necessitates reengineering medical AI development cycles to integrate ethical considerations at the architectural level. For instance, federated learning systems—which align with the EU's privacy principles—could be designed to inherently prioritize equity by weighting data from underrepresented populations more heavily during model training. Similarly, surgical AI systems could embed ethical circuit breakers that log override rationales during emergencies, creating datasets to refine both technical reliability and moral decision-making protocols. These innovations would operationalize bibliometric analysis derived recommendations for human override mechanisms while addressing the technical-social interdisciplinary gap through co-designed solutions.

The path forward hinges on global collaboration frameworks that transcend current regional fragmentation. Building on the AI Safety Summit's groundwork, an International Consortium for Medical AI Ethics could harmonize standards while preserving cultural specificity through subsidiary ethics committees. This consortium would maintain a living repository of failure modes and audit protocols, informed by mandatory incident reporting akin to aviation safety systems. By integrating the EU's risk-based approach, the US's dynamic monitoring ethos, and Canada's emphasis on appealability, such a framework would transform ethical compliance from a bureaucratic hurdle into a catalyst for innovation—ensuring AI's transformative potential serves not just clinical efficiency but medicine's enduring commitment to human dignity.

CONCLUSION

Contributions

This study makes three significant contributions to the evolving discourse on AI ethics in medicine. First, it addresses a critical gap in the literature by systematically analyzing the intersection of AI, ethics, and medical innovation—a triad that has been extensively studied in pairwise combinations (e.g. AI-ethics or AI-medicine) but rarely as an integrated framework. By employing Citespace-based bibliometric analysis, the research uncovers latent connections and thematic voids across 15 years of scholarship, revealing how fragmented discussions of algorithmic fairness, patient autonomy, and clinical efficacy coalesce into underrecognized ethical dilemmas unique to AI-driven healthcare. More critically, our findings underscore the imperative to reframe health technologies as tools for global equity rather than mere efficiency enhancers.

Second, the study advances beyond theoretical debates by translating publication trends map, dominant thematic clusters, burst terms maps and timeline charts into actionable ethical guidelines tailored for real-world implementation. These guidelines bridge the gap between abstract principles (e.g. transparency) and technical execution (e.g. real-time monitoring protocols), offering policymakers and developers a roadmap to operationalize ethics across AI's lifecycle. This approach aligns with recent calls for "ethics-by-design" frameworks in global health technologies, ensuring that innovations like AI-enabled diagnostic tools are culturally adapted to avoid exacerbating inequities in low- and middle-income countries.

Third, the research reveals an urgent need for "Global localization (glocal)" governance models that harmonize global ethical standards with local sociotechnical realities and provides a cross-cultural policy analysis, contrasting regional frameworks like the EU's risk-based AI Act with North America's emphasis on dynamic compliance, thereby identifying transferable strategies for harmonizing ethical standards without stifling innovation. For example, integrating Western algorithmic transparency mandates with Eastern emphasis on systemic governance could foster AI systems that address both individual rights and collective welfare in diverse contexts. By grounding its findings in both bibliometric trends and regulatory realities, the study equips stakeholders to navigate the tension between technological ambition and ethical restraint.

Fourth, the unresolved tension between AI's efficiency gains and medicine's humanistic ethos calls for a redefinition of success metrics in healthcare innovation. Current frameworks, including the U.S. FDA's emphasis on clinical validation and the UK's algorithmic audits, predominantly measure technical efficacy rather than ethical impact. To bridge this gap, ethical-technical benchmarks should be developed, quantifying outcomes such as trust erosion in marginalized communities or longitudinal patient autonomy preservation. These metrics, informed by the study's identified knowledge gaps in societal impacts, could be integrated into regulatory approval processes, incentivizing developers to prioritize equity alongside accuracy. For instance, AI diagnostic tools seeking market approval could be required to demonstrate not only 95% accuracy but also evidence of reducing disparities in misdiagnosis rates across racial or socioeconomic groups.

This study further contributes to the discourse by pioneering a methodological synthesis that bridges bibliometric rigor with policy-relevant insights. Unlike prior works that treat technical, ethical, and clinical dimensions in isolation, our triadic framework operationalizes their interdependence through actionable metrics. For instance, the integration of WoS and CNKI datasets not only maps regional disparities but also identifies synergistic ethical priorities, such as combining Western algorithmic accountability mechanisms with Eastern systemic governance models. This approach offers policymakers a blueprint for designing hybrid regulations that respect cultural specificity while advancing global equity—a critical need as AI permeates diverse healthcare ecosystems.

Additionally, the research introduces novel evaluative criteria for ethical AI deployment, such as longitudinal trust metrics and patient autonomy indices, which transcend conventional compliance-based assessments. By embedding these metrics into regulatory frameworks—e.g., requiring AI tools to demonstrate reductions in diagnostic disparities alongside accuracy—the study redefines success in healthcare innovation. Furthermore, the emphasis on participatory validation protocols challenges the status quo by positioning patients as co-designers rather than passive beneficiaries, fostering inclusive AI development. These contributions collectively advance the vision of AI as a tool for humanistic medicine, where technological progress and ethical imperatives evolve in tandem.

The path forward is neither linear nor prescriptive. It demands humility to recognize that ethical frameworks will perpetually lag behind technological capabilities, yet courage to insist that innovation serves humanity's highest aspirations. As AI reshapes the boundaries of medical possibility, the lessons from this study—rooted in bibliometric rigor and policy analysis—must catalyze a paradigm shift from ethics as constraint to ethics as compass. Only then can we ensure that the algorithms guiding tomorrow's healthcare decisions embody not just computational intelligence, but moral wisdom.

Limitations

While this study provides critical insights into the ethical challenges of AI-driven medical innovations, several limitations underscore the need for cautious interpretation and future refinement. First, the bibliometric methodology, though robust in mapping scholarly trends, inherently prioritizes quantifiable patterns over qualitative nuances. By relying on CiteSpace's keyword clustering and citation networks, the analysis may inadvertently marginalize emerging or unconventional ethical discourses that lack established terminology or citation traction. For instance, grassroots initiatives in low-resource settings advocating for community-centric AI governance—often published in non-indexed regional journals or gray literature—are underrepresented in WoS and CNKI. This omission risks reinforcing a Eurocentric and Sinocentric bias in ethical discourse, overlooking indigenous epistemologies that could enrich global frameworks. Furthermore, the exclusion of non-English and non-Chinese publications (e.g., African or South American scholarship) limits the study's cross-cultural validity, as ethical priorities in these regions—such as oral consent traditions or collective decision-making—remain unaddressed.

Second, the 2010–2025 timeframe introduces methodological ambiguities. While the inclusion of publications up to 2025 aims to capture emergent trends, the predictive classification of post-2023 literature remains speculative. Rapid advancements in generative AI, quantum computing, and neurosymbolic systems—developments that could radically redefine medical ethics—are not yet fully reflected in academic databases. For example, the ethical implications of AI systems capable of real-time genetic editing or brain-computer interfaces, emerging post-2023, are absent from the analysis. This temporal gap underscores the challenge of maintaining ethical frameworks' relevance in an era of exponential technological change.

Third, the proposed ethical guidelines, though theoretically grounded, lack empirical validation. The absence of case studies in diverse healthcare ecosystems—ranging from high-income hospitals with advanced AI infrastructure to LMIC clinics reliant on intermittent connectivity—limits the framework's operational applicability. For instance, recommendations for "participatory validation protocols" assume equitable access to digital literacy and stakeholder engagement mechanisms, which may be unfeasible in regions with entrenched power imbalances or limited internet access. Without testing these guidelines in contexts where cultural hierarchies or resource scarcity dominate (e.g., patriarchal societies where patients defer to clinicians), their universal feasibility remains unproven. Similarly, the emphasis on blockchain-audited decision trails and real-time monitoring presupposes institutional capacity and funding, ignoring infrastructural barriers in under-resourced settings.

Fourth, while the study acknowledges cross-cultural ethical divergences, it insufficiently addresses how structural inequities—such as global digital divides or colonial legacies in healthcare—constrain the implementation of "glocalized" frameworks. For example, AI systems designed with Western transparency standards may clash with LMIC realities where data privacy laws are underdeveloped or unenforced. Moreover, the analysis does not critically examine the geopolitical dynamics influencing ethical standardization. Dominant AI governance narratives, often shaped by high-income countries, risk perpetuating neocolonial patterns where LMICs adopt externally imposed frameworks ill-suited to local realities. The study's reliance on WoS and CNKI data inadvertently mirrors this asymmetry, as both platforms disproportionately represent scholarship from economically powerful regions.

These limitations collectively highlight the tension between theoretical rigor and real-world applicability. Future research must prioritize empirical, context-sensitive validation of ethical guidelines, engage underrepresented voices in framework co-creation, and establish agile governance structures that evolve alongside AI's trajectory. Only through such iterative, inclusive efforts can ethical frameworks transcend academic idealism to meaningfully safeguard patient welfare in a digitized medical landscape.

REFERENCES

Adhikari, S., Ahmed, I., Bajracharya, D., Khanal, B., Solomon, C., Jayaratne, K., Al Mamum, K. A., Talukder, M. S. H., Shakya, S., Manandhar, S., & Memon, Z. A. (2025). Transforming healthcare through just, equitable and quality driven artificial intelligence solutions in South Asia. *NPJ Digital Medicine*, *8*(1), 139. Advance online publication. DOI: 10.1038/s41746-025-01534-0 PMID: 40038520

Barragan-Montero, A., Javaid, U., Valdes, G., Nguyen, D., Desbordes, P., Macq, B., Willems, S., Vandewinckele, L., Holmstrom, M., Lofman, F., Michiels, S., Souris, K., Sterpin, E., & Lee, J. A. (2021). Artificial intelligence and machine learning for medical imaging: A technology review. *Physica Medica : PM : An International Journal Devoted to the Applications of Physics to Medicine and Biology : Official Journal of the Italian Association of Biomedical Physics (AIFB)*, *83*, 242–256. DOI: 10.1016/j.ejmp.2021.04.016 PMID: 33979715

Bouderhem, R. (2024). Shaping the future of AI in healthcare through ethics and governance. *Humanities & Social Sciences Communications*, *11*(1), 416. Advance online publication. DOI: 10.1057/s41599-024-02894-w

Cath, C. (2018). Governing artificial intelligence: ethical, legal and technical opportunities and challenges Introduction [Editorial Material]. *Philosophical Transactions of the Royal Society a-Mathematical Physical and Engineering Sciences, 376*(2133), 8, Article 20180080. https://doi.org/DOI: 10.1098/rsta.2018.0080

Char, D. S., Shah, N. H., & Magnus, D. (2018). Implementing Machine Learning in Health Care - Addressing Ethical Challenges. *The New England Journal of Medicine*, *378*(11), 981–983. DOI: 10.1056/NEJMp1714229 PMID: 29539284

Chen, C. (2016). *CiteSpace: A Practical Guide for Mapping Scientific Literature*. CiteSpace: A Practical Guide for Mapping Scientific Literature.

Chen, C. (2020). How to Use CiteSpace (c) 2015-2020.

Chen, C. M. (2006). CiteSpace II: Detecting and visualizing emerging trends and transient patterns in scientific literature. *Journal of the American Society for Information Science and Technology*, *57*(3), 359–377. DOI: 10.1002/asi.20317

Chin, M. H., Afsar-Manesh, N., Bierman, A. S., Chang, C. S. E., Colón-Rodríguez, C. J., Dullabh, P., Duran, D. G., Fair, M., Hernandez-Boussard, T., Hightower, M., Jain, A., Jordan, W. B., Konya, S., Moore, R. H., Moore, T. T., Rodriguez, R., Shaheen, G., Snyder, L. P., Srinivasan, M., & Ohno-Machado, L. (2023). Guiding Principles to Address the Impact of Algorithm Bias on Racial and Ethnic Disparities in Health and Health Care. *JAMA Network Open*, *6*(12), e2345050. Advance online publication. DOI: 10.1001/jamanetworkopen.2023.45050 PMID: 38100101

Dalton-Brown, S. (2020). The Ethics of Medical AI and the Physician-Patient Relationship. *Cambridge Quarterly of Healthcare Ethics, 29*(1), 115-121, Article Pii s0963180119000847. https://doi.org/DOI: 10.1017/S0963180119000847

Ding, X., & Yang, Z. (2022). Knowledge mapping of platform research: A visual analysis using VOSviewer and CiteSpace. *Electronic Commerce Research*, *22*(3), 787–809. DOI: 10.1007/s10660-020-09410-7

Drew, D. A., Nguyen, L. H., Steves, C. J., Menni, C., Freydin, M., Varsavsky, T., Sudre, C. H., Cardoso, M. J., Ourselin, S., Wolf, J., Spector, T. D., & Chan, A. T. (2020). Rapid implementation of mobile technology for real-time epidemiology of COVID-19. *Science, 368*(6497), 1362-+. https://doi.org/DOI: 10.1126/science.abc0473

Federico, C. A., & Trotsyuk, A. A. (2024). Biomedical Data Science, Artificial Intelligence, and Ethics: Navigating Challenges in the Face of Explosive Growth. *Annual Review of Biomedical Data Science*, *7*(1), 104553. Advance online publication. DOI: 10.1146/annurev-biodatasci-102623-104553 PMID: 38598860

Gaviria-Marin, M., Merigó, J. M., & Baier-Fuentes, H. (2019). Knowledge management: A global examination based on bibliometric analysis. *Technological Forecasting and Social Change*, *140*, 194–220. DOI: 10.1016/j.techfore.2018.07.006

Geng, Y. Q., Xiang, Q. J., Gao, J. A., Yan, Y., & Li, J. Y. (2024). Progress and framework of clean energy production: Bibliometric analysis from 2002 to 2022. *Energy Strategy Reviews*, *52*, 101270. Advance online publication. DOI: 10.1016/j.esr.2023.101270

Gerke, S., Yeung, S. R., & Cohen, I. G. (2020). Ethical and Legal Aspects of Ambient Intelligence in Hospitals. *Journal of the American Medical Association*, *323*(7), 601–602. DOI: 10.1001/jama.2019.21699 PMID: 31977033

Goirand, M., Austin, E., & Clay-Williams, R. (2021). Implementing Ethics in Healthcare AI-Based Applications: A Scoping Review. *Science and Engineering Ethics*, *27*(5), 61. Advance online publication. DOI: 10.1007/s11948-021-00336-3 PMID: 34480239

Manyazewal, T., Woldeamanuel, Y., Blumberg, H. M., Fekadu, A., & Marconi, V. C. (2021). The potential use of digital health technologies in the African context: A systematic review of evidence from Ethiopia. *NPJ Digital Medicine*, *4*(1), 125. Advance online publication. DOI: 10.1038/s41746-021-00487-4 PMID: 34404895

McLennan, S., Fiske, A., Tigard, D., Müller, R., Haddadin, S., & Buyx, A. (2022). Embedded ethics: A proposal for integrating ethics into the development of medical AI. *BMC Medical Ethics*, *23*(1), 6. Advance online publication. DOI: 10.1186/s12910-022-00746-3 PMID: 35081955

Merigó, J. M., & Yang, J. B. (2017). A bibliometric analysis of operations research and management science. *Omega*, *73*, 37–48. DOI: 10.1016/j.omega.2016.12.004

Mittelstadt, B. (2019). Principles alone cannot guarantee ethical AI. *Nature Machine Intelligence*, *1*(11), 501–507. DOI: 10.1038/s42256-019-0114-4

Moodley, K. (2024). Artificial intelligence (AI) or augmented intelligence? How big data and AI are transforming healthcare: Challenges and opportunities. *Samj South African Medical Journal*, *114*(1), 16–20. DOI: 10.7196/SAMJ.2024.v114i2.1631 PMID: 38525617

Obermeyer, Z., Powers, B., Vogeli, C., & Mullainathan, S. (2019). Dissecting racial bias in an algorithm used to manage the health of populations. *Science, 366*(6464), 447-+, Article aax2342. https://doi.org/DOI: 10.1126/science.aax2342

Ploug, T., & Holm, S. (2020). The four dimensions of contestable AI diagnostics - A patient-centric approach to explainable AI. *Artificial Intelligence in Medicine*, *107*, 101901. Advance online publication. DOI: 10.1016/j.artmed.2020.101901 PMID: 32828448

Rajkomar, A., Hardt, M., Howell, M. D., Corrado, G., & Chin, M. H. (2018). Ensuring Fairness in Machine Learning to Advance Health Equity. *Annals of Internal Medicine, 169*(12), 866-+. https://doi.org/DOI: 10.7326/M18-1990

Reddy, S., Allan, S., Coghlan, S., & Cooper, P. (2020). A governance model for the application of AI in health care. *Journal of the American Medical Informatics Association : JAMIA*, *27*(3), 491–497. DOI: 10.1093/jamia/ocz192 PMID: 31682262

Saheb, T., Saheb, T., & Carpenter, D. O. (2021). Mapping research strands of ethics of artificial intelligence in healthcare: A bibliometric and content analysis. *Computers in Biology and Medicine*, *135*, 104660. Advance online publication. DOI: 10.1016/j.compbiomed.2021.104660 PMID: 34346319

Su, X., Li, X., & Kang, Y. (2019). A Bibliometric Analysis of Research on Intangible Cultural Heritage Using CiteSpace. *SAGE Open, 2019*(4). https://doi.org/doi: DOI: 10.1177/2158244019840119

Topol, E. J. (2019). High-performance medicine: The convergence of human and artificial intelligence. *Nature Medicine, 25*(1), 44–56. DOI: 10.1038/s41591-018-0300-7 PMID: 30617339

Tuzov, V., & Lin, F. (2024). Two paths of balancing technology and ethics: A comparative study on AI governance in China and Germany. *Telecommunications Policy, 48*(10), 102850. Advance online publication. DOI: 10.1016/j.telpol.2024.102850

van Kolfschooten, H., & van Oirschot, J. (2024). The EU Artificial Intelligence Act (2024): Implications for healthcare. *Health Policy (Amsterdam), 149*, 105152. Advance online publication. DOI: 10.1016/j.healthpol.2024.105152 PMID: 39244818

Varnosfaderani, S. M., & Forouzanfar, M. (2024). The Role of AI in Hospitals and Clinics: Transforming Healthcare in the 21st Century. *Bioengineering (Basel, Switzerland), 11*(4), 337. Advance online publication. DOI: 10.3390/bioengineering11040337 PMID: 38671759

Wang, C. Y., Liu, S. R., Yang, H., Guo, J. L., Wu, Y. X., & Liu, J. L. (2023). Ethical Considerations of Using ChatGPT in Health Care. *Journal of Medical Internet Research, 25*, e48009. Advance online publication. DOI: 10.2196/48009 PMID: 37566454

Wang, Y., Li, Y., Chen, Y., Lu, S., & Yu, P. (2024). The Role of Emerging Technologies in Modernizing the Healthcare Industry: Case Studies from China. *European Academic Journal - II CHINA, 1*(1). https://eaj.ebujournals.lu/index.php/EAJ_II/article/view/112

Yu, P., Lu, S., Long, Z., Chen, Y., Qian, J., & Shah, Z. A. (2024). Exploring Ethical Considerations in Utilizing Generative AI for Global Knowledge Sharing in Higher Education. In Yu, P., Mulli, J., Syed, Z. A. S., & Umme, L. (Eds.), *Facilitating Global Collaboration and Knowledge Sharing in Higher Education With Generative AI* (pp. 1–27). IGI Global., DOI: 10.4018/979-8-3693-0487-7.ch001

Yu, P., & Xu, Y. (2022). Public-Private Partnership for Healthcare in China: The Effectiveness on the Regional Cities of Healthcare Service. In Akkaya, B., Jermsittiparsert, K., & Gunsel, A. (Eds.), *Handbook of Research on Current Trends in Asian Economics, Business, and Administration* (pp. 328–348). IGI Global., DOI: 10.4018/978-1-7998-8486-6.ch018

Yu, P., Xue, W., & Mahendran, R. (2022). The Development and Impact of China's Digital Transformation in the Medical Industry. In Rodrigues, M. A., & Proença, J. F. (Eds.), *Impact of Digital Transformation on the Development of New Business Models and Consumer Experience* (pp. 97–128). IGI Global., DOI: 10.4018/978-1-7998-9179-6.ch006

Zhuang, Q. D., Hussein, M. K., Ariffin, N. F. M., & Yunos, M. Y. M. (2022). Landscape character: A knowledge mapping analysis using CiteSpace. *International Journal of Environmental Science and Technology*, *19*(10), 10477–10492. DOI: 10.1007/s13762-022-04279-5

Chapter 10

The Regulatory Challenges From the Intersection of AI and Blockchain Technology in Healthcare:

A Case Study of BurstIQ

Eleftheria Panagiotopoulou
http://orcid.org/0009-0006-5218-8481
University College London, UK

Mohan P. M. Mishra
FinJuris, UAE

ABSTRACT

Artificial intelligence (AI) and blockchain convergence is a paradigm shift in the current delivery of healthcare services, essentially changing how medical information is processed, secured, and used in any clinical setting around the globe. The once optional intersection is progressively becoming a necessity to build scalable, ethical, patient-centric digital health systems. This chapter uses a qualitative methodology – focusing on the case study of BurstIQ – to examine the regulatory challenges that arise from this convergence. The findings reveal that AI-blockchain systems introduce an unprecedented level of regulatory complexity that current frameworks are ill-equipped to deal with. The incorporation process demands trust in the systems, construction compliance, and stakeholders' active involvement. This chapter

DOI: 10.4018/979-8-2600-2238-2.ch010

proposes a unified governance paradigm in which AI-blockchain is regulated as interconnected architectures, prioritising privacy-preserving and compliant infrastructure that allows innovation while maintaining existing regulatory relationships.

1. INTRODUCTION

A convergence of artificial intelligence (AI) and blockchain in healthcare represents a transformational evolution with far-reaching consequences for the global medical landscape. Both of these two cutting-edge technologies, one unique for its capabilities and one not so unique but remarkable for its ability to excel at its one capability, are being increasingly used in concert to solve problems that are long-standing for healthcare delivery, data management and system security. This is because AI has developed complex analytical models for diagnostic, predictive analytics and automation in decision making, whereas blockchain has enabled immutable, transparent and secure information exchange (Bathula et al., 2024). The once optional intersection is progressively becoming a necessity to build scalable, ethical, patient-driven digital health systems.

The complementary strengths of AI and blockchain are both dawning simultaneously. Blockchain proposes certain mechanisms for securing high-quality, large volumes of data utilised by AI with integrity, traceability and decentralisation (Al-abdulatif et al., 2022). The synergy among the components of this system supports real-time diagnostics, remote patient monitoring and decentralised data governance, building trust among patients, providers and regulators (Saeed et al., 2022). The datasets used by AI models are secure through the security offered by blockchain, and provenance and auditability are required in sensitive use cases such as clinical trials and Electronic Health Records (EHRs) (Tahir et al., 2024). By pairing these two up, it moves from a technical synergy to a systemic one for using health information.

Nevertheless, with opportunity comes regulatory tension between innovation and compliance. Among the sectors subject to the highest degree of global regulatory scrutiny, healthcare requires new technologies to conform to well-defined ethical, patient safety and data protection standards. AI models, specifically deep learning algorithms, often work as a black box due to the lack of explainability, accountability, and how bias can be mitigated (Hassija et al., 2023). Although immutability is valuable for tamper- resistance, blockchain directly clashes with laws such as the European General Data Protection Regulation (GDPR) that codify the right to be forgotten (Tandon et al., 2020). There is a need for a regulatory approach that balances the innovation curtailment mindset with the desire to protect public health interests.

The healthcare sector has been selected as a focal domain for the convergence of AI and blockchain, particularly due to the intrinsic nature of the features of the sector. First, it is considerably data-intensive. Vast amounts of data are generated by all healthcare systems from numerous sources (electronic records, imaging systems, genomics, wearable technologies). The heterogeneity of such data demands robust systems for data curation, privacy and interoperability. Blockchain's decentralised consensus (i.e., the rule of agreeing in a network) and smart contracts (i.e., automated digital contracts) provide a safe and traceable manner for health data transactions, and likewise, AI can analyse these health data for diagnostics and prediction (Sun et al., 2022). Second, healthcare is critical in life. In this domain, any type of technological error can have catastrophic implications. As such, any digital system should, at the least, be highly resilient, transparent and reasonably ethically validated. The speed and adaptability of AI, combined with the strength of data lineage with blockchain and cryptographic assurance, and traceable data lineage, make it vital for early detection in emergencies along with decision support (Agbo et al., 2019). The interplay in this system improves both clinical precision, which is very important in situations such as pandemics or critical care units, and system reliability. Third, healthcare also plays a sensitive role ethically. Matters relating to data consent, patient rights, equal access and unfair treatment by algorithms are significant areas in the discussion of digital health technology.

With blockchain, patients can control their access to their medical data and designers of AI solutions should be careful not to repeat or make health inequities even greater (Tahir et al., 2024). By using cryptography and AI ethics, these technologies are designed to help future digital health systems promote fairness. This convergence has significant effects everywhere in the world. Health institutions worldwide that deal with elderly populations, frequent health issues and post-pandemic recovery need steadier support based on strong, new digital infrastructures (Stoumpos et al., 2023). Experts have seen nations exploring regulatory sandboxes to work with AI and blockchain at the same time. However, there are still significant challenges in creating laws that treat them as part of the same system (Alabdulatif et al., 2022; Bathula et al., 2024). In particular, emerging economies could move past their typical infrastructure challenges by adopting mobile health, telemedicine and data exchange linked to AI-blockchain.

This chapter employs a qualitative study methodology to examine the multifaceted regulatory challenges arising from the intersection of AI and blockchain technology in healthcare applications, with the aim of developing concepts and policy lessons from a single rich case — BurstIQ —and not to claim that the findings are numerically representative of all firms. More specifically, BurstIQ is used to examine how companies that combine these technologies navigate current regulatory frameworks while balancing innovation and compliance. BurstIQ is a leading US-based provider of network data solutions in healthcare, leveraging both blockchain and AI to offer secure, ethical, and interoperable data ecosystems (BurstIQ, 2025a). A concise overview of the company is presented in Table 1.

Table 1. BurstIQ Snapshot: Blockchain and AI in Healthcare

Attribute	Summary
Founded	2015 in Denver, Colorado (USA)
Nature of Business	Private—health technology company. It provides secure, interoperable health data exchange. Its flagship platform is LifeGraph —a permissioned blockchain network linking patients, providers, and researchers through tokenised data ownership.
Core Technologies	Blockchain and AI
Governance Model	Patient-driven data control using cryptographic keys
Regulatory Alignment	Designed to support HIPAA, GDPR, HITECH
Primary Use Cases	Insurer data management, clinical research sharing and life-science collaboration

The analysis draws on two primary sources of evidence, including firstly official regulatory frameworks such as GDPR, HIPAA, the EU AI Act and the NIST AI risk management framework, and secondly a semi-structured expert interview conducted (in 2025 – anonymised) with a senior representative from BurstIQ to validate the platform-level regulatory navigation. By using this mixed-source methodological approach, triangulation of regulatory theory, practical implementation and organisational experience was achieved, offering grounded insights into the governance complexities of AI and blockchain in healthcare. The chapter commences by providing an overview of the technological and regulatory dimensions of AI and blockchain in healthcare. It subsequently examines the in-depth case study of BurstIQ to evaluate real-world implementation, compliance approaches and challenges.

2. TECHNOLOGICAL OVERVIEW

2.1 Blockchain in Healthcare

2.1.1 Introduction to Blockchain

Blockchain is a public ledger with all transactions stored in a list of blocks, with key features including decentralisation, persistence, pseudonymity and automatability (Zheng et al., 2017). Distributed ledger technology is the foundation of blockchain, offering a consensus mechanism through a network of computers, facilitating peer-to-peer transactions without the need for a centralised authority to update and maintain information generated by the transactions. Blockchain offers in healthcare applications a strong structure for streamlined healthcare data management operations, ensuring that treatment histories, patient data and clinical transactions can be recorded immutably and accessed transparently, through decentralised storage, immutability, transparency and flexible data access (Al Omar et al., 2019; Esposito et al., 2018; Hasselgren et al., 2020). Thus, this enhances trust and reduces data manipulation across institutions and providers (Chukwu & Garg, 2020).

The two main types of blockchain are permissioned and permissionless. A permissioned or private blockchain, in which only approved participants can join and validate, is typically controlled by an organisation or a group. It is increasingly utilised in healthcare. Permissionless blockchains are public, allowing anyone to join, use, or help maintain them (Michael et al., 2018).

In blockchain, asymmetric cryptography mechanisms are used to ensure the authenticity of transactions, with each user holding a pair of cryptographic keys: a private (i.e., highly confidential) key and a public key (Zheng et al., 2017). This mechanism in healthcare enables both patients and clinicians to digitally sign consent forms, prescriptions, or record updates, ensuring that each action is verifiable and non-repudiable.

In healthcare environments, consensus choice is governed less by latency alone and more by finality, governance, particularly validator accountability and privacy-law-aligned auditability. Table 4 (see Appendix) summarises various mechanisms for achieving consensus among nodes that are occasionally "untrustworthy" in blockchain networks and their applicability to healthcare.

2.1.2 The Layered Architecture of Blockchain

Blockchain is predominantly structured into two models: an ecosystem-based approach with layers ranked from 0 to 3, and a protocol stack approach showing how the technology functions end-to-end from physical devices to user interfaces (Birje et al., 2022) (Figure 1). Ecosystem-Based Model blockchain systems are designed with a layered architecture that organises software systems into multiple levels, with each level responsible for different functions, ranging from low-level commitment and consensus protocols to high-level application interfaces, providing significant benefits in scalability, modularity, security, and interoperability. This is highly significant in the healthcare context as it enhances scalability, interoperability and security, given the high volume of sensitive data that needs to be exchanged across different systems, institutions, and jurisdictions. The Protocol Stack Model, on the other hand, is similar to the OSI networking model, including the Hardware, Data, Network, Consensus, and Application layers.

Figure 1. Blockchain Layered Architecture for Healthcare Systems With Policy Interfaces

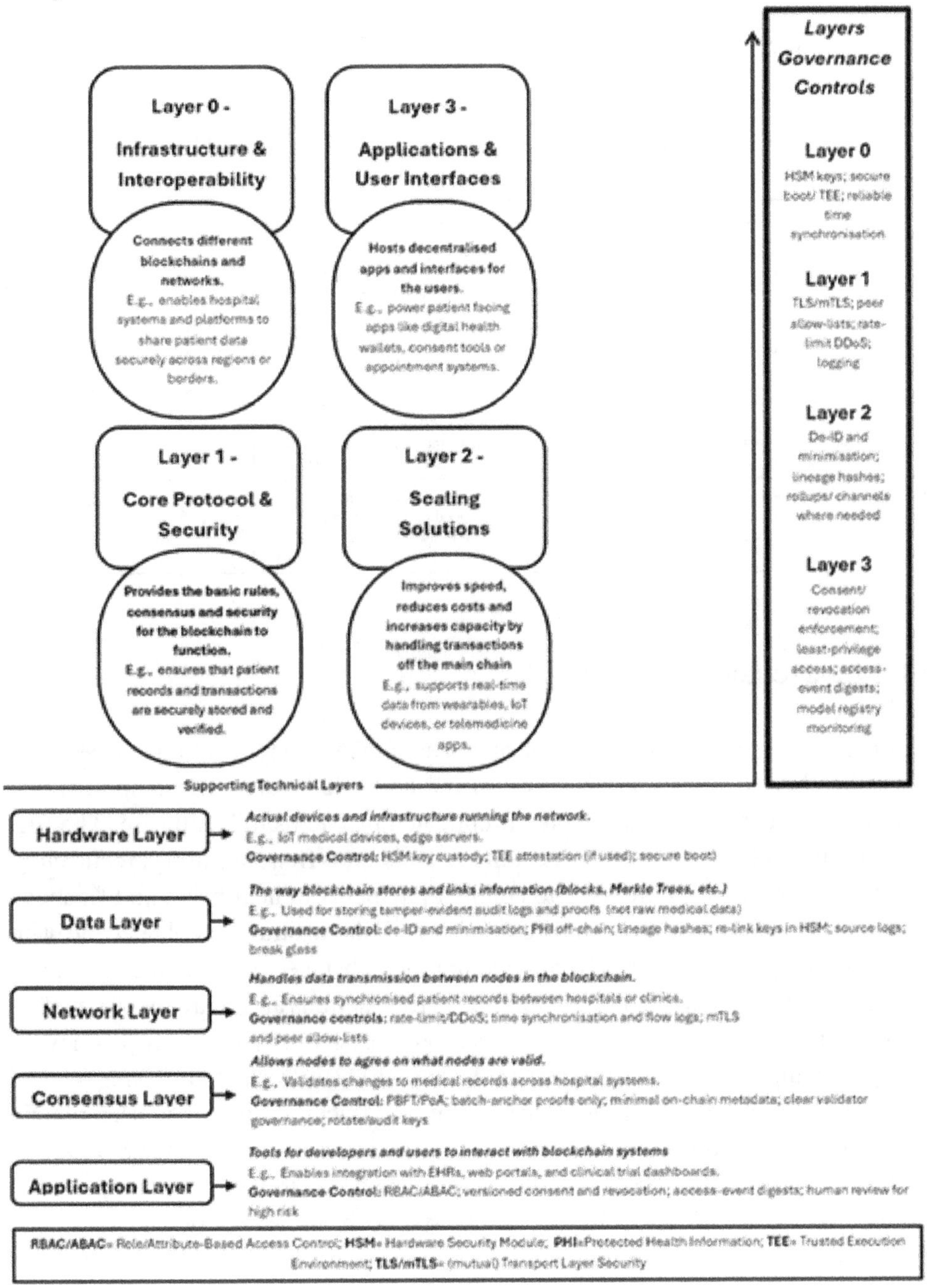

Table 2 maps the technical layers presented in Figure 1 to governance steps and audit artefacts, specifying the decision that needs to be made in each layer, and the evidence retained on (i.e., proof on the ledger) and off (i.e., documents stored privately) the chain.

Table 2. Healthcare Layered Governance: Actions, Evidence (Off-chain), Proofs (On-Chain)

	Decision to Set	**Evidence Retained (off-chain)**	**Proofs Recorded (on-chain)**
L0	Key-custody establishment; clock-synchronisation policies	Key inventory; rotation records; time-synchronisation reports; secure-start/attestation report	N/A
L1	What evidence is recorded, and how often needs to be defined; connections only from approved peers over encrypted links should be allowed	Approved-peer list; certificate register; connection/flow logs; recording and anchoring manifest	Consent-receipt IDs; access-event digests (e.g., who, when, purpose); policy/version hashes
L2	Before sharing, require de-identification and data minimisation; each model/dataset should be assigned a verifiable lineage fingerprint	De-identification method; risk review; lineage register; controlled re-link /key custody note	Dataset/model lineage hashes
L3	Version consent with revocation should be enforced; brief access summaries for audit; least-privilege access; register and monitor AI models where used	Consent records and revocation trail; model cards with validation/ monitoring reports; access logs	Consent-receipt IDs; model-artefact hash; access-event digests

2.1.3 Blockchain Evolution

Since its invention, the history of blockchain technology has transformed how data is handled in healthcare, because of the multiple levels of development that have been achieved in solving more complicated problems in healthcare. The first version of the technology was Blockchain 1.0, which was first used in cryptocurrency, where digital currencies are used to conduct payments in healthcare and financial activities of medical systems (Khezr et al., 2019). This substrate established the principle of cryptography that will be applied in more advanced levels in the healthcare sector. Cryptocurrencies enable decentralised transactions and share many benefits, including but not limited to lower transaction fees, security and transparency on money tracking and anonymity (Zakarneh et al., 2022). Blockchain 1.0 has several applications across different industries, but in Healthcare, it has been used mainly for payments and transaction monitoring, from companies such as the "My Doctor Medical Group" in San Francisco, allowing its patients to pay, for example, with Bitcoin (My Doctor Medical Group, 2021). Despite the great benefits of Blockchain 1.0, it also faced significant challenges, including but not limited to high investment risk and volatility (Zakarneh et al., 2022). Bitcoin's limited resources could no longer meet the general application requirements, with the high demand for transition to decentralisation, signifying the introduction of Ethereum and Blockchain

2.0, which addressed many of Bitcoin's scripting deficiencies such as consistency, openness, fast transactions, paperless operations, and elimination of a vast network of intermediaries (Raskin, 2016).

Blockchain 2.0 applications and smart contracts are used in healthcare to tokenise patient records, automating insurance claims. Smart contracts have been especially useful in managing consents by calling up immutability and transparency in a fair agreement between patients and healthcare providers, which satisfy compliance rules and preserve patient autonomy. For example, MediBloc is a patient data access and decentralised clinical pathway (MediBloc Limited, 2025). Blockchain 2.0, although sharing many benefits compared to Blockchain 1.0, faces challenges such as scalability issues, high gas fees, as well as being exposed to transaction vulnerabilities and privacy concerns (Vukoli, 2017). Despite the Blockchain 2.0 advancements, the demand for scalability and interoperability led to the creation of Layer 2 solutions (e.g., rollups) and Layer 0 frameworks (e.g., Polkadot), opening the way for the Blockchain 3.0 era.

The emergence of Blockchain 3.0-5.0 has seen remarkable innovations in areas of decentralised finance (DeFi), creation of health insurance, central bank digital currencies (CBDCs) in dispensing government health payments, and asset tokens such as intellectual property and medical equipment (Shaikh et al., 2025). These advances have led to end-to-end ecosystems allowing health stakeholders to enter into safe, transparent financial transactions and comply with regulations. Blockchain in healthcare has also proved exceptionally efficient in various realms. One of the key applications is medical record integrity and access control because blockchain provides an immutable ledger that guarantees data authenticity and the ability to grant access on a granular basis (Bathula et al., 2024). Tracking drugs and vaccines in supply chains has been relatively successful, with solutions such as BRUINChain already demonstrating a 100 per cent traceability and counterfeit detection rate (Shaikh et al., 2025). Moreover, self-sovereign identity systems have also enabled patients to own their data, which has changed the paradigm of provider-controlled systems to a patient-driven system.

2.1.4 Blockchain Applications in Healthcare

Building on the classifications proposed by Haleem et al. (2021) and Attaran (2022) blockchain applications in healthcare can be structured into five thematic areas, including (i) health data management and record keeping; (ii) clinical research and evidence generation; (iii) security, safety and validation; (iv) patient monitoring and access control; (v) and operational efficiency and financial management (Figure 2). For health data management and record keeping, blockchain offers features such as storing individual patient information, maintaining health records, minimising data transformation, and displaying information. For instance, healthcare providers can seamlessly match patient records, including lab tests, assessments or surveys, to the original tamper-proof version stored in blockchain, thus enhancing the integrity and verification of clinical study data (Aggarwal et al., 2021; De Aguiar et al., 2020; Ejaz et al., 2021). For clinical research and evidence generation, blockchain can offer features such as analysing the effects of a particular procedure, supporting clinical trials and creating research initiatives. For instance, blockchain in clinical trials is used to prevent false results and fragmented data misaligned with research objectives, thus improving trust and integrity in clinical trials (Gökalp et al., 2018; Leeming et al., 2019). Blockchain in healthcare, as one of its fundamental features, offers safety, transparency, security and identification of false content, addressing medication validity, and drug traceability problems (Nguyen et al., 2021; Tandon et al., 2020). Last but not least, blockchain in healthcare can help with patient monitoring by enabling secure, real-time monitoring of medical equipment availability, bed usage, room conditions, and supply levels (Mamoshina et al., 2017; Ray et al., 2020).

Figure 2. Blockchain Applications in Healthcare and Challenges.

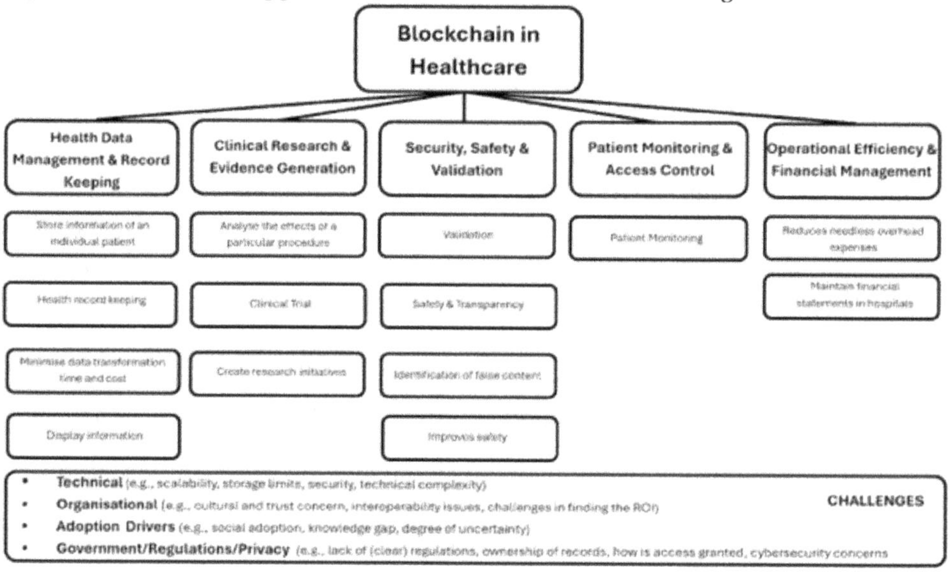

Despite its promising features, the application of blockchain in healthcare is constrained by a series of technical challenges such as scalability, storage limits, security and technical capabilities issues (Gordon & Catalini, 2018; Ichikawa et al., 2017); organisational, such as cultural and trust concerns, interoperability and challenges in finding the ROI (Deloitte, 2016; Roehrs et al., 2017); adoption drivers, such as social adoption, knowledge gap, degree of uncertainty; regulation-government and privacy issues, including the lack of (clear) regulation (Yaeger et al., 2019), ownership of records, how the access is granted and cybersecurity concerns.

2.2 AI in Healthcare

2.2.1 Introduction to AI

AI is the simulation of human intelligence in machines programmed to think and act like humans, designed to analyse data, learn from it, and perform tasks that typically require human cognition, such as problem-solving, decision-making, visual perception, and language translation (Schank & Abelson, 1977; Trappl, 1986). The main two categories of AI include the Narrow AI – weak AI – designed to handle a specific task or narrow range of tasks, with the prominent examples of Siri or Alexa; and the General-AI-strong-AI- a hypothetical form of AI that would have the capability to perform any cognitive task that a human can do, possessing self- awareness and consciousness, making decisions and solving problems across multiple domains without needing human intervention.

Key technologies behind AI include Machine Learning (ML), Deep Learning (DL) and Natural Language Processing (NLP) (Halper, 2017). ML, as a subset of AI, focuses on the development of algorithms that allow computers to learn from data without explicit programming. They include supervising learning where an algorithm is trained on a labelled dataset, with the system learning to mapping input data to the correct output; unsupervised learning, which predominantly works with unlabelled data and aims to find hidden patterns or intrinsic structures on the data; reinforcement learning, where an agent learns to make decisions by interacting with an environment and receiving rewards or penalties based on its actions. DL, as a subset of ML, uses neural networks with many layers to model complex patterns in data. Convolutional Neural Networks are used predominantly for vision tasks, such as image classification, and object detection, while Recurrent Neural Networks are used for processing sequential data, such as time series or speech, with strong memory capabilities. NLP allows machines not just to understand human language but also to interpret and generate it too, combining linguistics and computer science to process and analyse large amounts of natural language data.

AI's history can be traced back to the 1950s, with its term being used first by John McCarthy in 1955 (Trappl, 1986). Between the 1950s and 1970s, research on AI was focused on symbolic AI, involving creating algorithms that simulate human reasoning. Between the 1970s and 1990s, AI experienced a decline due to limited computational power and the inability to deliver its promises, leading to decreased funding and research. Between the 1990s and the 2010s, AI started to experience a renaissance, due to the rise of big data and more powerful computing hardware. Practical applications of AI have started appearing, including, for example, speech recognition, with the progress of ML, neural networks, and NLP technologies. After 2010, AI marked its modern era, with powering technologies such as chatbots and AI-driven recommendation systems, while DL and reinforcement learning became the most dominant techniques driving AI's success.

2.2.2 AI Applications in Healthcare

AI has turned out to be a game-changer in healthcare services development, dramatically transforming the accuracy of diagnostics, customisation of treatment, and its efficacy. The most sophisticated machine learning methods of AI can be used in a diagnostic setting and give the best results in radiology, pathology, and genomics (Alowais et al., 2023). In particular, AI mammogram analysis has produced a reduction in false positives of 5.7% and false negatives of 9.4%, respectively, and skin cancer detection based on convolutional neural networks has the same accuracy as a dermatologist.

Furthermore, predictive analytics tools have transformed hospital allocation and disease outbreak management resources. The AI machines use the massive datasets in electronic health records to predict readmissions of patients, enhance their care pathways, and predict resource allocation (Dixon et al., 2024). NLP technologies have made it easier to manage electronic health records by retrieving valuable insights and enhancing clinical decision-making by assessing the content of unstructured clinical notes (Faiyazuddin et al., 2025).

AI can be applied in healthcare through robotic surgery, drug discovery, and virtual nursing assistants, creating intelligent healthcare ecosystems. Pharmaceutical research has been made faster with machine learning algorithms in predicting the molecular behaviour, optimising trial schemes, and possible identification of drug candidates (Alowais et al., 2023). Nursing assistants using AI can continuously track and guide patients, which can be helpful in remote care and monitoring chronic diseases. However, the significant issues that can be raised are the scale, sensitivity, and explainability questions. The scale issue has to deal with large pools of care data, and retaining real-time responsiveness to support critical care applications (Mennella et al., 2024). The relevant sensitivity issues include safeguarding patient confidentiality without compromising the ability to analyse all data to train AI models. Explainability issues are created due to AI's "black box" nature, where complicated algorithms create accurate results without an obvious decision-making process between healthcare professionals and patients.

Figure 3. AI Applications in Healthcare & Challenges.

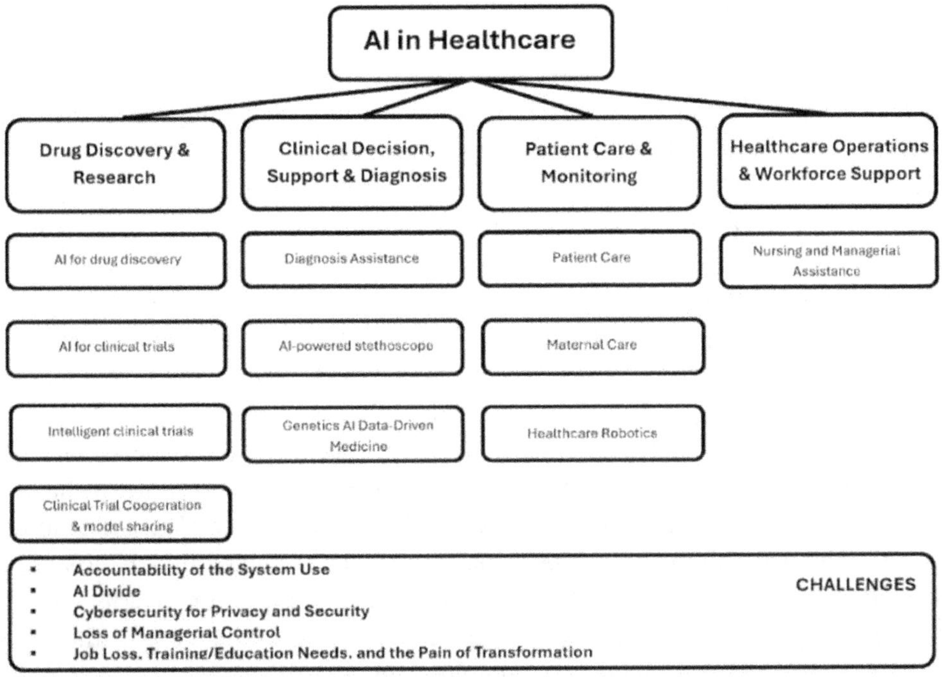

Drawing on the work of Lee and Yoon (2021) and Shaheen (2021), AI applications in healthcare can be organised into four main areas, including (i) drug discovery research, (ii) clinical decisions support and diagnosis, (iii) patient care and monitoring and (iv) healthcare operations and workforce support (Figure 3). More specifically, AI's popularity in drug discovery offers several benefits, including identifying drugs, supporting clinical trials, and facilitating cooperation and model sharing. For instance, as noted by Mayorga-Ruiz et al. (2019), the impact of human error might be decreased in data collection, allowing for a smoother system integration by using AI. In addition, AI supports the overall patient diagnosis, offers an AI-powered stethoscope, with the readings being able to be taken even in a noisy environment, allowing for a more accurate diagnosis (Prabu, 2021), and supports genetics AI data- driven medicine supporting precision and agility of genetic disease detection (Hummel & Braun, 2020). It is also important in patient care and monitoring, as it enhances patient care and monitoring, and supports ongoing patient care. Additionally, it offers healthcare robotics, such as exoskeleton robots that assist patients with paralysis (Shi et al., 2019), while also providing nursing and managerial assistance (Shaheen, 2021).

AI has been widely praised for its significant advantages as noted by an increasing number of authors and these advantages have been broadly classified by Sharma (2024) into four categories: (i) growth and profits benefits such as stakeholder engagement, value-co-creation, productivity, fostering innovation reliability, quality of service, and network expansion; (ii) performance ease and comfort benefits such accuracy speed, time and cost saving, computation and decision making; (iii) safety benefits, such as real-time monitoring, robotic assistance in dangerous occupation tasks; and (iv) sustainability benefits such as optimal research utilisation, equality, transparency, energy saving and job creation. Nevertheless, the adoption of AI has raised specific concerns which have been broadly classified into three categories: (i) trust, such as privacy breach, cybersecurity (Safavi & Kalis, 2019) error, bias, misuse, or inexplicability, unexpected machine action, technology readiness and technology robustness and transparency, and AI divide - considering that the success of the AI-enabled technology/ system and the patient it also depends on trust as stressed by Lupton (2018); (ii) ethical concerns, such as unemployment, job replacement, human skill loss (Lee & Yoon, 2021) inequality social anxiety, human control, redundancy or man-machine symbiosis and the accountability of the system for medical errors (Abomhara & Køien, 2015) (iii) disruption concerns such as change is supply-demand actors and operations, power shift, change in institutional structures, change in culture and demand for different skillset.

In line with recent health-AI governance frameworks such as the EU AI Act/ ONC transparency and WHO guidance, health trust depends on fairness and explainability (i.e., plain language reasons for outputs), human oversight (i.e., clinicians can challenge or override), safety and effectiveness (i.e., publish short evaluation summaries), transparency and control (i.e., consent exercise with who accessed what, when and for what purpose), clear redress for complaints and outcomes and inclusion (i.e., accessible design and equity monitoring). As evidenced by empirical studies (Busch et al., 2025; Scipion et al., 2025; Tun et al., 2025), patients and clinicians report higher trust and a greater willingness to use AI in healthcare when systems are explainable, demonstrate safety and effectiveness, and retain human oversight. Nevertheless, adoption still depends on workflow fit and supportive conditions such as training governance.

2.3 The Synergic Value of Blockchain and AI in Healthcare

The collaboration of AI and blockchain in the healthcare space includes focusing on how to increase the accuracy of healthcare data, what to do with the use of analytics and breaking up large centralised healthcare systems into a series of smaller units (Omidian, 2024). While AI thrives on good data, blockchain helps keep that data untampered (Tagde et al., 2021); hence, these technologies work together best. More specifically, blockchain works to improve AI simplicity and auditability through immutable records of the AI decision-making processes, training data used in the models, and outputs provided by the algorithms (Kasralikar et al., 2025). This integration allows healthcare providers to identify recommendations made by the AI based on their input data and thus go back to them and be responsible or meet the regulatory requirements.

On the other hand, AI makes blockchain more scalable in terms of intelligent shardings, predictive consensus, and optimisation of smart contracts. The AI algorithms can forecast network overload, streamline transaction settlement, and improve the blockchain channel on large-scale healthcare deployments (Solaiman & Awad, 2025). As an example, federated learning on blockchain-based infrastructure using the capabilities of AI enables the shared training of models across institutions in the healthcare industry without intrusion into privacy and without the loss of institutional control.

Moreover, concrete applications explain how this convergence can change everything. The decision-making process of AI prediction models records unchangeable results on blockchain ledgers, thus creating audit trails. The patient monitoring systems use AI to do a real-time analysis, and blockchain provides data integrity and the management of patient consent (Bathula et al., 2024). This combination is especially valuable in precision medicine, where AI would use the information contained in genomic data, and blockchain would retain secure and trackable records containing genetic information and results of the treatments. With blockchain, patients are in charge of who can view their health records, and AI makes diagnoses and treatment decisions using each patient's health data (Xie et al., 2021). To illustrate, with chronic disease management, AI examines data from wearables, and blockchain is used to protect privacy everywhere data are stored, making the infrastructure ready for early intervention and future clinical and regulatory requirements (Krittanawong et al., 2019; Xie et al., 2021).

There are still many significant challenges that come with integrating these things. Because these technologies are both heavy on computing power, there are questions about making them run on a larger scale and how much energy they use. Furthermore, the combination makes it even harder to address issues like algorithmic bias and how consent is obtained for some patients since blockchain does not allow data to be deleted according to GDPR (Krittanawong et al., 2019). Also, since there are no standardised procedures for bringing blockchain technology together with AI, it is more difficult for different systems to interact and for regulations to be followed (Tagde et al., 2021). These two technologies have regulatory conditions of uncertainty, interoperability problems, and limitations in scaling, which need to be addressed in a coordinated manner (Tagde et al., 2021). Establishing trust will be a significant factor because the healthcare stakeholders need to have confidence in the accuracy of AI algorithms and their blockchain security measures. The intersection, therefore, demands holistic governance structures concerning technical, ethical, and regulatory options to allow the best use of integrated AI-blockchain healthcare systems. In addition, the different platforms that support the blockchain and various AI frameworks lack interoperability, which hampers data flow and system integration in the healthcare environment. Given the existence of these challenges, it becomes clear that strong technical capabilities should be linked with thorough ethics and legal standards to make the best use of AI and blockchain in healthcare.

Indicators of readiness include having a data flow map, conducting standard interoperability tests, and implementing key management practices, such as periodic rotation, backup and restore (OECD, 2022). Maintaining clear documentation of test reports and key management logs supports and encourages continuity and compliance, thereby minimising operational and regulatory risks.

3. REGULATORY LANDSCAPE

3.1 Existing Governance of Blockchain

Current governance of blockchain in healthcare points to a worldwide regulatory system that is difficult to unite and relies on various jurisdictions making their own rules for something decentralised. According to Corte-Real et al. (2024), there are significant differences in the systems to protect data, by comparing European GDPR to other attempts such as the United States (Health Insurance Portability and Accountability Act, or HIPAA), California (Consumer Privacy Act, or CCPA), Canada (Personal Information Protection and Electronic Documents Act, or PIPEDA), Australia (Privacy Act of 1988), Japan (Act on the Protection of Personal Information, or APPI) and Brazil (Lei Geral de Protecao de Dados). The existence of these differences in regulation indicates that there are competing requirements that blockchain applications must address in a fluid regulatory environment. Solving this issue primarily involves distinguishing between new innovation desires and legal and moral rules. The EU's GDPR is considered an excellent personal data protection system that highlights data reduction, clear information and the right to have data removed (Hoofnagle et al., 2019). Nevertheless, the two key features of blockchain—immutability (i.e., the state of being unchangeable) and sharing data without a central authority (i.e., decentralisation)—make many of these demands challenging (Shuaib et al., 2021). Instead, the US employs a general sector approach, as outlined in the Health Insurance Portability and Accountability Act (HIPAA), which lacks blockchain sections and is limited in its actions regarding data sharing outside the country and pseudonymous ledgers (Ahmed et al., 2025). The Federal

Trade Commission clarified and expanded breach notification requirements for consumer health apps in 2024, making an architecture with off-chain PHI and on-chain proofs more defensible (Federal Trade Commission, 2024).

Comprehensive regulation of blockchain is hindered by the fact that there is no global harmonisation. The Markets in Crypto-Assets (MiCA) framework adopted by the EU to harmonise laws on crypto is very different from the approach taken by the U.S. Securities and Exchange Commission (SEC) and Financial Crimes Enforcement Network (FinCEN), which mainly handle finance compliance and anti-money laundering (AML) issues (Wronka, 2024). On the other hand, Japan and Singapore in the Asia-Pacific area have adopted hybrids that mix creativity with risk control, though these frameworks are usually incompatible with the data rules used in the United States and Europe (Corte-Real et al., 2024). Due to this fragmentation, blockchain healthcare applications, particularly those involving distributed identities or international patient data sharing, face significant risks.

Several MENA health authorities are already testing AI and data-intensive health solutions in supervised compliance-first sandboxes (Ministry of Health - Saudi Arabia, 2024), such as the Dubai Health Data Sandbox (Sandbox Dubai, 2025), mirroring the EU approach of trialling in controlled environments. Since requirements on purpose and data location are strictly enforced under the UAE PDPL (2025), even in innovation settings, UAE health blockchains should provide policy-level on-chain proofs and keep identifiable data off-chain (Government of the United Arab Emirates, 2025).

Blockchain's pseudonymity and contribution to decentralised finance (DeFi) introduce several unique issues. Public blockchain networks guarantee security, but participation is anonymous, making it challenging to conduct standard AML and KYC compliance in healthcare and insurance (Buterin et al., 2023). DeFi protocols are increasingly associated with financial services, enabling people to bypass traditional billing methods for health services. As a result, these applications escape proper regulation since the organisations that handle health and finance rules are divided. Because blockchain networks often cross boundaries, it is challenging to enforce data residency rules or ensure that audit trails comply with regulations in each country (Kasyapa & Vanmathi, 2024).

Critical gaps emerge when sector-specific regulations are reconciled with the immutable nature of blockchain, particularly when these regulations are examined in isolation on a sector-by-sector basis. The U.S. has HIPAA for personal health information, but that does not work in distributed ledgers, which require decentralised data validation; they are not adaptable (Shojaei et al., 2024). However, in the EU, GDPR's Article 17, known as the 'right to be forgotten', conflicts directly with the design of the blockchain, whose nature resists data deletion (Sabiri et al., 2025). There are difficulties associated with using smart contracts as a central point of storage due to the slowness of the local network and hefty storage costs, but these can be solved with off-chain storage (i.e., documents stored privately) or via a zero-knowledge proof (i.e., verify a rule without revealing the data) – both of which are technically very tricky and inconsistent to implement. As highlighted by Ettaloui et al. (2023), there is a built-in conflict between the permanence of the blockchain and the necessity of regulation in healthcare, specifically citing the difference between the GDPR right to be forgotten and inherent unchangeable record designations of the blockchain itself. The incompatibilities impose the emergence of such new concepts as off-chain storage and cryptographic techniques needed to ensure regulatory compliance and maintain blockchain security benefits. Permanence is the core of blockchain's contradictions, and healthcare's legal obligation to provide corrective or erasable data also shows one of its regulatory contradictions (Shuaib et al., 2021).

However, the lack of blockchain-specific regulatory frameworks for healthcare compounds the question of non-compliance while hindering innovation in attaining blockchain adoption in the healthcare sector. Now that most laws were designed for static databases and not dynamic, immutable ledgers with the ability to facilitate real-time global data exchange, it is clear that a new way of regulating distributed, immutable health-data environments must be introduced. Efforts to bridge this gap include adaptive regulatory mechanisms that adapt to emerging privacy-preserving technologies, including Privacy Pools that help users demonstrate compliance without revealing transaction histories (Buterin et al., 2023). In addition, blockchain system interoperability needs to take into consideration the national and international legal requirements for the protection of patient rights and to ensure ethical standards in digital health transformation. Without alignment, regulatory uncertainty can very much curtail the promise of blockchain in healthcare.

Moving beyond the US and the EU, health data governance across regions such as Africa, Asia-Pacific, and the Gulf differs in terms of oversight style, scope, and cross-border controls. On the one hand, a similar pattern across these regions is to keep patient-identifying data off the blockchain and to anchor only non-identifying evidence (e.g., consent-receipt identifiers, brief-access-event summaries—who/when/purpose, without identifiers—and dataset/model lineage fingerprints supporting audit and accountability without relocating data). The Nigeria Data Protection Act 2023 follows a GDPR-style model, so blockchain health projects in Africa should store PHI off-chain to avoid conflicts with erasure and purpose rules (Federal Republic of Nigeria, 2023). On the other hand, for instance, the EU's data governance is more comprehensive and rights-centric, compared to the US, which is more sectoral and enforcement-led, while APAC is more heterogeneous and interoperability-oriented, Gulf's is pro-innovative with conditional transfers, and finally, Africa's is emerging and more localised (see Appendix, Table 5).

3.2 Existing Governance of AI

With the rapid adoption of AI into healthcare, there has been a need for wide and comprehensive frameworks for governance to ensure ethical, transparent and accountable AI deployment. These frameworks are lynchpins of necessary emerging regulation—the European Union's (EU) AI Act and the United States' (US) National Institute of Standards and Technology's (NIST) AI Risk Management Framework (AI RMF)—which are pioneering efforts to find the right balance between innovation and ethical oversight. The EU AI Act is based on a risk-based classification system that separates AI applications based on their potential danger to essential rights and security, with stringent necessities for 'high-risk' AI frameworks, for example, those found in computerised medical clinics (Aboy et al., 2024). In the meantime, the NIST AI RMF takes more of a voluntary and flexible approach that nudges organisations to govern AI risks at the outset by means of functions such as governance, mapping, measurement and management of an AI system over its lifecycle (NIST, 2023). A convergence in both frameworks is needed for explainable, accountable and human-supervised models that can deal with AI complexity and adaptability risks (Cheong, 2024; Novelli et al., 2023). Both represent evolving regulatory strategies designed to ensure trustworthiness in the deployment of AI whilst at the same time enabling innovation.

Existing AI governance regimes based on transparency and explainability, aiming to ensure that users and stakeholders can understand and contest AI decision-making processes, are trying to address this issue. According to Cheong (2024), transparency is essential to protect individual and societal well-being as it helps users understand and challenge algorithmic decisions. In healthcare, for example, where diagnostics and treatment recommendations can have a massive difference to patients via AI, this is particularly critical. The so-called "black box" nature, particularly of deep learning systems, however, makes transparency less straightforward and complicated (Cheong, 2024). In order to correct this, regulatory initiatives are expected to mandate that developers include interpretable explanations and documentation in their AI models describing model design and decision logic. These same demands are explicitly incorporated in the EU AI Act, which mandates conformity assessments, post-market monitoring, and human-in-the-loop supervision mechanisms for high-risk AI used as medical devices (Aboy et al., 2024; Santra et al., 2024). The measures attempt to achieve an equally challenging balance between transparency and intellectual property protection, which often hampers disclosure.

In AI governance, accountability requires the explicit assignment of responsibility for AI system outcomes, which is a challenging undertaking due to the sociotechnical, complex and distributed nature of AI. Answerability, authority recognition and power limitation are proposed by Novelli et al. (2023) as an 'architecture' of accountability that requires multi-stakeholder engagement in the oversight function. The EU AI Act operationalises accountability by requiring AI "providers" or "users" to adopt specific actions, including the creation of risk management plans, and enables enforcement through audits and penalties (Aboy et al., 2024; Novelli et al., 2023). Additionally, organisational governance is identified as the foundational function comprising accountability across all stages of the AI lifecycle described in the NIST AI RMF (NIST, 2023). This governance includes reporting, monitoring for bias and redress in case of negative impact. In this way, taken together, these approaches make accountability not merely a legal label but a process that should be continuously scrutinised and supervised in a specific context (Iniesta, 2023; Novelli et al., 2023).

One significant challenge with AI regulation is the 'regulatory lag' because AI algorithms are dynamic and adaptive in ways that traditional laws are not. This is the context of AI-enabled combination medical devices, with the iterative learning model updating post-deployment, complicating a pre-market approval and conformity assessment (Santra et al., 2024). This stream of work, however, tries to offset this challenge in the US Food and Drug Administration's (FDA) 'evolving' framework where 'predetermined change control plans' are introduced, permitting specific interventions in AI which do not require new submissions, as long as safety and performance are retained (Santra et al., 2024). Similarly, the EU AI Act anticipates post-market surveillance and continuous compliance with respect to such dynamic risks (Aboy et al., 2024). Despite this, both frameworks recognise that regulators are always behind in utilising AI innovation due to the safety issues of public health, and it is essential to have some flexible, risk-based and human-centred regulatory models (Carapinha et al., 2024; NIST, 2023).

Model and dataset fingerprints, along with evaluation-report hashes and change-approval IDs, can be utilised as on-chain proofs to support transparency and post-market monitoring, as required by current health-AI rules.

3.3 Combined Regulatory Challenges

Integration of AI and blockchain in healthcare brings with it multifold regulatory challenges beyond those already faced by these technologies used in isolation. A preeminent problem exists because there is no coherent regulatory framework for AI or blockchain, taken separately, and there is none for the two systems together. AI systems need to be enforced through algorithm transparency, bias mitigation and dynamic adaptability, as with blockchain, which emphasises immutability, decentralisation and data integrity, which typically clash with classical data governance requirements (Kalenzi, 2022; Kuznetsov et al., 2024). For instance, the fact that AI requires the modification of data to fix mistakes or eliminate biased inputs in conflict with blockchain's immutable ledger has created regulatory tension that is making compliance difficult (Zhuk, 2025). The nature of this fragmentation results in oversight gaps cross-sectorally as different regulatory bodies govern the technology for AI and blockchain, with potential jurisdictional mismatches that stymie effective governance (Bharanitharan & Kaur, 2024).

In addition, the paradox of innovation and conformity is a barrier to technological developments. Kalenzi (2022) reports that various industry actors are calling for either self-regulation to help the cause of innovation or more government regulation to promote safety and ethical practices. This debate means further deeper problems about balancing technological innovations and safety measures, particularly regarding life-supporting technological medical equipment.

An additional important problem concerns the allocation of liability and accountability in combined AI–blockchain systems. In healthcare, where errors and harm driven by AI applications, as well as data security and provenance, are handled by blockchain, locating accountability for errors and harm is complicated. Unlike traditional software, where a developer or operator may be held accountable, the autonomous decision-making of AI, coupled with the decentralised data storage of blockchain, spreads and distributes accountability across multiple stakeholders (Kuznetsov et al., 2024; OECD, 2024a). An example is where, for instance, an AI algorithm that recommends a treatment based on blockchain-sealed patient records causes adverse effects, leaving one uncertain as to whether the AI developer, blockchain provider, healthcare institution, the proprietor of the blockchain-sealed patient records or further data contributors bear the legal responsibility (Bharanitharan & Kaur, 2024). With this diffusion of liability, however, current frameworks are insufficient to offer novel legal interpretations or adaptive regulatory approaches (Zhuk, 2025).

Adding to these challenges are jurisdictional inconsistencies caused by blockchain networks and AI applications' global and distributed nature. While Blockchain's immutable records clash with regional data protection laws such as the European Union's GDPR, where it comes down to the right to be forgotten when data about individuals needs to be erased upon individuals' request (Kuznetsov et al., 2024; OECD, 2024a), the immutable ledgers do not allow to do so. The problem is compounded when AI algorithms have to be trained and validated on complete datasets, which disallows compliance with privacy mandates. In addition, the divergence of regulation between countries introduces compliance costs to multinational healthcare providers that use AI blockchain solutions because these providers must negotiate a variety of overlapping and conflicting data sovereignty laws (OECD, 2024a; Zhuk, 2025). These jurisdictional tensions make harmonising standards and acting globally to protect patient privacy difficult to do in an integrated way under a unified regulatory policy.

The rapid pace of innovation in AI and blockchain technologies only adds fuel to tensions between innovation promotion and regulatory compliance. The regulatory frameworks often run behind technological advances, and they have become outdated or over-restrictive (Kalenzi, 2022). For example, dynamic learning models of AI require constant oversight, which cannot be achieved through a traditional control hierarchy. Similarly, blockchain systems are based on decentralised consensus mechanisms (Bharanitharan & Kaur, 2024). Tension has been proposed to be reconciled utilising regulatory sandboxes or adaptive governance models, where the former would allow for controlled experimentation in a sandbox environment while the latter regulates how changes are applied and customises to technical requirements and sustainability constraints (OECD, 2024a). While these adaptive approaches to regulation integrate these approaches in the context of two technologies, that integration has not been driven to a point sufficient to close regulatory gaps or avoid excessive burdens that stifle innovation.

AI and blockchain in healthcare pose combined regulatory challenges of fragmented governance, unclear liability allocation, territorial dispute and innovation versus compliance tension. These problems necessitate the development of multi-stakeholder frameworks that bring all stakeholders together to treat AI blockchain systems as a unified entity, rather than disjointed components. There is also a strong advocacy for agile, transparent and interoperable regulatory mechanisms that align with the distinctive characteristics of the two technologies, subject to patient rights and system integrity protection (Kalenzi, 2022; Kuznetsov et al., 2024; OECD, 2024a). To achieve the potential of AI-blockchain healthcare integrations, it is imperative to achieve such comprehensive regulatory evolution in order to ensure both innovation and societal trust. Also, as observed by Corte-Real et al. (2024), the privacy legislation, which involves the right to destroy or alter information, directly conflicts with the immutability of blockchain technology. This jurisdictional and moral conflict, such as between the GDPR right to be forgotten and blockchain immutability, cannot be addressed without new technical paradigms, such as off-chain storage and cryptographic solutions, in a world where the jurisdictions applied do not all necessarily coincide. Consequently, AI-blockchain convergence in healthcare is still characterised by a lack of clarity, jurisdictional issues, and technical incompatibilities beyond the scope of the existing frameworks that have regulated them. New regulation forms that may do the same are needed.

4. CASE STUDY: BURSTIQ

4.1 Background

BurstIQ appears as a one-of-a-kind healthcare technology venture that effectively demonstrates how AI and blockchain technologies should naturally come together in practical market dynamics in the clinical setting. The company was launched in 2015 by CEO Frank Ricotta and Co-Founder Brian Jackson, who developed the company out of the simple frustration with data privacy violations, to which Ricotta is famous for saying, "I just got sick and tired of people stealing my data" (BurstIQ, 2024). This individual's drive became an organisational mission to change healthcare management through innovative use of technology in managing data.

This Denver-based firm has displayed outstanding growth and sustainability, being financially independent since 2016 and raising 5.5 million dollars in Series A funding with Elsewhere Partners as the lead investor (Pennic, 2019). Besides, the strategic expansion measure initiated by BurstIQ can be traced in recent moves on the Amazon Web Services Partner Network, where the LifeGraph platform is now available in AWS Marketplace and more accessible to the cloud consumer group (BurstIQ, 2025a). The company has a core philosophy anchored upon three main aspects: the appreciation of data as an artefact of human experience, the adherence to dignity as a core human right, and the ability of people to use their information to an advantage (BurstIQ, 2024).

BurstIQ strategically chose healthcare as its primary domain, recognising it as the "Everest of data" due to its complex and sensitive nature, which demanded robust technological solutions (BurstIQ, 2024). This deliberate focus on healthcare's data challenges has enabled the company to develop comprehensive solutions applicable across multiple industries while maintaining specialised expertise in life-critical applications. The company's vision encompasses "a world where billions of Life-Graphs empower meaningful human-to-business interactions, foster collaboration, and inspire innovation," positioning them at the forefront of the patient-driven data management revolution.

4.2 Implementation Overview

BurstIQ's integrated solution focuses on its proprietary LifeGraph platform, a strategic combination of blockchain, AI, and knowledge graphs to solve complementary healthcare ecosystem problems and deliver the highest data value. The platform's architecture establishes a holistic data management system with blockchain offering secure, transparent, and immutable underpinnings to managing health data that ensures privacy, regulatory compliance, and finer access control rules.

This technological integration is a multi-layered method in which blockchain ensures the integrity and verification of all health data. In contrast, knowledge graphs organise and relate health data to be interoperable across heterogeneous healthcare systems. AI then uses these structured data sets to develop actionable intelligence, aid clinical decision-making efforts, and help in predictive and preventive medical care efforts. This combination design ensures that each technology will complement the other because the blockchain will make AI more transparent and auditable. AI will make blockchain more scalable with intelligent optimisation algorithms.

Additionally, the consent management system in the platform shows high-level integration of blockchain and AI capabilities as a smart contract prioritises patients' rights. These cryptographically secured smart contracts enable patients to take control, grant, alter, or revoke access to their information in real-time so that only agreed-upon data is involved in training AI models and clinical use of such models. Furthermore, BurstIQ guarantees full interoperability among healthcare systems with the support of the industry standards, such as REST APIs, FHIR, and HL7 protocols, so that data can be freely exchanged irrespective of the technological fundamentals. The platform transforms the static and siloed data into dynamic interactive ecosystems where organisations can fully utilise their data whilst upholding high privacy and security norms throughout the data life cycle.

4.3 Regulatory Navigation

The compliance strategy employed by BurstIQ implies the advanced techniques of understanding highly complex healthcare and data protection regulations that vary across the jurisdictional systems. It has a SOC 2 Type II compliance certification and it has consistently maintained compliance over the past 7 years with a strong, assured dedication to privacy practices, security, availability, and confidentiality (BurstIQ, 2025b). Although the security practices that provide exceptional underpinning to this certification are good, the organisation acknowledges that SOC 2 certification is not a guarantee of conformity with other special requirements and regulations, including HIPAA or GDPR, which have a distinctive framework of the compliance procedure.

Consequently, BurstIQ has developed the LifeGraph platform, where comprehensive compliance has been made vigilant, including privacy and security practices at the platform level, using blockchain technology. The approach enables organisations to put in place data environments that ensure that regulatory requirements like the principle of data protection by design and default of GDPR, as well as the highly technical healthcare privacy requirements of HIPAA, are met, and integrate them to be mutually compatible. The platform has blockchain-based capabilities that can support compliance with the strict privacy-related laws of various jurisdictions and dynamically adapt to the regulatory environment.

Moreover, the regulatory identification process within the company includes a close cooperation with partner organisations to get a clear picture of subtle regulatory requirements and design platform features to adhere to industry best practices, including SOC 2 Type II and the NIST frameworks. BurstIQ adds a blockchain-based mechanism of consent, automated compliance with smart contracts, and a transparent and privacy-protecting framework to keep the total regulatory environment in line. These technologies offer verifiable audit trails, dynamic consent, automated policy enforcement, and user-centric control over personal data in a manner that also provides regulatory compliance assurance and enhanced stakeholder trust. Interestingly, the company regards regulatory ambiguity as an element of participation by actively meeting compliance requirements instead of making adjustments. BurstIQ includes various regulatory requirements considerations in its base platform design, therefore resolving regulatory issues before they arise, achieving long-term frameworks to move into the variable regulations environment, and staying innovatively charged.

4.4 Lessons Learned

The experience that BurstIQ has already acquired proves the crucial facts about the future of working with AI and blockchain and compliance with regulations in the healthcare ecosystem. The most critical strategic discovery of the company is that trust must serve as a guide in formulating and executing any system. They have found that organisations can be respected and revered by stakeholders and regulating agents by developing systems to provoke trust at every point of operation and providing proofs that they can be trusted.

The company also discovered that privacy and security are not add-ons to healthcare technology applications but are existential requirements rather than options. The main regulatory compliance principles demanded by HIPAA, GDPR, and other similar regulations should be ingrained into platform architecture and not implemented as overlays using separate systems. Such an architectural form of integration avoids introducing complexity, lessens the vulnerability exposure, removes the number of possible failure points, and makes the compliance process more straightforward to maintain in an ever-fluctuating regulatory environment.

Additionally, BurstIQ found out that the platforms explicitly designed to achieve compliance allow companies to transform rapidly and risk-free without jeopardising the safety of patients and compromising sensitive health information. This integrated and compliance-based strategy makes operational processes and interactions smoother, minimises organisational risk exposure, and helps to ensure that patient rights protection remains at the core of technological advancement and promotion initiatives. The effects of COVID-19 experienced by the company only hastened their platform development, showing the necessity of a flexible technology infrastructure that allows them to react to the unforeseen changes in the environment and regulatory requirements. Nonetheless, major obstacles were faced concerning stakeholder education on the advantages of blockchain technology and on the reluctance to use new technologies. Thus, particular communication strategies must be developed, emphasising value creation instead of technical aspects. The ability of the company to focus on the benefits of the blockchain to data privacy and security instead of detailing the inner workings has been paramount in its stakeholder engagement and uptake of the technology in various healthcare settings.

International gaps, workflow resistance and unclear regulation are the primary (organisational) challenges that should be mitigated by clarifying data-governance roles, planning for portability to avoid vendor lock-in and engaging users at an early stage. As noted by Borges do Nascimento et al. (2023), adoption barriers are often organisational, including psychological constraints, infrastructure and technical constraints, and workload-related issues. Nevertheless, role-appropriate training, attention to perceived usefulness and multi-stakeholder incentives consistently enable uptake (World Health Organization, 2021). Ultimately, these findings align with broader socio-technical literature that links non-adoption and scale difficulties to organisational fit and context, and with global guidance that emphasises governance capability and workforce development. Testbed experiences and Sandbox reports show the same pattern, including that uptake improves when users see clear safeguards, observable compliance steps, and role-appropriate training (World Bank, 2025).

In Europe and the Gulf, there are seen comparable initiatives showing the same regulatory pattern, such as health and AI sandboxes operating in supervised, time-bounded environments, with the requirement of participants keeping identifiable health data off-chain or to be de-identified, along with using predefined artefacts to evidence compliance rather than putting the patient records on a ledger. This is consistent with the EDPB's 2025 draft Guidelines on processing personal data through blockchain, which stress data minimisation and off-chain storage for GDPR purposes, and with Dubai's Health Data/Healthcare Sandbox model, which tests data-driven innovations under adaptive regulatory oversight (EDPB, 2025a; 2025b; Sandbox Dubai, 2025).

5. STAKEHOLDER DYNAMICS AND GOVERNANCE

Within the governance environment of AI-blockchain convergence of healthcare, the power of various stakeholders developing divergent strategic goals interacts with the overall regulatory process. As custodians of primary data, healthcare institutions have operational efficiency and patient safety as their primary concerns, and they deal with the pressures of compliance requirements that lead them to more risk-averse approaches in favour of existing regulatory frameworks than new technological solutions (Mennella et al., 2024). At the same time, technology providers such as BurstIQ are also pursuing proactive steps to ensure transparency and trust, which is clearly stated in their compliance success, with seven years of SOC 2 Type II accreditation.

In addition, regulators act under disjointed jurisdiction, which introduces inconsistent regulation measures that cannot capitalise on the interconnected nature of AI-blockchain systems. The AI Act regulation presented by the European Union places medical devices with AI features in the high-risk category, which activates the comprehensive obligation sets, and the blockchain governance is not concentrated in any regulation (Aboy et al., 2024). This regulatory disintegration has allowed the technology companies to forum shop and find the jurisdiction with friendlier regulations, which dilutes consistent international regulation.

Additionally, as patients, end-users are in a paradoxical state; on the one hand, they want to pay more attention to privacy and safety and expect better results in healthcare; on the other hand, they have little knowledge about blockchain. The experience of BurstIQ shows that the education of stakeholders becomes a priority, as the unwillingness to embrace new technologies needs particular communication strategies, which should be aimed at highlighting the reality of the possible advantages, but not on the technical complexity. Also, healthcare professionals become both users and gatekeepers of adoption as their acceptance or opposition to AI-blockchain would shape adoption, especially where questions of transparency and explainability remain unaddressed (Williamson & Prybutok, 2024). Therefore, governance becomes a negotiated process instead of top-down regulation, where stakeholder relationships will dictate implementation success. As the case study shows, achieving regulatory harmony requires companies to collaborate in their dealings, collaborating with their partner organisations to comprehend refined regulatory needs.

6. STRATEGIC AND POLICY IMPLICATIONS

This regulatory navigation experience provides valuable empirical evidence to inform the development of an agile, risk-based regulatory framework that efficiently supports innovation promotion and patient protection simultaneously. Given that adoption capacity is uneven across healthcare settings, particularly in low-infrastructure emerging economies, policy guidance should require routine bias and subgroup—

performance checks and ensure accessibility options (e.g., telehealth deployment) so that blockchain/AI solutions do not reinforce existing health inequities.

Table 3 turns the case findings into actionable guidance, covering the key tensions derived from BurstIQ's regulatory navigation experience, the corresponding responses and the actors responsible for each action point. Although these actions are drawn from a single, data-rich case, comparable sandbox and pilot experiences point to the same regulatory tensions, which support the transferability of the policy proposals.

Table 3. BurstIQ-derived Policy Actions

Insights from BurstIQ	Policy Action	Primary Actor(s)
Operational costs are increased due to integration, change management, and privacy/security. ROI improves when access is faster and audit findings are fewer	An evidence-first approach should be adopted. This includes keeping PHI off-chain, recording non-identifying evidence, and prioritising duplicate-reduction projects to recover integration costs	Healthcare providers, IT managers, vendors
Blockchain and AI were treated as a single technological architecture.	One governance-risk-compliance process should be run with clear accountability for the combined AI-Blockchain stack	Regulators, hospital and programme managers and CIO/ CDO
Compliance was evidenced through controlled conditions	Regulatory sandboxes should be used with safety criteria to allow firms to demonstrate compliance on real workflow before scaling up	Regulators, vendor compliance leaders and provider managers
Trust and adoption required privacy-by-design and stakeholder communication, not technical detail.	Privacy and security should be embedded into the platform design, and run stakeholder education to explain value and control	Vendors, clinical managers and patient-engagement teams
Capability had to be built by the providers to assess AI-Blockchain and to procure long-term compliant platforms	In-house training and assessment should be created with a shift to procurement to privacy-preserving, compliance-proven platforms	Healthcare providers, procurement, and training managers
Regulatory arbitrage risk was created due to cross-border/ jurisdictional variation	Risk-based evaluation should be applied, focusing on use and patient impact, and on cross-border coordination to align approaches	Policymaker, national regulators and health-system executives
Some settings have lower adoption capacity due to, for example, a lack of infrastructure or skills	Bias and subgroup checks should be added, along with mobile/telehealth access, and guidance should be given	Healthcare providers and policymakers

System integration, change management and privacy and security controls introduce operational costs (OECD, 2024b). Faster, safer access to data, fewer duplicate records, and fewer audit findings accelerate returns on investment. For health providers, the main cost drivers include integration with legacy EHR/HIS systems, data preparation and quality work, alignment with security upgrades to meet health data laws, and staff training, all of which need to be budgeted into pilots (Rathore et al., 2025). The new governance paradigm should evolve into an integrated style of regulation that acknowledges that blockchain-AI systems should be regarded as a single set of technological architectures instead of separate blocks (Kasralikar et al., 2025). This paradigm shift also requires regulatory sandboxes that facilitate experimental conditions without risk but under safety criteria, where these companies will prove that they comply using practice instead of theory.

Technology companies ought to implement progressive regulatory measures that integrate considerations of compliance into major platform design in place of external restrictions. The success of BurstIQ reveals that privacy and security should become core design requirements, and the company's strategy to directly embed regulatory compliance into blockchain architecture via novel cryptographic technologies offers a path that can be followed and applied by other companies in the industry. Moreover, companies should consider launching stakeholder educational campaigns, as introducing new technology requires technical superiority, user knowledge, and the creation of a trust relationship.

Healthcare providers need strategic frameworks that enable them to utilise AI-blockchain while dealing with the risk of operations and regulatory requirements. The evidence indicates that organisations must focus on platforms with a proven compliance history and privacy-preserving architecture that allows innovation while maintaining existing regulatory relationships. Moreover, healthcare organisations must establish in-house competencies in assessing AI-blockchain solutions. Training should be tailored to the different roles (e.g., clinical users, policy owners, and system administrators) supported by scenario-based exercises after major releases, with clear documentation of participation and scenario outcomes serving as evidence of operational readiness. Building on this capability, procurement can shift to long-term technology relationships, which will help align with regulatory frameworks over time and ensure safety, interoperability, and auditability.

Policy makers should initiate flexible regulatory structures that can embrace the swift technological changes but still provide the needed safeguards. This necessitates establishing risk-based evaluation methodologies that measure the AI-blockchain systems in their healthcare use and possible impact on patients, not technological sophistication (Kalenzi, 2022). In addition, global regulatory coordination mechanisms are required to deal with cross-border data transfer and consistent regulatory approaches to jurisdiction, such that regulatory arbitrage is avoided, yet healthcare globally promotes innovation. The strategic imperative is to develop competitive regulatory environments that support responsible innovation, setting up incentives to align and not burden compliance.

7. CONCLUSION

This in-depth exploration of the convergence between AI and blockchain in healthcare using the BurstIQ case study sheds light on the transformational opportunities and regulatory complexity that continue to define this technological point of contact. The theoretical evaluation provides evidence that although the AI and the blockchain technologies have a set of complementary capabilities between them, together they introduce an unprecedented level of regulatory complexity that current frameworks are ill-equipped to deal with. Regulatory landscape analysis demonstrates structural strains between the promotion of innovation and enforcement of compliance based on diverse governance frameworks that lead to jurisdictional overlaps and inconsistent regulation and supervision. These issues become especially sharp when laws such as the right to be forgotten within GDPR cannot be fitted to the structure of blockchains, requiring radical technical innovations and adaptations to the rules and regulations. Practical lessons on the case of BurstIQ narrative show that the sound design of the AI-blockchain incorporation process demands reliance or trust in the systems, built-in compliance, and stakeholders' active involvement. In the review of stakeholder dynamics, governance dynamics can be seen to be negotiated involvements between the healthcare institutions, the technology providers, regulators, and the patients, with differing goals, which ultimately determine the outcomes of various implementation actions. As the future unfolds, implementing AI and blockchain in healthcare requires a logical development of regulations that should strike the right balance between encouraging new frontiers and safeguarding patient healthcare. The standardisation of these trust duties across regions, along with the "proofs-only, patient-data-off-chain" pattern, provides auditable assurance without exposing PHI.

REFERENCES

Abomhara, M., & Køien, G. M. (2015). Cyber security and the internet of things: Vulnerabilities, threats, intruders and attacks. *Journal of Cyber Security and Mobility*, *4*(1), 65–88. DOI: 10.13052/jcsm2245-1439.414

Aboy, M., Minssen, T., & Vayena, E. (2024). Navigating the EU AI Act: Implications for regulated digital medical products. npj. *Digital Medicine*, *7*(1), 237. Advance online publication. DOI: 10.1038/s41746-024-01232-3 PMID: 39242831

Agbo, C., Mahmoud, Q., & Eklund, J. (2019). Blockchain technology in healthcare: A systematic review. *Health Care*, *7*(2), 56. Advance online publication. DOI: 10.3390/healthcare7020056 PMID: 30987333

Aggarwal, S., Kumar, N., Alhussein, M., & Muhammad, G. (2021). Blockchain-based UAV path planning for healthcare 4.0: Current challenges and the way ahead. *IEEE Network*, *35*(1), 20–29. DOI: 10.1109/MNET.011.2000069

Ahmed, A., Shahzad, A., Naseem, A., Ali, S., & Ahmad, I. (2025). Evaluating the effectiveness of data governance frameworks in ensuring security and privacy of healthcare data: A quantitative analysis of ISO standards, GDPR, and HIPAA in blockchain technology. *PLoS One*, *20*(5), e0324285. Advance online publication. DOI: 10.1371/journal.pone.0324285 PMID: 40408373

AI Verify Foundations; IMDA; PDPC. (2024, May 29). Model AI Governance Framework for Generative AI.

Al Omar, A., Bhuiyan, M. Z. A., Basu, A., Kiyomoto, S., & Rahman, M. S. (2019). Privacy-friendly platform for healthcare data in cloud based on blockchain environment. *Future Generation Computer Systems*, *95*, 511–521. DOI: 10.1016/j.future.2018.12.044

Alabdulatif, A., Khalil, I., & Rahman, M. S. (2022). Security of blockchain and AI-empowered smart healthcare: Application-based analysis. *Applied Sciences (Basel, Switzerland)*, *12*(21), 11039. Advance online publication. DOI: 10.3390/app122111039

Alowais, S. A., Alghamdi, S. S., Alsuhebany, N., Alqahtani, T., Alshaya, A., Almohareb, S. N., Aldairem, A., Alrashed, M., Saleh, K. B., Badreldin, H. A., Yami, A., Harbi, S. A., & Albekairy, A. M. (2023). Revolutionising healthcare: The role of artificial intelligence in clinical practice. *BMC Medical Education*, *23*(1), 1–15. DOI: 10.1186/s12909-023-04698-z PMID: 36593450

Attaran, M. (2022). Blockchain technology in healthcare: Challenges and opportunities. *International Journal of Healthcare Management*, *15*(1), 70–83. DOI: 10.1080/20479700.2020.1843887

Bachani, V., & Bhattacharjya, A. (2022). Preferential delegated proof of stake (PDPoS)—Modified DPoS with two layers towards scalability and higher TPS. *Symmetry*, *15*(1), 4. DOI: 10.3390/sym15010004

Bathula, A., Gupta, S. K., Merugu, S., Saba, L., Khanna, N. N., Laird, J. R., Sanagala, S. S., Singh, R., Garg, D., Fouda, M. M., & Suri, J. S. (2024). Blockchain, artificial intelligence, and healthcare: The tripod of future—A narrative review. *Artificial Intelligence Review*, *57*(9), 238. DOI: 10.1007/s10462-024-10873-5

Bharanitharan, K., & Kaur, G. (2024). The double-edged sword: Legal implications of AI errors and blockchain in finance. *European Economic Letters*, *14*(2). Advance online publication. DOI: 10.52783/eel.v14i2.1637

Birje, M. N., Goudar, R. H., Rakshitha, C. M., & Tapale, M. T. (2022, July). A review on layered architecture and application domains of blockchain technology. In *2022 International Conference on Electrical, Computer and Energy Technologies (ICECET)* (pp. 1–5). IEEE. DOI: 10.1109/ICECET55527.2022.9872729

Borges do Nascimento, I. J., Abdulazeem, H., Vasanthan, L. T., Martinez, E. Z., Zucoloto, M. L., Østengaard, L., Azzopardi-Muscat, N., Zapata, T., & Novillo-Ortiz, D. (2023). Barriers and facilitators to utilizing digital health technologies by healthcare professionals. npj. *Digital Medicine*, *6*(1), 161. PMID: 37723240

Burst IQ. (2024). About BurstIQ. https://burstiq.com/about-burstiq/

Burst IQ. (2025a). BurstIQ joins the AWS Partner Network to bring AI-ready data management solutions to cloud customers. PR Newswire. https://www.prnewswire.com/news-releases/burstiq-joins-the-aws-partner-network-to-bring-ai-ready-data-management-solutions-to-cloud-customers-302477982.html

Burst IQ. (2025b). BurstIQ completes its sixth annual independent SOC 2 type II audit, continuing a legacy of best-in-class data security. https://burstiq.com/burstiq-completes-its-sixth-annual-independent-soc-2-type-ii-audit-continuing-a-legacy-of-best-in-class-data-security/

Busch, F., Hoffmann, L., Xu, L., Zhang, L. J., Hu, B., García-Juárez, I., Toapanta-Yanchapaxi, L. N., Gorelik, N., Gorelik, V., Rodriguez-Granillo, G. A., Ferrarotti, C., Cuong, N. N., Thi, C. A. P., Tuncel, M., Kaya, G., Solis-Barquero, S. M., Mendez Avila, M. C., Ivanova, N. G., Kitamura, F. C., & Zhang, S. (2025). Multinational attitudes toward AI in healthcare and diagnostics among hospital patients. *JAMA Network Open*, *8*(6), e2514452. DOI: 10.1001/jamanetworkopen.2025.14452 PMID: 40493367

Buterin, V., Illum, J., Nadler, M., Schär, F., & Soleimani, A. (2023). Blockchain privacy and regulatory compliance: Towards a practical equilibrium. Blockchain. *SSRN*, *5*(1), 100176. Advance online publication. DOI: 10.2139/ssrn.4563364

Carapinha, J., Botes, D., & Carapinha, R. (2024). Balancing innovation and ethics in AI governance for health technology assessment. *Journal of Medical Economics*, *27*(1), 754–757. Advance online publication. DOI: 10.1080/13696998.2024.2352821 PMID: 38711204

Cason, D., Fynn, E., Milosevic, N., Milosevic, Z., Buchman, E., & Pedone, F. (2021, September). The design, architecture and performance of the Tendermint blockchain network. In 2021 40th International Symposium on Reliable Distributed Systems (SRDS) (pp. 23–33). IEEE. DOI: 10.1109/SRDS53918.2021.00012

Chen, L., Xu, L., Shah, N., Gao, Z., Lu, Y., & Shi, W. (2017, October). On security analysis of proof-of-elapsed-time (PoET). In *International Symposium on Stabilization, Safety, and Security of Distributed Systems* (pp. 282–297). Springer.

Cheong, B. C. (2024). Transparency and accountability in AI systems: Safeguarding wellbeing in the age of algorithmic decision-making. *Frontiers in Human Dynamics*, *6*, 1421273. Advance online publication. DOI: 10.3389/fhumd.2024.1421273

Chukwu, E., & Garg, L. (2020). A systematic review of blockchain in healthcare: Frameworks, prototypes, and implementations. *IEEE Access : Practical Innovations, Open Solutions*, *8*, 21196–21214. DOI: 10.1109/ACCESS.2020.2969881

Corte-Real, A., Nunes, T., & da Cunha, P. R. (2024). Reflections about blockchain in health data sharing: Navigating a disruptive technology. *International Journal of Environmental Research and Public Health*, *21*(2), 230. Advance online publication. DOI: 10.3390/ijerph21020230 PMID: 38397719

De Aguiar, E. J., Faiçal, B. S., Krishnamachari, B., & Ueyama, J. (2020). A survey of blockchain-based strategies for healthcare. *ACM Computing Surveys*, *53*(2), 27.

De Angelis, S., Aniello, L., Baldoni, R., Lombardi, F., Margheri, A., & Sassone, V. (2018). PBFT vs proof-of-authority: Applying the CAP theorem to permissioned blockchain. In *CEUR Workshop Proceedings* (Vol. 2058). CEUR-WS.

Deloitte. (2016). Blockchain: Opportunities for healthcare. https://www2.deloitte.com/content/dam/Deloitte/us/Documents/public-sector/us-blockchain-opportunities-for-health-care.pdf

Dixon, D., Sattar, H., Moros, N., Kesireddy, S. R., Ahsan, H., Lakkimsetti, M., Fatima, M., Doshi, D., Sadhu, K., & Hassan, M. J. (2024). Unveiling the influence of AI predictive analytics on patient outcomes: A comprehensive narrative review. *Cureus, 16*(5). Advance online publication. DOI: 10.7759/cureus.59954 PMID: 38854327

Ejaz, M., Kumar, T., Kovacevic, I., Ylianttila, M., & Harjula, E. (2021). Health-blockedge: Blockchain-edge framework for reliable low-latency digital healthcare applications. *Sensors (Basel), 21*(7), 2502. DOI: 10.3390/s21072502 PMID: 33916700

Esposito, C., De Santis, A., Tortora, G., Chang, H., & Choo, K. K. R. (2018). Blockchain: A panacea for healthcare cloud-based data security and privacy? *IEEE Cloud Computing*, *5*(1), 31–37. DOI: 10.1109/MCC.2018.011791712

Ettaloui, N., Arezki, S., & Gadi, T. (2023). An overview of blockchain-based electronic health records and compliance with GDPR and HIPAA. 2, 166. DOI: 10.56294/dm2023166

European Data Protection Board. (2025a). EDPB adopts guidelines on processing personal data through blockchains and is ready to cooperate with AI office on guidelines on AI Act and EU data protection law. https://www.edpb.europa.eu/news/news/2025/edpb-adopts-guidelines-processing-personal-data-through-blockchains-and-ready_en

European Data Protection Board. (2025b). Guidelines, recommendations, best practices. https://www.edpb.europa.eu/our-work-tools/general-guidance/guidelines-recommendations-best-practices_en

European Union. (2024). Regulation (EU) 2024/1689 of 13 June 2024 laying down harmonised rules on artificial intelligence (Artificial Intelligence Act). Official Journal of the European Union.

European Union. (2025). Regulation (EU) 2025/327 of 11 February 2025 on the European Health Data Space. Official Journal of the European Union.

Faiyazuddin, M., Syed, A. G., Siddiqui, R. K., Mehta, R., Khatib, M. N., Gaidhane, S., Zahiruddin, Q. S., Hussain, A., & Sah, R. (2025). The impact of artificial intelligence on healthcare: A comprehensive review of advancements in diagnostics, treatment, and operational efficiency. *Health Science Reports*, *8*(1), e70312. Advance online publication. DOI: 10.1002/hsr2.70312 PMID: 39763580

Federal Republic of Nigeria. (2023). Nigeria Data Protection Act, 2023.

Federal Trade Commission. (2024, May 30). Health Breach Notification Rule—Final rule (amendments). *Federal Register*.

Gervais, A., Karame, G. O., Wüst, K., Glykantzis, V., Ritzdorf, H., & Capkun, S. (2016, October). On the security and performance of proof of work blockchains. In *Proceedings of the 2016 ACM SIGSAC Conference on Computer and Communications Security* (pp. 3–16). DOI: 10.1145/2976749.2978341

Gökalp, E., Gökalp, M. O., Çoban, S., & Eren, P. E. (2018). Analysing opportunities and challenges of integrated blockchain technologies in healthcare. In Eurosymposium on Systems Analysis and Design (pp. 174–183). DOI: 10.1007/978-3-030-00060-8_13

Gordon, W. J., & Catalini, C. (2018). Blockchain technology for healthcare: Facilitating the transition to patient-driven interoperability. *Computational and Structural Biotechnology Journal*, *16*, 224–230. DOI: 10.1016/j.csbj.2018.06.003 PMID: 30069284

Government of the United Arab Emirates. (2025, July 7). Data protection laws—UAE PDPL overview.

Haleem, A., Javaid, M., Singh, R. P., Suman, R., & Rab, S. (2021). Blockchain technology applications in healthcare: An overview. *International Journal of Intelligent Networks*, *2*, 130–139. DOI: 10.1016/j.ijin.2021.09.005

Halper, F. (2017). Advanced analytics: Moving toward AI, machine learning, and natural language processing (TDWI Best Practices Report).

Hasselgren, A., Kralevska, K., Gligoroski, D., Pedersen, S. A., & Faxvaag, A. (2020). Blockchain in healthcare and health sciences—A scoping review. *International Journal of Medical Informatics*, *134*, 104040. DOI: 10.1016/j.ijmedinf.2019.104040 PMID: 31865055

Hassija, V., Chamola, V., Mahapatra, A., Singal, A., Goel, D., Huang, K., Scardapane, S., Spinelli, I., Mahmud, M., & Hussain, A. (2023). Interpreting black-box models: A review on explainable artificial intelligence. *Cognitive Computation*, *16*(1), 45–74. Advance online publication. DOI: 10.1007/s12559-023-10179-8

Hoofnagle, C. J., van der Sloot, B., & Borgesius, F. Z. (2019). The European Union general data protection regulation: What it is and what it means. *Information & Communications Technology Law*, *28*(1), 65–98. DOI: 10.1080/13600834.2019.1573501

Hummel, P., & Braun, M. (2020). Just data? Solidarity and justice in data-driven medicine. *Life Sciences, Society and Policy*, *16*(1), 8. DOI: 10.1186/s40504-020-00101-7 PMID: 32839878

Ichikawa, D., Kashiyama, M., & Ueno, T. (2017). Tamper-resistant mobile health using blockchain technology. *JMIR mHealth and uHealth*, *5*(7), e7938. DOI: 10.2196/mhealth.7938 PMID: 28747296

Iniesta, R. (2023). The human role to guarantee an ethical AI in healthcare: A five-facts approach. *AI and Ethics*. Advance online publication. DOI: 10.1007/s43681-023-00353-x

Kalenzi, C. (2022). Artificial intelligence and blockchain: How should emerging technologies be governed? *Frontiers in Research Metrics and Analytics*, *7*, 801549. Advance online publication. DOI: 10.3389/frma.2022.801549 PMID: 35224423

Karantias, K., Kiayias, A., & Zindros, D. (2020, February). *Proof-of-burn. In International Conference on Financial Cryptography and Data Security* (pp. 523–540). Springer.

Kasralikar, P., Polu, O. R., Chamarthi, B., Veer Samara Sihman Bharattej Rupavath, R., Patel, S., & Tumati, R. (2025). Blockchain for securing AI-driven healthcare systems: A systematic review and future research perspectives. *Cureus*. Advance online publication. DOI: 10.7759/cureus.83136 PMID: 40438823

Kasyapa, M. S. B., & Vanmathi, C. (2024). Blockchain integration in healthcare: A comprehensive investigation of use cases, performance issues, and mitigation strategies. *Frontiers in Digital Health*, *6*, 1359858. Advance online publication. DOI: 10.3389/fdgth.2024.1359858 PMID: 38736708

Khezr, S., Moniruzzaman, M., Yassine, A., & Benlamri, R. (2019). Blockchain technology in healthcare: A comprehensive review and directions for future research. *Applied Sciences (Basel, Switzerland)*, *9*(9), 1736. Advance online publication. DOI: 10.3390/app9091736

Krittanawong, C., Rogers, A. J., Aydar, M., Choi, E., Johnson, K. W., Wang, Z., & Narayan, S. M. (2019). Integrating blockchain technology with artificial intelligence for cardiovascular medicine. *Nature Reviews. Cardiology*, *17*(1), 1–3. DOI: 10.1038/s41569-019-0294-y PMID: 31605093

Kuznetsov, A., Sernani, P., Romeo, L., Frontoni, E., & Mancini, A. (2024). On the integration of artificial intelligence and blockchain technology: A perspective about security. *IEEE Access : Practical Innovations, Open Solutions*, *12*, 3881–3897. Advance online publication. DOI: 10.1109/ACCESS.2023.3349019

Lee, D., & Yoon, S. N. (2021). Application of artificial intelligence-based technologies in the healthcare industry: Opportunities and challenges. *International Journal of Environmental Research and Public Health*, *18*(1), 271. DOI: 10.3390/ijerph18010271 PMID: 33401373

Leeming, G., Cunningham, J., & Ainsworth, J. (2019). A ledger of me: Personalizing healthcare using blockchain technology. *Frontiers in Medicine*, *6*, 171. DOI: 10.3389/fmed.2019.00171 PMID: 31396516

Li, W., Andreina, S., Bohli, J. M., & Karame, G. (2017, September). Securing proof-of-stake blockchain protocols. In *International Workshop on Data Privacy Management* (pp. 297–315). Springer.

Lupton, M. (2018). Some ethical and legal consequences of the application of artificial intelligence in the field of medicine. Trends in Medicine, 18(4), Article 100147.

Mamoshina, P., Ojomoko, L., Yanovich, Y., Ostrovski, A., Botezatu, A., Prikhodko, P., Izumchenko, E., Aliper, A., Romantsov, K., Zhebrak, A., Ogu, I. O., & Zhavoronkov, A. (2017). Converging blockchain and next-generation artificial intelligence technologies to decentralize and accelerate biomedical research and healthcare. *Oncotarget*, *9*(5), 5665–5690. DOI: 10.18632/oncotarget.22345 PMID: 29464026

Mayorga-Ruiz, I., Jiménez-Pastor, A., Fos-Guarinos, B., López-González, R., García-Castro, F., & Alberich-Bayarri, Á. (2019). The role of AI in clinical trials. In *Artificial intelligence in medical imaging: Opportunities, applications and risks* (pp. 231–243). Springer. DOI: 10.1007/978-3-319-94878-2_16

MediBloc Limited. (2025). Own your health data. It's rightfully yours. https://medibloc.com/

Mennella, C., Maniscalco, U., Di Pietro, G., & Esposito, M. (2024). Ethical and regulatory challenges of AI technologies in healthcare: A narrative review. *Heliyon*, *10*(4), e26297. Advance online publication. DOI: 10.1016/j.heliyon.2024.e26297 PMID: 38384518

Michael, J., Cohn, A. L. A. N., & Butcher, J. R. (2018). Blockchain technology. *The Journal*, *1*(7), 1–11.

Ministry of Economy, Trade and Industry. (Japan) & Personal Information Protection Commission (Japan). (2024, May 7). Global CBPR Forum.

Ministry of Health Saudi Arabia. (2024). To promote healthcare transformation... MOH calls for participation in the healthcare sandbox. https://www.moh.gov.sa/en/Ministry/MediaCenter/News/Pages/News-2024-08-20-001.aspx

My Doctor Medical Group. (2021). Bitcoin and cryptocurrency. https://mydoctorsf.com/bitcoin/

National Institute of Standards and Technology (NIST). (2023). *Artificial Intelligence Risk Management Framework (AI RMF 1.0)*. U.S. Department of Commerce., DOI: 10.6028/NIST.AI.100-1

Nguyen, D. C., Pathirana, P. N., Ding, M., & Seneviratne, A. (2021). BEdgeHealth: A decentralized architecture for edge-based IoMT networks using blockchain. *IEEE Internet of Things Journal*, *8*(14), 11743–11757. DOI: 10.1109/JIOT.2021.3058953

Nigeria Data Protection Commission. (2023). Nigeria Data Protection Act (NDPA) 2023.

Novelli, C., Taddeo, M., & Floridi, L. (2023). Accountability in artificial intelligence: What it is and how it works. *AI & Society*, *39*(1), 1871–1882. Advance online publication. DOI: 10.1007/s00146-023-01635-y

OECD. (2022). Going digital guide to data governance policy making. OECD Publishing. https://www.oecd.org/en/publications/going-digital-guide-to-data-governance-policy-making_40d53904-en.html

OECD. (2024a). *Regulatory approaches to artificial intelligence in finance (OECD Artificial Intelligence Papers, No. 24)*. OECD Publishing.

OECD. (2024b). Collective action for responsible AI in health (OECD Artificial Intelligence Papers, No. 10). OECD Publishing. https://www.oecd.org/en/publications/collective-action-for-responsible-ai-in-health_f2050177-en.html

Office of the National Coordinator for Health IT. (2024, January 9). Health Data, Technology, and Interoperability (HTO-1) Final Rule. *Federal Register*, *89*, 1192.

Omidian, H. (2024). Synergizing blockchain and artificial intelligence to enhance healthcare. *Drug Discovery Today*, *29*(9), 104111. DOI: 10.1016/j.drudis.2024.104111 PMID: 39034026

Onireti, O., Zhang, L., & Imran, M. A. (2019, December). On the viable area of wireless practical Byzantine fault tolerance (PBFT) blockchain networks. In *2019 IEEE Global Communications Conference (GLOBECOM)* (pp. 1–6). IEEE. DOI: 10.1109/GLOBECOM38437.2019.9013778

Pennic, J. (2019). Healthcare blockchain startup BurstIQ nabs $5.5M for HIPAA-compliant blockchain platform. HIT Consultant. https://hitconsultant.net/2019/10/01/burstiq-hipaa-compliant-blockchain-platform-funding/

Prabu, A. (2021). SmartScope: An AI-powered digital auscultation device to detect cardiopulmonary diseases. *Authorea Preprints.*

Raskin, M. (2016). Law and legality of smart contracts. *Georgetown Law Technology Review, 1*, 305.

Rathore, N., Kumari, A., Patel, M., Chudasama, A., Bhalani, D., Tanwar, S., & Al-abdulatif, A. (2025). Synergy of AI and blockchain to secure electronic healthcare records. *Security and Privacy, 8*(1), e463. DOI: 10.1002/spy2.463

Ray, P. P., Dash, D., Salah, K., & Kumar, N. (2020). Blockchain for IoT-based healthcare: Background, consensus, platforms, and use cases. *IEEE Systems Journal, 15*(1), 85–94. DOI: 10.1109/JSYST.2020.2963840

Roehrs, A., Da Costa, C. A., & da Rosa Righi, R. (2017). OmniPHR: A distributed architecture model to integrate personal health records. *Journal of Biomedical Informatics, 71*, 70–81. DOI: 10.1016/j.jbi.2017.05.012 PMID: 28545835

Sabiri, K., Sousa, F., & Rocha, T. (2025). A systematic review of privacy-preserving blockchain applications in healthcare. *Multimedia Tools and Applications, 84*(32), 39925–39980. Advance online publication. DOI: 10.1007/s11042-024-20541-z

Saeed, H., Malik, H., Bashir, U., Ahmad, A., Riaz, S., Ilyas, M., Bukhari, W. A., & Khan, M. I. A. (2022). Blockchain technology in healthcare: A systematic review. *PLoS One, 17*(4), e0266462. DOI: 10.1371/journal.pone.0266462 PMID: 35404955

Safavi, K., & Kalis, B. (2019). How AI can change the future of healthcare. *Harvard Business Review.*

Sandbox Dubai. (2025). We are Sandbox Dubai—Healthcare Sandbox. https://www.sandboxdubai.gov.ae/sandboxes/health-care-sandbox

Santra, S., Kukreja, P., Saxena, K., Gandhi, S., & Singh, O. V. (2024). Navigating regulatory and policy challenges for AI enabled combination devices. *Frontiers in Medical Technology, 6*, 1473350. Advance online publication. DOI: 10.3389/fmedt.2024.1473350 PMID: 39669903

Saudi Data & AI Authority (SDAIA). (2023, April 23). Personal Data Protection Law (PDPL).

Saudi Data & AI Authority (SDAIA). (2023). Implementing regulations of the Personal Data Protection Law.

Schank, R. C., & Abelson, R. P. (1977). *Scripts, plans, goals, and understanding: An inquiry into human knowledge structures*. Lawrence Erlbaum.

Scipion, C. E., Manchester, M. A., Federman, A., Wang, Y., & Arias, J. J. (2025). Barriers to and facilitators of clinician acceptance and use of artificial intelligence in healthcare settings: A scoping review. *BMJ Open*, *15*(4), e092624. DOI: 10.1136/bmjopen-2024-092624 PMID: 40233955

Shaheen, M. Y. (2021). Applications of artificial intelligence (AI) in healthcare: A review. ScienceOpen *Preprints*.

Shaikh, M., Memon, S. A., Ebrahimi, A., & Wiil, U. K. (2025). A systematic literature review for blockchain-based healthcare implementations. *Health Care*, *13*(9), 1087. Advance online publication. DOI: 10.3390/healthcare13091087 PMID: 40361865

Sharma, S. (2024). Benefits or concerns of AI: A multistakeholder responsibility. *Futures*, *157*, 103328. DOI: 10.1016/j.futures.2024.103328

Shi, D., Zhang, W., Zhang, W., & Ding, X. (2019). A review on lower limb rehabilitation exoskeleton robots. *Chinese Journal of Mechanical Engineering*, *32*(1), 1–11. DOI: 10.1186/s10033-019-0389-8

Shojaei, P., Gjorgievska, E. V., & Chow, Y.-W. (2024). Security and privacy of technologies in health information systems: A systematic literature review. *Computers*, *13*(2), 41. Advance online publication. DOI: 10.3390/computers13020041

Shuaib, M., Alam, S., Shabbir Alam, M., & Shahnawaz Nasir, M. (2021). Compliance with HIPAA and GDPR in blockchain-based electronic health record. *Materials Today: Proceedings*. Advance online publication. DOI: 10.1016/j.matpr.2021.03.059

Solaiman, E., & Awad, C. (2025). Trust and dependability in blockchain & AI based MedIoT applications: Research challenges and future directions. https://doi.org//arXiv.2501.02647DOI: 10.48550

Stoumpos, A. I., Kitsios, F., & Talias, M. A. (2023). Digital transformation in healthcare: Technology acceptance and its applications. *International Journal of Environmental Research and Public Health*, *20*(4), 3407. DOI: 10.3390/ijerph20043407 PMID: 36834105

Sun, Z., Han, D., Li, D., Wang, X., Chang, C.-C., & Wu, Z. (2022). A blockchain-based secure storage scheme for medical information. EURASIP Journal on Wireless Communications and Networking, 2022(1). DOI: 10.1186/s13638-022-02122-6

Tagde, P., Tagde, S., Bhattacharya, T., Tagde, P., Chopra, H., Akter, R., Kaushik, D., & Rahman, M. (2021). Blockchain and artificial intelligence technology in e-Health. *Environmental Science and Pollution Research International, 28*(38), 52810–52831. DOI: 10.1007/s11356-021-16223-0 PMID: 34476701

Tahir, U. A., Barber, J. L., Cruz, D. E., Kars, M. E., Deng, S., Tuftin, B., Gillman, M. G., Benson, M. D., Robbins, J. M., Chen, Z. Z., Rao, P., Katz, D. H., Farrell, L., Sofer, T., Hall, M. E., Ekunwe, L., Tracy, R. P., Durda, P., Taylor, K. D., & Gerszten, R. E. (2024). Proteogenomic analysis integrated with electronic health records data reveals disease-associated variants in Black Americans. *The Journal of Clinical Investigation, 134*(21), e181802. DOI: 10.1172/JCI181802 PMID: 39316441

Tandon, A., Dhir, A., Islam, N., & Mäntymäki, M. (2020). Blockchain in healthcare: A systematic literature review, synthesizing framework and future research agenda. *Computers in Industry, 122*, 103290. Advance online publication. DOI: 10.1016/j.compind.2020.103290

Trappl, R. (Ed.). (1986). *Impacts of artificial intelligence: Scientific, technological, military, economic, societal, cultural, and political* (2nd ed.). Elsevier Science.

Tun, H. M., Rahman, H. A., Naing, L., & Malik, O. A. (2025). Trust in artificial intelligence–based clinical decision support systems among healthcare workers: Systematic review. *Journal of Medical Internet Research, 27*, e69678. DOI: 10.2196/69678 PMID: 40772775

Vukoli, M., (2017). *Rethinking Permissioned Blockchains*. In the ACM Workshop.

Williamson, S. M., & Prybutok, V. (2024). Balancing privacy and progress: A review of privacy challenges, systemic oversight, and patient perceptions in AI-driven healthcare. *Applied Sciences (Basel, Switzerland), 14*(2), 675. Advance online publication. DOI: 10.3390/app14020675

World Bank. (2025). Regulatory sandboxes for digital health. https://documents.worldbank.org/en/publication/documents-reports/documentdetail/099011825011040830

World Health Organization. (2021). Global strategy on digital health 2020–2025. https://www.who.int/publications/i/item/9789240020924

Wronka, C. (2024). Crypto-asset regulatory landscape: A comparative analysis of the crypto-asset regulation in the UK and Germany. *Journal of Asset Management, 25*(4), 417–426. Advance online publication. DOI: 10.1057/s41260-024-00358-z

Xie, Y., Lu, L., Gao, F., He, S., Zhao, H., Fang, Y., Yang, J., An, Y., Ye, Z., & Dong, Z. (2021). Integration of artificial intelligence, blockchain, and wearable technology for chronic disease management: A new paradigm in smart healthcare. *Current Medical Science*, *41*(6), 1123–1133. DOI: 10.1007/s11596-021-2485-0 PMID: 34950987

Yaeger, K., Martini, M., Rasouli, J., & Costa, A. (2019). Emerging blockchain technology solutions for modern healthcare infrastructure. *Journal of Scientific Innovation in Medicine*, *2*(1), 1. DOI: 10.29024/jsim.7

Zakarneh, S. K., Qaroush, Z., & Dawabsheh, A. (2022). Cryptocurrencies advantages and disadvantages: A review. *International Journal of Applied Sciences and Smart Technologies*, *4*(1), 1–20. DOI: 10.24071/ijasst.v5i1.4611

Zheng, Z., Xie, S., Dai, H., Chen, X., & Wang, H. (2017, June). An overview of blockchain technology: Architecture, consensus, and future trends. In 2017 IEEE International Congress on Big Data (BigData Congress) (pp. 557–564). IEEE.

Zhuk, A. (2025). Beyond the blockchain hype: Addressing legal and regulatory challenges. *SN Social Sciences*, *5*(2), 11. Advance online publication. DOI: 10.1007/s43545-024-01044-y

APPENDIX

Table 4. Consensus Mechanisms for Healthcare Data Governance.

Mechanism	Performance (Finality & Latency)	Governance & Identity	Healthcare/ Compliance Fit	Citation
Proof of Work (PoW)	Probabilistic finality; seconds-minutes	Open Permissionless; anonymous miners	Strong integrity/audit trail; very high energy; PHI off-chain; generally unsuitable for clinical consortia- use only for public anchoring if needed.	(Gervais et al., 2016)
Proof of Stake (PoS)	Economic/probabilistic finality; seconds-minutes	Open with economic staking; validator incentives via stake	Energy-efficient; suitable for public discovery/timestamping; keep sensitive data off-chain; ensure auditability outside the ledger	(Li et al., 2017)
Delegated Proof of Stake (DPoS)	Fast economic finality; seconds	Elected delegates; voting governance	High performance; governance/ liability must be explicit; PHI off-chain; suitable if delegate accountability is clear	(Bachani & Bhattacharjya, 2022)
Proof of Authority (PoA)	Deterministic finality; sub-second to seconds	Whitelisted authorities; identity-linked validators	Strong accountability and auditability in permissioned networks; good fit for regulated consortia; PHI off-chain	(De Angelis et al., 2018)
Practical BFT (PBFT)	Deterministic finality; sub-second to seconds	Validator committee; known nodes	Ideal for hospital networks/ HIEs; strong audit trails and clear controller roles; PHI off-chain	(Onireti et al., 2019)
Proof of Elapsed Time (PoET)	Lottery via trusted hardware; seconds	Permissioned; relies on TEEs	Low energy; depends on trust in hardware attestation-document TEE controls; PHI off-chain	(Chen et al., 2017)
Proof of Burn (PoB)	Economic finality; variable	Public permissionless; participants burn coins for rights	Rarely relevant to healthcare data assurance; more about token economics than compliance; generally not recommended for consortia	(Karantias et al., 2020)
Tendermint (BFT)	Deterministic immediate finality; seconds	Validator set; stake-weighted BFT	Strong for application-specific chains; fast, auditable commits; PHI off-chain; good operational fit for permissioned health data networks	(Cason et al., 2021)

Table 5. Comparative Summary of Regional Regulatory Instruments, Focus Area and Proofs-only Rationales

Region	Current Instrument	Regulatory Focus	Proofs-only Rationale
EU	(EU. 2024 AI Act; EU, 2025 EHDS)	Focuses on rights and is considered comprehensive for AI, combining preventive and after-the-fact oversight measures and strict data-transfer safeguards	Consent-receipts ID, brief access-event summaries (e.g., who/when/purpose, no identifiers) and dataset/model lineage fingerprints can be used for audit needs while honouring erasure and minimisation. Identifiable patient data remains off the ledger.
US	(ONC,2024; FTC, 2024 HBNR)	It is sectoral and enforcement-led, with strong after-the-fact oversight and fragmented transfer rules	It provides limited access and demonstrates consent without redistributing patient data, and supports audits across both HIPAA and non-HIPAA settings without moving records. Proof includes: consent-receipt IDs, purpose-scoped access digests, model artefact fingerprints used in clinical decision support
Asia-Pacific	(AIVerify/IMDAPDPC, 2024;METI/PPC,2024 CBPR)	They are considered diverse but interoperability-oriented, risk-based, with guarded outbound transfers	Audit can be completed through standardised evidence (e.g., cross-jurisdiction consent-receipt IDs, access event digest, lineage fingerprints) while data remains in the country, thus erasing cross-jurisdiction exchange
Middle East (Gulf region and UAE)	(SDAIA, 2023 PDPL & Implementing Regulations; UAE, 2025 PDLP Overview)	Innovative, with clear accountability and sandboxing, conditional for cross-border transfers	Oversights and recognition across borders are anchored to evidence (e.g., consent-receipt IDs, access-event digests, provider attestation hash showing approved partner/peer list version and lineage fingerprints) without exposing patient data to network participants
Africa	(NDPC, 2023 NDPA; African Union, 2024 Data Policy Framework)	Emerging frameworks with variable capacity and frequent localisation	Auditability is achieved through small, verifiable evidence (e.g., consent receipt ID, minimal-access digests, dataset lineage fingerprints for registries, and policy/version hashes for the localisation policy in force) and minimal data movement, while keeping identifiable patient data local

Compilation of References

Aanuoluwapo, C. D.-O., Olawade, D. B., Yanuoluwa, O. O., Famujimi, M. E., Olawumi, T. T., & Esan, D. T. (2024). Nursing in the Digital Age: Harnessing telemedicine for enhanced patient care. *Informatics and Health*, *1*(2), 100–110. DOI: 10.1016/j.infoh.2024.07.003

Abbafati, C., Abbas, K. M., Abbasi, M., Abbasifard, M., Abbasi-Kangevari, M., Abbastabar, H., Abd-Allah, F., Abdelalim, A., Abdollahi, M., Abdollahpour, I., Abedi, A., Abedi, P., Abegaz, K. H., Abolhassani, H., Abosetugn, A. E., Aboyans, V., Abrams, E. M., Abreu, L. G., Abrigo, M. R. M., & Murray, C. J. L. (2020). Global burden of 369 diseases and injuries in 204 countries and territories, 1990–2019: A systematic analysis for the Global Burden of Disease Study 2019. *Lancet*, *396*(10258), 1204–1222. DOI: 10.1016/S0140-6736(20)30925-9

Abbo, C. (2011). Profiles and outcome of traditional healing practices for severe mental illnesses in two districts of Eastern Uganda. *Global Health Action*, *4*. Advance online publication. DOI: 10.3402/gha.v4i0.7117

Abd-Alrazaq, A. A., Rababeh, A., Alajlani, M., Bewick, B. M., & Househ, M. (2020). Effectiveness and safety of using chatbots to improve mental health: Systematic review and meta-analysis. *Journal of Medical Internet Research*, *22*(7), 1–17. DOI: 10.2196/16021

Abel, G., Atherton, H., Sussex, J., Akter, N., Aminu, A. Q., Bak, W., Bryce, C., Clark, C. E., Cockcroft, E., Evans, H., Gkousis, E., Jenkins, G., Jenkinson, C., Khan, N., Lambert, J., Leach, B., Marriott, C., Newbould, J., Parkinson, S., & Campbell, J. L. (2024). Current experience and future potential of facilitating access to digital NHS primary care services in England: The Di-Facto mixed-methods study. *Health and Social Care Delivery Research*, *12*(32), 1–197. DOI: 10.3310/JKYT5803 PMID: 39324475

Abodunrin, L. O., & Makanjuola, T. A. (2009). Knowledge and Perception of E-Health and Telemedicine among Health Professionals in LAUTECH Teaching Hospital, Osogbo, Nigeria. *International Journal of Health Research*, *2*(1), 51–58. DOI: 10.4314/ijhr.v2i1.55388

Abomhara, M., & Køien, G. M. (2015). Cyber security and the internet of things: Vulnerabilities, threats, intruders and attacks. *Journal of Cyber Security and Mobility*, *4*(1), 65–88. DOI: 10.13052/jcsm2245-1439.414

Abouzid, M. R., Elshafei, S. M., Elkhawas, I., & Elbana, M. K. (2022). Applications for telemedicine in the Middle East and North Africa region: Benefits gained and challenges faced. *Cureus*, *14*(7), e26611. Advance online publication. DOI: 10.7759/cureus.26611 PMID: 35936169

Aboy, M., Minssen, T., & Vayena, E. (2024). Navigating the EU AI Act: Implications for regulated digital medical products. npj. *Digital Medicine*, *7*(1), 237. Advance online publication. DOI: 10.1038/s41746-024-01232-3 PMID: 39242831

Adambounou, K., Farin, F., Boucher, A., Adjenou, K. V., Gbeassor, M., N'dakena, K., Vincent, N., Adesina, A., Chumba, D., Nelson, A. M., Orem, J., Roberts, D. J., Wabinga, H., Wilson, M., Adong, G., Odoyo, C., & Ondulo, J. (2024). Factors influencing the successful implementation of eHealth in healthcare facilities in developing countries: A scoping review. Journal of Science. *Innovation and Creativity*, *3*(2), 8–17.

Adegbite, T. (2021). 'Telemedicine – A Panacea for Nigeria's Healthcare Ills?' https://www.thisdaylive.com/index.php/2021/03/21/telemedicine-a-panacea-for-nigeriashealthcare-ills

Adem, J. B., Zeleke, T., Walle, A. D., Atinafu, W. T., Tilahun, K. N., Melaku, M. S., & Kebede, S. D. (2023). Awareness and readiness of mental healthcare providers to implement telemental health services and associated factors at public referral hospitals in Addis Ababa City, Ethiopia. *BMJ Open*, *13*(7), 1–13. DOI: 10.1136/bmjopen-2022-069671

Adewale, O. S. (2004). An internet-based telemedicine system in Nigeria. *International Journal of Information Management*, *24*(3), 221–234. DOI: 10.1016/j.ijinfomgt.2003.12.014

Adhikari, S., Ahmed, I., Bajracharya, D., Khanal, B., Solomon, C., Jayaratne, K., Al Mamum, K. A., Talukder, M. S. H., Shakya, S., Manandhar, S., & Memon, Z. A. (2025). Transforming healthcare through just, equitable and quality driven artificial intelligence solutions in South Asia. *NPJ Digital Medicine*, *8*(1), 139. Advance online publication. DOI: 10.1038/s41746-025-01534-0 PMID: 40038520

Adiukwu, F., Ojeahere, M., Adesokun, O., & Babalola, G. (2022). Mental health distress during the COVID-19 pandemic in Nigeria: Need for psychological intervention. *South African Journal of Psychiatry, 28*, 1–6. DOI: 10.4102/sajpsychiatry.v28i0.1550

Afrizal, S. H., Handayani, P. W., Hidayanto, A. N., Eryando, T., Budiharsana, M., & Martha, E. (2019). Barriers and challenges to primary health care information system (PHCIS) adoption from health management perspective: A qualitative study. *Informatics in Medicine Unlocked, 17*, 100198. Advance online publication. DOI: 10.1016/j.imu.2019.100198

Agbeyangi, A. O., & Lukose, J. M. (2025). Telemedicine Adoption and Prospects in Sub-Sahara Africa: A Systematic Review with a Focus on South Africa, Kenya, and Nigeria. *Healthcare (Switzerland), 13*(7), 1–25. DOI: 10.3390/healthcare13070762

Agbo, C., Mahmoud, Q., & Eklund, J. (2019). Blockchain technology in healthcare: A systematic review. *Health Care, 7*(2), 56. Advance online publication. DOI: 10.3390/healthcare7020056 PMID: 30987333

Aggarwal, S., Kumar, N., Alhussein, M., & Muhammad, G. (2021). Blockchain-based UAV path planning for healthcare 4.0: Current challenges and the way ahead. *IEEE Network, 35*(1), 20–29. DOI: 10.1109/MNET.011.2000069

Agyepong, I. A., Sewankambo, N., Binagwaho, A., Coll-Seck, A. M., Corrah, T., Ezeh, A., Fekadu, A., Kilonzo, N., Lamptey, P., Masiye, F., Mayosi, B., Mboup, S., Muyembe, J. J., Pate, M., Sidibe, M., Simons, B., Tlou, S., Gheorghe, A., Legido-Quigley, H., & Piot, P. (2017). The path to longer and healthier lives for all Africans by 2030: The Lancet Commission on the future of health in sub-Saharan Africa. *Lancet, 390*(10114), 2803–2859. DOI: 10.1016/S0140-6736(17)31509-X

Ahanwa, E. S., & Okoloma, H. C. (2023). Telehealth in Nigeria: A Legal Perspective. [IJOLACLE]. *International Journal of Law and Clinical Legal Education, 4*, 136–143.

Ahmed, A., Shahzad, A., Naseem, A., Ali, S., & Ahmad, I. (2025). Evaluating the effectiveness of data governance frameworks in ensuring security and privacy of healthcare data: A quantitative analysis of ISO standards, GDPR, and HIPAA in blockchain technology. *PLoS One, 20*(5), e0324285. Advance online publication. DOI: 10.1371/journal.pone.0324285 PMID: 40408373

Ahmed, F., & Nisar, N. (2010). Public-private partnership scenario in the health care system of Pakistan, *EMHJ-. Eastern Mediterranean Health Journal, 16*(8), 910–912. DOI: 10.26719/2010.16.8.910

AI Verify Foundations; IMDA; PDPC. (2024, May 29). Model AI Governance Framework for Generative AI.

Akdere, M., Top, M., & Tekingündüz, S. (2020). Examining patient perceptions of service quality in Turkish hospitals: The SERVPERF model. *Total Quality Management & Business Excellence*, *31*(3–4), 342–352. DOI: 10.1080/14783363.2018.1427501

Akintosin, J. (2015). The status of telemedicine in Africa: The role of broadband. http://nuviun.com/content/ the-status-of-telemedicine-in-africa/

Akkem, Y., Biswas, S. K., & Varanasi, A. (2024). A comprehensive review of synthetic data generation in smart farming by using variational autoencoder and generative adversarial network. *Engineering Applications of Artificial Intelligence*, *131*, 107881. DOI: 10.1016/j.engappai.2024.107881

Al Kuwaiti, A., Nazer, K., Al-Reedy, A., Al-Shehri, S., Al-Muhanna, A., Subbarayalu, A. V., Al Muhanna, D., & Al-Muhanna, F. A. (2023). A Review of the Role of Artificial Intelligence in Healthcare. *Journal of Personalized Medicine*, *13*(6), 951. Advance online publication. DOI: 10.3390/jpm13060951 PMID: 37373940

Al Omar, A., Bhuiyan, M. Z. A., Basu, A., Kiyomoto, S., & Rahman, M. S. (2019). Privacy-friendly platform for healthcare data in cloud based on blockchain environment. *Future Generation Computer Systems*, *95*, 511–521. DOI: 10.1016/j.future.2018.12.044

Alabdulatif, A., Khalil, I., & Rahman, M. S. (2022). Security of blockchain and AI-empowered smart healthcare: Application-based analysis. *Applied Sciences (Basel, Switzerland)*, *12*(21), 11039. Advance online publication. DOI: 10.3390/app122111039

Alboraie, M., Allam, M. A., Youssef, N., Abdalgaber, M., El-Raey, F., Abdeen, N., Mahdy, R. E., Elshaarawy, O., Elgebaly, A., Haydara, T., Abd-Elsalam, S., Nassar, Y. A., Shabana, H., & Zaky, S. (2021). Knowledge, applicability, and barriers of telemedicine in Egypt: A national survey. *International Journal of Telemedicine and Applications*, *2021*, 5565652. Advance online publication. DOI: 10.1155/2021/5565652 PMID: 34211550

Alborie, H. M., & Damanhouri, A. M. S. (2013). Patients' satisfaction of service quality in Saudi hospitals: A SERVQUAL analysis. *International Journal of Health Care Quality Assurance*, *26*(1), 20–30. DOI: 10.1108/09526861311288613

Aljafari, R., Soh, F., Setia, P., & Agarwal, R. (2023). The local environment matters: Evidence from digital healthcare services for patient engagement. *Journal of the Academy of Marketing Science*, *52*(5), 1343–1365. DOI: 10.1007/s11747-023-00972-0

Aljohani, A. M. (2023). Barriers and challenges to adopting telemedicine in Saudi Arabia.

AlNasser, S., & AlMuhaideb, S. (2024). Listening to patients: Advanced Arabic aspect-based sentiment analysis using transformer models towards better healthcare. *Big Data and Cognitive Computing*, *8*(11), 156. DOI: 10.3390/bdcc8110156

Alowais, S. A., Alghamdi, S. S., Alsuhebany, N., Alqahtani, T., Alshaya, A. I., Almohareb, S. N., Aldairem, A., Alrashed, M., Bin Saleh, K., Badreldin, H. A., Al Yami, M. S., Al Harbi, S., & Albekairy, A. M. (2023). Revolutionizing healthcare: The role of artificial intelligence in clinical practice. *BMC Medical Education*, *23*(1), 689. Advance online publication. DOI: 10.1186/s12909-023-04698-z PMID: 37740191

Alshuwaikhat, H. M., & Abussaud, L. Z. (2023). *Generative urban design for smart, sustainable resilience cities, IAIA conference. Malaysia, 9-11 May*. International Association for Impact Assessment.

Altuntas, S., Dereli, T., & Kaya, I. (2020). Monitoring patient dissatisfaction: A methodology based on SERVQUAL scale and statistical process control charts. *Total Quality Management & Business Excellence*, *31*(9–10), 978–1008. DOI: 10.1080/14783363.2018.1457434

Amann, J., Vayena, E., Ormond, K. E., Frey, D., Madai, V. I., & Blasimme, A. (2023). Expectations and attitudes towards medical artificial intelligence: A qualitative study in the field of stroke. *PLoS One*, *18*(1), e0279088. Advance online publication. DOI: 10.1371/journal.pone.0279088 PMID: 36630325

Anaiye, E. B., & Daudu, B. O. (2025). Medical Care and Patients' Health Correlation in Anyigba Community Health Sectors of Kogi East in Nigeria. *Tanzania Journal of Health Research*, *26*(4), 2277–2288. https://www.ajol.info/index.php/thrb/article/view/269962. DOI: 10.4314/thrb.v26i4.15

Anderson, N. H. (1971). Integration theory and attitude change. *Psychological Review*, *78*(3), 171–206. DOI: 10.1037/h0030834

Andres, B., Poler, R., Camarinha-Matos, L., & Afsarmanesh, H. (2017). A simulation approach to assess partners selected for a collaborative network. *International Journal of Simulation Modelling*, *16*(3), 399–411. DOI: 10.2507/IJSIMM16(3)3.382

Arksey, H., & O'Malley, L. (2005). Scoping studies: Towards a methodological framework. *International Journal of Social Research Methodology*, *8*(1), 19–32. DOI: 10.1080/1364557032000119616

Arora, A., Wright, A., Cheng, T. K. M., Khwaja, Z., & Seah, M. (2021). Innovation pathways in the NHS: An introductory review. *Therapeutic Innovation & Regulatory Science*, *55*(5), 1045–1058. DOI: 10.1007/s43441-021-00304-w PMID: 34009551

Asthana, S., Jones, R., & Sheaff, R. (2019). Why does the NHS struggle to adopt eHealth innovations? A review of macro, meso and micro factors. *BMC Health Services Research*, *19*(984), 1–7. DOI: 10.1186/s12913-019-4790-x PMID: 31864370

Atewologun, F., Adigun, O. A., Okesanya, O. J., Hassan, H. K., Olabode, O. N., Micheal, A. S., Ahmed, M. M., Ukoaka, B. M., Idris, N. B., Oso, T. A., & Lucero-Prisno, D. E. (2025). A comprehensive review of mental health services across selected countries in sub-Saharan Africa: Assessing progress, challenges, and future direction. *Discover Mental Health*, *5*(1). Advance online publication. DOI: 10.1007/s44192-025-00177-7

Attaran, M. (2022). Blockchain technology in healthcare: Challenges and opportunities. *International Journal of Healthcare Management*, *15*(1), 70–83. DOI: 10.1080/20479700.2020.1843887

Atujuna, M., Simpson, N., Ngobeni, M., Monese, T., Giovenco, D., Pike, C., Figerova, Z., Visser, M., Biriotti, M., Kydd, A., & Bekker, L. G. (2021). Khuluma: Using Participatory, Peer-Led and Digital Methods to Deliver Psychosocial Support to Young People Living With HIV in South Africa. *Frontiers in Reproductive Health*, *3*(July). Advance online publication. DOI: 10.3389/frph.2021.687677

Babacan, H. (2020). Public-private partnerships for global health. In Haring, R., Kickbusch, I., Ganten, D., & Moeti, M. (Eds.), *Handbook of Global Health*. Springer International Publishing., DOI: 10.1007/978-3-030-05325-3_117-1

Baballe, A. M., Ayagi, S. H., & Musa, U. F. (2023). Using artificial intelligence (AI) technology in the health sector has several goals. *Global Journal of Research in Engineering & Computer Sciences*, *3*(5), 31–35. DOI: 10.5281/zenodo.10048487

Bachani, V., & Bhattacharjya, A. (2022). Preferential delegated proof of stake (PDPoS)—Modified DPoS with two layers towards scalability and higher TPS. *Symmetry*, *15*(1), 4. DOI: 10.3390/sym15010004

Bainey, K. (2024). *AI-driven project management: Harnessing the power of artificial intelligence and ChatGPT to achieve peak productivity and success*. John Wiley & Sons.

Barragan-Montero, A., Javaid, U., Valdes, G., Nguyen, D., Desbordes, P., Macq, B., Willems, S., Vandewinckele, L., Holmstrom, M., Lofman, F., Michiels, S., Souris, K., Sterpin, E., & Lee, J. A. (2021). Artificial intelligence and machine learning for medical imaging: A technology review. *Physica Medica : PM : An International Journal Devoted to the Applications of Physics to Medicine and Biology : Official Journal of the Italian Association of Biomedical Physics (AIFB)*, *83*, 242–256. DOI: 10.1016/j.ejmp.2021.04.016 PMID: 33979715

Bathula, A., Gupta, S. K., Merugu, S., Saba, L., Khanna, N. N., Laird, J. R., Sanagala, S. S., Singh, R., Garg, D., Fouda, M. M., & Suri, J. S. (2024). Blockchain, artificial intelligence, and healthcare: The tripod of future—A narrative review. *Artificial Intelligence Review*, *57*(9), 238. DOI: 10.1007/s10462-024-10873-5

Ben-Zeev, D., Agorinya, J., Beaulieu, A., Sottie, E. Q., Larsen, A., Attah, D. A., Bedard-Gilligan, M., Ohene, S., Collins, P. Y., Lindgren, K. P., Ofori-Atta, A., Kaysen, D., & Obeng, K. (2025). Sexual trauma and interest in mobile health among women with mental illness in Ghana. Internet Interventions, 40(October 2024), 100829. DOI: 10.1016/j.invent.2025.100829

Ben-Zeev, D., Meller, S., Snyder, J., Attah, D. A., Albright, L., Le, H., Asafo, S. M., Collins, P. Y., & Ofori-Atta, A. (2021). A digital toolkit (m-healer) to improve care and reduce human rights abuses against people with mental illness in west africa: User-centered design, development, and usability study. *JMIR Mental Health*, *8*(7). Advance online publication. DOI: 10.2196/28526

Berhe, K. T., Gesesew, H. A., & Ward, P. R. (2024). Traditional healing practices, factors influencing to access the practices and its complementary effect on mental health in sub-Saharan Africa: A systematic review. *BMJ Open*, *14*(9). Advance online publication. DOI: 10.1136/bmjopen-2023-083004

Bharanitharan, K., & Kaur, G. (2024). The double-edged sword: Legal implications of AI errors and blockchain in finance. *European Economic Letters*, *14*(2). Advance online publication. DOI: 10.52783/eel.v14i2.1637

Bhaskar, S., Bradley, S., Chattu, V. K., Adisesh, A., Nurtazina, A., Kyrykbayeva, S., Sakhamuri, S., Yaya, S., Sunil, T., Thomas, P., Mucci, V., Moguilner, S., Israel-Korn, S., Alacapa, J., Mishra, A., Pandya, S., Schroeder, S., Atreja, A., Banach, M., & Ray, D. (2020). Telemedicine across the globe—Position paper from the COVID-19 Pandemic Health System Resilience PROGRAM (REPROGRAM) International Consortium (Part 1). *Frontiers in Public Health*, *8*, 556720. Advance online publication. DOI: 10.3389/fpubh.2020.556720 PMID: 33178656

Birhane, A. (2021). Algorithmic injustice: A relational ethics approach. *Patterns (New York, N.Y.)*, *2*(2), 100205. DOI: 10.1016/j.patter.2021.100205

Birje, M. N., Goudar, R. H., Rakshitha, C. M., & Tapale, M. T. (2022, July). A review on layered architecture and application domains of blockchain technology. In *2022 International Conference on Electrical, Computer and Energy Technologies (ICECET)* (pp. 1–5). IEEE. DOI: 10.1109/ICECET55527.2022.9872729

Blandford, A., Wesson, J., Amalberti, R., AlHazme, R., & Allwihan, R. (2020). Opportunities and challenges for telehealth within, and beyond, a pandemic. *The Lancet. Global Health*, *8*(11), e1364–e1365. DOI: 10.1016/S2214-109X(20)30362-4 PMID: 32791119

Blease, C., Kaptchuk, T. J., Bernstein, M. H., Mandl, K. D., Halamka, J. D., & DesRoches, C. M. (2019). Artificial intelligence and the future of primary care: Exploratory qualitative study of UK general practitioners' views. *Journal of Medical Internet Research*, *21*(3), e12802. DOI: 10.2196/12802 PMID: 30892270

Bloomfield, P. (2006). The challenging business of long-term public-private partnerships: Reflections on local experience. *Public Administration Review*, *66*(3), 400–411. DOI: 10.1111/j.1540-6210.2006.00597.x

Boardman, A. E., Greve, C., & Hodge, G. A. (2015). Comparative analyses of infrastructure public-private partnerships. *Journal of Comparative Policy Analysis*, *17*(5), 441–447. DOI: 10.1080/13876988.2015.1052611

Boehringer Ingelheim. (2023). Utilisation of data science to identify the system impact of COVID-19 on the cardiometabolic pathway, and identifying opportunities for transformation across Greater Manchester. https://www.boehringer-ingelheim.com/uk/partnering/working-together/partnering-interests/collaborative-working/greater-manchester-utilisation-data-science

Bond, P. (1999). Globalization, pharmaceutical pricing, and South African health policy: Managing confrontation with US firms and politicians. *International Journal of Health Services*, *29*(4), 765–792. DOI: 10.2190/4MA6-53E3-LE1X-C1YY

Bord, J. D., Burke, W., & Dudzinski, D. M. D. M. (2023). Confidentiality. https://depts.washington.edu/bhdept/ethics-medicine/bioethicstopics/detail/58

Borges do Nascimento, I. J., Abdulazeem, H., Vasanthan, L. T., Martinez, E. Z., Zucoloto, M. L., Østengaard, L., Azzopardi-Muscat, N., Zapata, T., & Novillo-Ortiz, D. (2023). Barriers and facilitators to utilizing digital health technologies by healthcare professionals. *NPJ Digital Medicine*, *6*(1), 161. DOI: 10.1038/s41746-023-00899-4 PMID: 37723240

Borges do Nascimento, I. J., Abdulazeem, H., Vasanthan, L. T., Martinez, E. Z., Zucoloto, M. L., Østengaard, L., Azzopardi-Muscat, N., Zapata, T., & Novillo-Ortiz, D. (2023). Barriers and facilitators to utilizing digital health technologies by healthcare professionals. npj. *Digital Medicine*, *6*(1), 161. PMID: 37723240

Borges, A. P., Rodrigues, P., Brochado, A., & Sousa, A. (2025). Mindfulness as a mediating mechanism between health importance and positive mental well-being. *International Journal of Pharmaceutical and Healthcare Marketing*, *19*(3), 773–793. Advance online publication. DOI: 10.1108/IJPHM-07-2024-0069

Borowy, M. (2025). Generative AI as a driver of trust in innovation. *Building Trust in the Generative Artificial Intelligence Era*, 53-66.

Botes, M. (2025). Regulatory challenges of digital health: The case of mental health applications and personal data in South Africa. *Frontiers in Pharmacology*, *16*(April), 1–7. DOI: 10.3389/fphar.2025.1498600

Botti, A., & Monda, A. (2020). Sustainable value co-creation and digital health: The case of Trentino eHealth ecosystem. *Sustainability (Basel)*, *12*(13), 5263. Advance online publication. DOI: 10.3390/su12135263

Bouderhem, R. (2024). Shaping the future of AI in healthcare through ethics and governance. *Humanities & Social Sciences Communications*, *11*(1), 416. Advance online publication. DOI: 10.1057/s41599-024-02894-w

Bourgeois, D. M., Phantumvanit, P., Llodra, J. C., Horn, V., Carlile, M., & Eiselé, J. L. (2014). Rationale for the prevention of oral diseases in primary health care: An international collaborative study in oral health education. *International Dental Journal*, *64*, 1–11. DOI: 10.1111/idj.12126

Bowers, M. R., Swan, J. E., & Koehler, W. F. (1994). What attributes determine quality and satisfaction with health care delivery? *Health Care Management Review*, *19*(4), 49–55. DOI: 10.1097/00004010-199401940-00006

Bowser, D. M., Shepard, D. S., Nandakumar, A., Okunogbe, A., Morrill, T., Halasa-Rappel, Y., & Oluwayemisi, E. (2018). Cost effectiveness of mobile health for antenatal care and facility births in Nigeria. *Annals of Global Health*, *84*(4), 592–602. DOI: 10.29024/aogh.2364 PMID: 30779506

Bramer, W. M., de Jonge, G. B., Rethlefsen, M. L., Mast, F., & Kleijnen, J. (2018). A systematic approach to searching: An efficient and complete method to develop literature searches. *Journal of the Medical Library Association: JMLA*, *106*(4), 531–541. DOI: 10.5195/jmla.2018.283 PMID: 30271302

Breuer, J., Bishop, L., & Kinder-Kurlanda, K. (2020). The practical and ethical challenges in acquiring and sharing digital trace data: Negotiating public-private partnerships. *New Media & Society*, *22*(11), 2058–2080. DOI: 10.1177/1461444820924622

Bridoux, F., & Stoelhorst, J. W. (2022). Stakeholder theory, strategy, and organization: Past, present, and future. *Strategic Organization*, *20*(4), 797–809. DOI: 10.1177/14761270221127628

Briggs, A. D. M., Göpfert, A., Thorlby, R., Allwood, D., & Alderwick, H. (2020). Integrated health and care systems in England: Can they help prevent disease? *Integrated Healthcare Journal*, *2*(11), e000013. Advance online publication. DOI: 10.1136/ihj-2019-000013 PMID: 37441304

Brinkerhoff, J. M. (2002). Assessing and improving partnership relationships and outcomes: A proposed framework. *Evaluation and Program Planning*, *25*(3), 215–231. DOI: 10.1016/S0149-7189(02)00017-4

Bucci, S., Berry, N., Morris, R., Berry, K., Haddock, G., Lewis, S., & Edge, D. (2019). "They are not hard-to-reach clients. We have just got hard-to-reach services." Staff views of digital health tools in specialist mental health services. *Frontiers in Psychiatry*, *10*, 344. Advance online publication. DOI: 10.3389/fpsyt.2019.00344 PMID: 31133906

Bucci, S., Schwannauer, M., & Berry, N. (2019). The digital revolution and its impact on mental health care. Psychology and Psychotherapy: Theory. *Psychology and Psychotherapy*, *92*(2), 277–297. DOI: 10.1111/papt.12222 PMID: 30924316

Buck, C., Doctor, E., Hennrich, J., Jöhnk, J., & Eymann, T. (2022). General practitioners' attitudes toward artificial intelligence–enabled systems: Interview study. *Journal of Medical Internet Research*, *24*(1), e28916. DOI: 10.2196/28916 PMID: 35084342

Buckingham, S. A., Walker, T., & Morrissey, K. (2022). The feasibility and acceptability of digital technology for health and wellbeing in social housing residents in Cornwall: A qualitative scoping study. *Digital Health*, *8*, 1–12. DOI: 10.1177/20552076221074124 PMID: 35096410

Burst IQ. (2024). About BurstIQ. https://burstiq.com/about-burstiq/

Burst IQ. (2025a). BurstIQ joins the AWS Partner Network to bring AI-ready data management solutions to cloud customers. PR Newswire. https://www.prnewswire.com/news-releases/burstiq-joins-the-aws-partner-network-to-bring-ai-ready-data-management-solutions-to-cloud-customers-302477982.html

Burst IQ. (2025b). BurstIQ completes its sixth annual independent SOC 2 type II audit, continuing a legacy of best-in-class data security. https://burstiq.com/burstiq-completes-its-sixth-annual-independent-soc-2-type-ii-audit-continuing-a-legacy-of-best-in-class-data-security/

Busch, F., Hoffmann, L., Xu, L., Zhang, L. J., Hu, B., García-Juárez, I., Toapanta-Yanchapaxi, L. N., Gorelik, N., Gorelik, V., Rodriguez-Granillo, G. A., Ferrarotti, C., Cuong, N. N., Thi, C. A. P., Tuncel, M., Kaya, G., Solis-Barquero, S. M., Mendez Avila, M. C., Ivanova, N. G., Kitamura, F. C., & Zhang, S. (2025). Multinational attitudes toward AI in healthcare and diagnostics among hospital patients. *JAMA Network Open*, *8*(6), e2514452. DOI: 10.1001/jamanetworkopen.2025.14452 PMID: 40493367

Buse, K., & Walt, G. (2000a). Global public-private partnerships: Part I-a new development in health? *Bulletin of the World Health Organization*, *78*, 549–561.

Buse, K., & Walt, G. (2000b). Global public-private partnerships: Part II-what are the health issues for global governance? *Bulletin of the World Health Organization*, *78*(5), 699–709.

Buterin, V., Illum, J., Nadler, M., Schär, F., & Soleimani, A. (2023). Blockchain privacy and regulatory compliance: Towards a practical equilibrium. Blockchain. *SSRN*, *5*(1), 100176. Advance online publication. DOI: 10.2139/ssrn.4563364

Caines, K., Buse, K., Carlson, C., De Loor, R., Druce, N., Grace, C., Pearson, M., Sancho, J., & Sadanandan, R. (2004). *Assessing the impact of global health partnerships*. DFID Health Resource Centre.

Cao, X., Rajagopalan, S., & Tong, C. (2024). Impact of vertical integration in a referral-based healthcare system. *Omega*, *12*, 102998. DOI: 10.1016/j.omega.2023.102998

Carapinha, J., Botes, D., & Carapinha, R. (2024). Balancing innovation and ethics in AI governance for health technology assessment. *Journal of Medical Economics*, *27*(1), 754–757. Advance online publication. DOI: 10.1080/13696998.2024.2352821 PMID: 38711204

Carlson, C., Druce, N., & Sadanandan, R. (2004). *Assessing the impact of global health partnerships. country case study report*. DFID Health Resource Centre.

Carter, S. M., Rogers, W., Win, K. T., Frazer, H., Richards, B., & Houssami, N. (2020). The ethical, legal and social implications of using artificial intelligence systems in breast cancer care. *The Breast : Official Journal of the European Society of Mastology*, *49*, 25–32. DOI: 10.1016/j.breast.2019.10.001 PMID: 31677530

Cartolovni, A., Tomicic, A., & Mosler, E. L. (2022). Ethical, legal, and social considerations of AI-based medical decision-support tools: A scoping review. *International Journal of Medical Informatics*, *161*, 104738. Advance online publication. DOI: 10.1016/j.ijmedinf.2022.104738 PMID: 35299098

Cascella, L. M. (2023). Risk Perspectives in Telehealth: Informed Consent. https://www.medpro.com/telemedicine-informedconsent

Cason, D., Fynn, E., Milosevic, N., Milosevic, Z., Buchman, E., & Pedone, F. (2021, September). The design, architecture and performance of the Tendermint blockchain network. In 2021 40th International Symposium on Reliable Distributed Systems (SRDS) (pp. 23–33). IEEE. DOI: 10.1109/SRDS53918.2021.00012

Casper, T. (2004). Updated discussion paper on the core business model of a mature global fund, *Ninth board meeting of the Global Fund*. Arusha, 18-19 November. Geneva: The Global Fund.

Cath, C. (2018). Governing artificial intelligence: ethical, legal and technical opportunities and challenges Introduction [Editorial Material]. *Philosophical Transactions of the Royal Society a-Mathematical Physical and Engineering Sciences, 376*(2133), 8, Article 20180080. https://doi.org/DOI: 10.1098/rsta.2018.0080

Cavadi, G. (2025). Strengthening resilience in healthcare organizations through an AI-enhanced performance management framework. https://tesidottorato.depositolegale.it/handle/20.500.14242/187860

CEPAL. (2022). Closing the Digital Divide: More and Better Funding for the Digital Transformation of Health in Latin America and the Caribbean. Transform Health, November, 1–5. https://transformhealthcoalition.org/wp-content/uploads/2023/08/Latin-America-Regional-Brief-English-v2.pdf?

Chanussot-Deprez, C., & Contreras-Ruiz, J. (2013). Telemedicine in wound care. *Advances in Skin & Wound Care*, *26*(2), 78–82. DOI: 10.1097/01.ASW.0000426717.59326.5f PMID: 23337648

Chao, J., Lu, B., Zhang, H., Zhu, L., Jin, H., & Liu, P. (2017). Healthcare system responsiveness in Jiangsu Province, China. *BMC Health Services Research, 17*(1), 31. DOI: 10.1186/s12913-017-1980-2

Char, D. S., Shah, N. H., & Magnus, D. (2018). Implementing Machine Learning in Health Care - Addressing Ethical Challenges. *The New England Journal of Medicine*, *378*(11), 981–983. DOI: 10.1056/NEJMp1714229 PMID: 29539284

Charles, C., & McNulty, S. (1999). Partnering for results: assessing the impact of inter-sectoral partnering. Academy for Educational Development and United States Agency for International Development., https://pdf.usaid.gov/pdf_docs/Pnacd344.pdf, Retrieved October 15, 1999, from.

Chaturvedi, U., Chauhan, S. B., & Singh, I. (2025). The impact of artificial intelligence on remote healthcare: Enhancing patient engagement, connectivity, and overcoming challenges. *Intelligent Pharmacy*, *3*(5), 323–329. DOI: 10.1016/j.ipha.2024.12.003

Chauhan, C., & Gullapalli, R. R. (2021). Ethics of AI in Pathology <i>Current Paradigms and Emerging Issues</i>. *The American Journal of Pathology*, *191*(10), 1673–1683. DOI: 10.1016/j.ajpath.2021.06.011 PMID: 34252382

Chauhan, M. (2023). Emerging Trends in Telemedicine and Remote Patient Monitoring: Improving Access to Healthcare Services. *International Research Journal of Basic and Clinical Studies*, *8*(3), 1–5.

Chen, C. (2016). *CiteSpace: A Practical Guide for Mapping Scientific Literature*. CiteSpace: A Practical Guide for Mapping Scientific Literature.

Chen, C. (2020). How to Use CiteSpace (c) 2015-2020.

Chen, A., Li, L. J., & Wang, J. S. (2016). The experiential elements of patient satisfaction using the phenomenological qualitative study. *Zhongguo Weisheng Zhiliang Guanli*, *9*(5), 1–4.

Chen, C. (2004). Searching for intellectual turning points: Progressive knowledge domain visualization. *Proceedings of the National Academy of Sciences of the United States of America*, *101*(suppl_1), 5303–5310. https://doi.org/doi:10.1073/pnas.0307513100. DOI: 10.1073/pnas.0307513100 PMID: 14724295

Chen, C. (2020). A Glimpse of the First Eight Months of the COVID-19 Literature on Microsoft Academic Graph: Themes, Citation Contexts, and Uncertainties [Methods]. *Frontiers in Research Metrics and Analytics*, *5*, 607286. Advance online publication. DOI: 10.3389/frma.2020.607286 PMID: 33870064

Chen, C. M. (2006). CiteSpace II: Detecting and visualizing emerging trends and transient patterns in scientific literature. *Journal of the American Society for Information Science and Technology*, *57*(3), 359–377. DOI: 10.1002/asi.20317

Chen, L., Xu, L., Shah, N., Gao, Z., Lu, Y., & Shi, W. (2017, October). On security analysis of proof-of-elapsed-time (PoET). In *International Symposium on Stabilization, Safety, and Security of Distributed Systems* (pp. 282–297). Springer.

Chen, T., & Gombay, C. (2024). Advantages and disadvantages of digital mental health initiatives in Nigeria - a qualitative interview study. *Journal of Mental Health (Abingdon, England)*, *33*(5), 613–618. DOI: 10.1080/09638237.2024.2361234

Chen, Z. (2009). Launch of the health-care reform plan in China. *Lancet*, *373*(9672), 1322–1324. DOI: 10.1016/S0140-6736(09)60753-4

Cheong, B. C. (2024). Transparency and accountability in AI systems: Safeguarding wellbeing in the age of algorithmic decision-making. *Frontiers in Human Dynamics*, *6*, 1421273. Advance online publication. DOI: 10.3389/fhumd.2024.1421273

Chin, M. H., Afsar-Manesh, N., Bierman, A. S., Chang, C. S. E., Colón-Rodríguez, C. J., Dullabh, P., Duran, D. G., Fair, M., Hernandez-Boussard, T., Hightower, M., Jain, A., Jordan, W. B., Konya, S., Moore, R. H., Moore, T. T., Rodriguez, R., Shaheen, G., Snyder, L. P., Srinivasan, M., & Ohno-Machado, L. (2023). Guiding Principles to Address the Impact of Algorithm Bias on Racial and Ethnic Disparities in Health and Health Care. *JAMA Network Open*, *6*(12), e2345050. Advance online publication. DOI: 10.1001/jamanetworkopen.2023.45050 PMID: 38100101

Chipps, J., Brysiewicz, P., & Mars, M. (2012). Effectiveness and feasibility of telepsychiatry in resource constrained environments? A systematic review of the evidence. *African Journal of Psychiatry (South Africa)*, *15*(4), 235–243. DOI: 10.4314/ajpsy.v15i4.30

Chipps, J., & Mars, M. (2012). Readiness of health-care institutions in KwaZulu-Natal to implement telepsychiatry. *Journal of Telemedicine and Telecare*, *18*(3), 133–137. DOI: 10.1258/jtt.2012.SFT103

Chipps, J., Ramlall, S., & Mars, M. (2012). A telepsychiatry model to support psychiatric outreach in the public sector in South Africa. *African Journal of Psychiatry (South Africa)*, *15*(4), 264–270. DOI: 10.4314/ajpsy. v15i4.34

Choy, K., & Lee, W. B. (2002). A generic tool for the selection and management of supplier relationships in an outsourced manufacturing environment: The application of case based reasoning. *Logistics Information Management*, *15*(4), 235–253. DOI: 10.1108/09576050210436093

Christoforaki, M., & Beyan, O. (2022). AI Ethics-A Bird's Eye View. *Applied Sciences (Basel, Switzerland)*, *12*(9), 4130. Advance online publication. DOI: 10.3390/app12094130

Chukwu, E., & Garg, L. (2020). A systematic review of blockchain in healthcare: Frameworks, prototypes, and implementations. *IEEE Access : Practical Innovations, Open Solutions*, *8*, 21196–21214. DOI: 10.1109/ACCESS.2020.2969881

Chukwu, E., Garg, L., Foday, E., Konomanyi, A., Wright, R., & Smart, F. (2022). Electricity, computing hardware, and internet infrastructures in health facilities in Sierra Leone: Field mapping study. *JMIR Medical Informatics*, *10*(2), e30040. DOI: 10.2196/30040 PMID: 35113026

Clausen, H., Ruud, T., Odden, S., Benth, J. Š., Heiervang, K. S., Stuen, H. K., & Landheim, A. (2020). Improved Rehabilitation Outcomes for Persons With and Without Problematic Substance Use After 2 Years With Assertive Community Treatment—A Prospective Study of Patients With Severe Mental Illness in 12 Norwegian ACT Teams. *Frontiers in Psychiatry*, *11*(December), 1–11. DOI: 10.3389/fpsyt.2020.607071

Cohen, S., & Wills, T. A. (1985). Stress, social support, and the buffering hypothesis. *Psychological Bulletin*, *98*(2), 310–357. DOI: 10.1037/0033-2909.98.2.310

Congo Medika, R. D. C. (n.d.). https://congomedika.com/

Congo, R. X. | Consultation vidéo Médecins locaux internationaux. (n.d.). https://www.congorx.com/

Contaldo, M. T., Pasceri, G., Vignati, G., Bracchi, L., Triggiani, S., & Carrafiello, G. (2024). AI in Radiology: Navigating Medical Responsibility. *Diagnostics (Basel)*, *14*(14), 1506. Advance online publication. DOI: 10.3390/diagnostics14141506 PMID: 39061643

Conway, M. D., Gupta, S., & Prakash, S. (2006). Building better partnerships for global health. *The McKinsey Quarterly*, •••, 1–8.

Cooper, R., Giangreco, A., Duffy, M., Finlayson, E., Hamilton, S., Swanson, M., Colligan, J., Gilliatt, J., McIvor, M., & Sage, E. K. (2022). Evaluation of myCOPD digital self-management technology in a remote and rural population: Real-world feasibility study. *Journal of Medical Internet Research*, *10*(2), e30782. Advance online publication. DOI: 10.2196/30782 PMID: 35129453

Corfmat, M., Martineau, J. T., & Régis, C. (2025). High-reward, high-risk technologies? An ethical and legal account of AI development in healthcare. *BMC Medical Ethics*, *26*(1), 4. Advance online publication. DOI: 10.1186/s12910-024-01158-1 PMID: 39815254

Corte-Real, A., Nunes, T., & da Cunha, P. R. (2024). Reflections about blockchain in health data sharing: Navigating a disruptive technology. *International Journal of Environmental Research and Public Health*, *21*(2), 230. Advance online publication. DOI: 10.3390/ijerph21020230 PMID: 38397719

Cox, C. M., Masiano, S., Mazenga, A., Stark, M., Udedi, M., Simon, K. R., Ahmed, S., Nyasulu, P., & Kim, M. H. (2024). Phone-based psychosocial counseling for people living with HIV: Feasibility, acceptability and impact on uptake of psychosocial counseling services in Malawi. *Global Mental Health (Cambridge, England), 11*. Advance online publication. DOI: 10.1017/gmh.2023.84

Craig, J., & Patterson, V. (2005). Introduction to the practice of telemedicine. *Journal of Telemedicine and Telecare, 11*(1), 3–9. DOI: 10.1177/1357633X0501100102

Crisp, N. (2025). Abolishing NHS England: Risks and opportunities. *BMJ (Clinical Research Ed.), 388*, r553. Advance online publication. DOI: 10.1136/bmj.r553 PMID: 40101921

Cronin, J. J.Jr, & Taylor, S. A. (1994). SERVPERF versus SERVQUAL: Reconciling performance-based and perceptions-minus-expectations measurement of service quality. *Journal of Marketing, 58*(2), 125–131. DOI: 10.1177/002224299405800110

Cu, A., Meister, S., Lefebvre, B., & Ridde, V. (2021). Assessing healthcare access using the Levesque's conceptual framework– a scoping review. *International Journal for Equity in Health, 20*(1), 1–14. DOI: 10.1186/s12939-021-01416-3

Cummins, T., Conrad, K., & Finkenstadt, D. (2025). *Beyond the table: Insights on negotiated terms, synthetic scenario simulations, and future competencies in contract management.*

Da Silva, M., Horsley, T., Singh, D., Da Silva, E., Ly, V., Thomas, B., Daniel, R. C., Chagal-Feferkorn, K. A., Iantomasi, S., White, K., Kent, A., & Flood, C. M. (2022). Legal concerns in health-related artificial intelligence: A scoping review protocol. *Systematic Reviews, 11*(1), 123. Advance online publication. DOI: 10.1186/s13643-022-01939-y PMID: 35715812

Dailami, M., & Klein, M. (1998). *Government support to private infrastructure projects in emerging markets.* World Bank Publications.

Dalton-Brown, S. (2020). The Ethics of Medical AI and the Physician-Patient Relationship. *Cambridge Quarterly of Healthcare Ethics, 29*(1), 115-121, Article Pii s0963180119000847. https://doi.org/DOI: 10.1017/S0963180119000847

Damschroder, L. J., Reardon, C. M., Widerquist, M. A. O., & Lowery, J. (2022). The updated Consolidated Framework for Implementation Research based on user feedback. *Implementation Science : IS, 17*(1), 1–16. DOI: 10.1186/s13012-022-01245-0

Darzi, A. (2024). *Independent investigation of the NHS in England.* UK Department of Health and Social Care, November 15. www.gov.uk/government/publications/independent-investigation-of-the-nhs-in-england

Daudu, B. O., Amodu, S. A., Ojochenemi, P. Y., & Anaiye, E. B. (2025). Leveraging Data-Driven Approaches: A Case Study on Enhancing Water Governance in Africa. In Agarwal, S., & Garg, M. C. (Eds.), *The Handbook of AI for Clean Water: Innovations in Treatment and Monitoring* (pp. 293–306). CRC Press., DOI: 10.1201/9781003600718-24

Daudu, B. O., & Osimen, G. U. (2025). Combatting Cyberthreats in African Digital Space with Artificial Intelligence. In Vajjhala, N. R., & Strange, K. D. (Eds.), *Cybersecurity in Knowledge Management: Cyberthreats and Solutions* (pp. 115–130). CRC Press., DOI: 10.1201/9781003498094-8

Daudu, B. O., Osimen, G. U., & Anaiye, E. B. (2024). Sustainable Smart Cities in African Digital Space. In Whig, P., Sharma, P., Aneja, N., Elngar, A. A., & Silva, N. (Eds.), *Artificial Intelligence and Machine Learning for Sustainable Development: Innovations, Challenges, and Applications* (pp. 100–111). CRC Press., DOI: 10.1201/9781003497189-8

Dave, S., Abraham, S., Ramkisson, R., Matheiken, S., Pillai, A. S., Reza, H., Bamrah, J. S., & Tracy, D. K. (2021). Digital psychiatry and Covid-19: The big bang effect for the NHS? *BJPsych Bulletin*, *45*(5), 259–263. DOI: 10.1192/bjb.2020.114 PMID: 33081867

De Aguiar, E. J., Faiçal, B. S., Krishnamachari, B., & Ueyama, J. (2020). A survey of blockchain-based strategies for healthcare. *ACM Computing Surveys*, *53*(2), 27.

De Angelis, S., Aniello, L., Baldoni, R., Lombardi, F., Margheri, A., & Sassone, V. (2018). PBFT vs proof-of-authority: Applying the CAP theorem to permissioned blockchain. In *CEUR Workshop Proceedings* (Vol. 2058). CEUR-WS.

de Haan, E., Padigar, M., El Kihal, S., Kübler, R., & Wieringa, J. E. (2024). Unstructured data research in business: Toward a structured approach. *Journal of Business Research*, *177*, 114655. DOI: 10.1016/j.jbusres.2024.114655

Deloitte. (2016). Blockchain: Opportunities for healthcare. https://www2.deloitte.com/content/dam/Deloitte/us/Documents/public-sector/us-blockchain-opportunities-for-health-care.pdf

Demirel, S., Kahraman-Gokalp, E., & Gündüz, U. (2025). From optimism to concern: Unveiling sentiments and perceptions surrounding ChatGPT on Twitter. *International Journal of Human-Computer Interaction*, *41*(12), 7292–7314. DOI: 10.1080/10447318.2024.2392964

Department for Science, Innovation and Technology. (2025). *AI opportunities action plan*. GOV.UK. January 13.

Department of Health & Social Care. (2022). Data saves lives: Reshaping health and social care with data. https://data.parliament.uk/DepositedPapers/Files/DEP2022-0485/Data_saves_lives_Reshaping_health_and_social_care_with_data.pdf

Dhakate, N., & Joshi, R. (2023). Classification of reviews of e-healthcare services to improve patient satisfaction: Insights from an emerging economy. *Journal of Business Research, 164*, 114015. DOI: 10.1016/j.jbusres.2023.114015

Dietvorst, E., Hillegers, M. H. J., Legerstee, J. S., De Vries, L. P., Vreeker, A., & Keijsers, L. (2024). Real-time personalized feedback in mHealth for adolescents. *Digital Health, 10*. Advance online publication. DOI: 10.1177/20552076241247937

Digital Health London. (2023). Rolling out a digital consent pilot for patients undergoing surgery. https://digitalhealth.london/rolling-out-a-digital-consent-pilot-for-patients-undergoing-surgery

Digital Health. (2021, July). ORCHA poll reveals public are willing to embrace digital to help NHS. https://www.digitalhealth.net/2021/07/orcha-poll-digital-nhs/

Ding, X., & Yang, Z. (2022). Knowledge mapping of platform research: A visual analysis using VOSviewer and CiteSpace. *Electronic Commerce Research, 22*(3), 787–809. DOI: 10.1007/s10660-020-09410-7

Dixon, D., Sattar, H., Moros, N., Kesireddy, S. R., Ahsan, H., Lakkimsetti, M., Fatima, M., Doshi, D., Sadhu, K., & Hassan, M. J. (2024). Unveiling the influence of AI predictive analytics on patient outcomes: A comprehensive narrative review. *Cureus, 16*(5). Advance online publication. DOI: 10.7759/cureus.59954 PMID: 38854327

Dlugatch, R., Georgieva, A., & Kerasidou, A. (2023). Trustworthy artificial intelligence and ethical design: Public perceptions of trustworthiness of an AI-based decision-support tool in the context of intrapartum care. *BMC Medical Ethics, 24*(1), 42. Advance online publication. DOI: 10.1186/s12910-023-00917-w PMID: 37340408

Dodoo, J. E., Al-Samarraie, H., & Alsswey, A. (2022). The development of telemedicine programs in Sub-Saharan Africa: Progress and associated challenges. *Health Technology (Hong Kong), 12*(1), 33–46. DOI: 10.1007/s12553-021-00626-7 PMID: 34849325

Dodoo, J. E., Al-Samarraie, H., & Alzahrani, A. I. (2021). Telemedicine use in Sub-Saharan Africa: Barriers and policy recommendations for Covid-19 and beyond. *International Journal of Medical Informatics, 151*, 104467. DOI: 10.1016/j.ijmedinf.2021.104467

Doukani, A., van Dalen, R., Valev, H., Njenga, A., Sera, F., & Chibanda, D. (2021). A community health volunteer delivered problem-solving therapy mobile application based on the Friendship Bench 'Inuka Coaching' in Kenya: A pilot cohort study. *Global Mental Health (Cambridge, England), 8*. Advance online publication. DOI: 10.1017/gmh.2021.3

Drew, D. A., Nguyen, L. H., Steves, C. J., Menni, C., Freydin, M., Varsavsky, T., Sudre, C. H., Cardoso, M. J., Ourselin, S., Wolf, J., Spector, T. D., & Chan, A. T. (2020). Rapid implementation of mobile technology for real-time epidemiology of COVID-19. *Science, 368*(6497), 1362-+. https://doi.org/DOI: 10.1126/science.abc0473

Durán, J. M., & Jongsma, K. R. (2021). Who is afraid of black box algorithms? On the epistemological and ethical basis of trust in medical AI. *Journal of Medical Ethics, 47*(5), 329–335. DOI: 10.1136/medethics-2020-106820 PMID: 33737318

Dwivedi, Y. K., Kshetri, N., Hughes, L., Slade, E. L., Jeyaraj, A., Kar, A. K., Baabdullah, A. M., Koohang, A., Raghavan, V., Ahuja, M., Albanna, H., Albashrawi, M. A., Al-Busaidi, A. S., Balakrishnan, J., Barlette, Y., Basu, S., Bose, I., Brooks, L., Buhalis, D., & Wright, R. (2023). "So what if ChatGPT wrote it?" Multidisciplinary perspectives on opportunities, challenges and implications of generative conversational AI for research, practice and policy. *International Journal of Information Management, 71*, 102642. DOI: 10.1016/j.ijinfomgt.2023.102642

Eapen, T. T., & Finkenstadt, D. J. (2025). Managing difficult conversations on new technology integration: The case of generative AI. *Strategy and Leadership, 53*(2), 174–187. DOI: 10.1108/SL-07-2024-0062

Economist Impact. (2024). *Unlocking enterprise AI: Opportunities and strategies*, November 22.

Ejaz, M., Kumar, T., Kovacevic, I., Ylianttila, M., & Harjula, E. (2021). Health-blockedge: Blockchain-edge framework for reliable low-latency digital healthcare applications. *Sensors (Basel), 21*(7), 2502. DOI: 10.3390/s21072502 PMID: 33916700

El Malouf, N., & Bahemia, H. (2025). Diffusion of Innovations: A review. In S. Papagiannidis (Ed), *TheoryHub Book*. https://open.ncl.ac.uk

Elendu, C., Amaechi, D. C., Elendu, T. C., Jingwa, K. A., Okoye, O. K., Okah, M. J., & Alimi, H. A. (2023). Ethical implications of AI and robotics in healthcare. *Revista de Medicina (São Paulo), 102*(50), e36671. DOI: 10.1097/MD.0000000000036671 PMID: 38115340

Eleuch, A. K. (2011). Healthcare service quality perception in Japan. *International Journal of Health Care Quality Assurance, 24*(6), 417–429. DOI: 10.1108/09526861111150680

Emmanuel, A. K., Abdul, S. O., Obasi, D. E., Jokoh, P. E., Omoze, E. M., Usoh, A. E., Ashimi, A. A., & Adisa, A. A. (2025). Investigating the challenges and opportunities of telemedicine in enhancing health care access in Nigeria. *Int J Clin Med Case Stud., 2*(1), 1004. DOI: 10.52768/3067-3852/1004

Engel, N., & van Lente, H. (2014). Organisational innovation and control practices: The case of public-private mix in tuberculosis control in India. *Sociology of Health & Illness, 36*(6), 917–931. DOI: 10.1111/1467-9566.12125

Esposito, C., De Santis, A., Tortora, G., Chang, H., & Choo, K. K. R. (2018). Blockchain: A panacea for healthcare cloud-based data security and privacy? *IEEE Cloud Computing, 5*(1), 31–37. DOI: 10.1109/MCC.2018.011791712

Ettaloui, N., Arezki, S., & Gadi, T. (2023). An overview of blockchain-based electronic health records and compliance with GDPR and HIPAA. 2, 166. DOI: 10.56294/dm2023166

European Data Protection Board. (2025a). EDPB adopts guidelines on processing personal data through blockchains and is ready to cooperate with AI office on guidelines on AI Act and EU data protection law. https://www.edpb.europa.eu/news/news/2025/edpb-adopts-guidelines-processing-personal-data-through-blockchains-and-ready_en

European Data Protection Board. (2025b). Guidelines, recommendations, best practices. https://www.edpb.europa.eu/our-work-tools/general-guidance/guidelines-recommendations-best-practices_en

European Union. (2024). Regulation (EU) 2024/1689 of 13 June 2024 laying down harmonised rules on artificial intelligence (Artificial Intelligence Act). Official Journal of the European Union.

European Union. (2025). Regulation (EU) 2025/327 of 11 February 2025 on the European Health Data Space. Official Journal of the European Union.

Evans, A. J., Krupinski, E. A., Weinstein, R. S., & Pantanowitz, L. (2015). 2014 American Telemedicine Association clinical guidelines for telepathology: Another important step in support of increased adoption of telepathology for patient care. *Journal of Pathology Informatics, 6*(1), 13. Advance online publication. DOI: 10.4103/2153-3539.153906 PMID: 25838965

Evans, B. J. (2023). Rules for robots, and why medical AI breaks them. *Journal of Law and the Biosciences*, *10*(1), lsad001. Advance online publication. DOI: 10.1093/jlb/lsad001 PMID: 36815975

Exner-Pirot, H. (2022). Challenges of Telehealth. https://openpress.usask.ca/northernhealthcare/chapter/chapter-25-challenges-totelehealth-implementation/

Ezeani, I. U., Okwuonu, G. C., Chukwuonye, I. I., & Nkpozi, M. O. (2022). The Impact of Telemedicine during the COVID-19 Pandemic in Nigeria: A Review. *Annals of Health Research*, *8*(4), 260–268. DOI: 10.30442/ahr.0804-02-177

Faiyazuddin, M., Syed, A. G., Siddiqui, R. K., Mehta, R., Khatib, M. N., Gaidhane, S., Zahiruddin, Q. S., Hussain, A., & Sah, R. (2025). The impact of artificial intelligence on healthcare: A comprehensive review of advancements in diagnostics, treatment, and operational efficiency. *Health Science Reports*, *8*(1), e70312. Advance online publication. DOI: 10.1002/hsr2.70312 PMID: 39763580

Fan, L.-H., Gao, L., Liu, X., Zhao, S. H., Mu, H., Li, Z., Shi, L., Wang, L., Jia, X., Ha, M., & Lou, F. (2017). Patients' perceptions of service quality in China: An investigation using the SERVQUAL model. *PLoS One*, *2*(12), e0190123. DOI: 10.1371/journal.pone.0190123

Farabi, H., Rezapour, A., Jahangiri, R., Jafari, A., Rashki Kemmak, A., & Nikjoo, S. (2020). Economic evaluation of the utilization of telemedicine for patients with cardiovascular disease: A systematic review. *Heart Failure Reviews*, *25*(6), 1063–1075. DOI: 10.1007/s10741-019-09864-4 PMID: 31760593

Fatima, T., Malik, S. A., & Shabbir, A. (2018). Hospital healthcare service quality, patient satisfaction and loyalty: An investigation in context of private healthcare systems. *International Journal of Quality & Reliability Management*, *35*(6), 1195–1214. https://doi.org/ https://doi.org/10.1108/IJQRM-02-2017-0031. DOI: 10.1108/IJQRM-02-2017-0031

Fazakarley, C. A., Breen, M., Leeson, P., Thompson, B., & Williamson, V. (2023). Experiences of using artificial intelligence in healthcare: A qualitative study of UK clinician and key stakeholder perspectives. *BMJ Open*, *13*(12), e076950. Advance online publication. DOI: 10.1136/bmjopen-2023-076950 PMID: 38081671

Federal Republic of Nigeria. (2023). Nigeria Data Protection Act, 2023.

Federal Trade Commission. (2024, May 30). Health Breach Notification Rule—Final rule (amendments). *Federal Register*.

Federico, C. A., & Trotsyuk, A. A. (2024). Biomedical Data Science, Artificial Intelligence, and Ethics: Navigating Challenges in the Face of Explosive Growth. *Annual Review of Biomedical Data Science*, *7*(1), 104553. Advance online publication. DOI: 10.1146/annurev-biodatasci-102623-104553 PMID: 38598860

Federspiel, F., Mitchell, R., Asokan, A., Umana, C., & McCoy, D. (2023). Threats by artificial intelligence to human health and human existence. *BMJ Global Health*, *8*(5), e010435. DOI: 10.1136/bmjgh-2022-010435

Feng, J., & Zhang, T. (2009). Comparison of models of ownership structure in the health care and its Chinese choice. *Jianghai Journal*, *6*, 74–79.

Fostina, P., Okon, E. U., & Chikaodili, A. I. (2024). Knowledge, Attitude, and Use of Telemedicine among Health Care Professionals in Federal Medical Center, Bayelsa State, Nigeria. GPH -. *International Journal of Health Sciences and Nursing*, *7*(05), 62–140. DOI: 10.5281/10.5281/zenodo.14237894

Fournier-Tombs, E., & McHardy, J. (2023). A Medical Ethics Framework for Conversational Artificial Intelligence. *Journal of Medical Internet Research*, *25*, e43068. Advance online publication. DOI: 10.2196/43068 PMID: 37224277

Frampton, S. B., & Guastellos, S. (2008). Honoring the life of a pioneer in patient-centered care: Harvey Picker (1915–2008). *The Patient*, *1*(2), 73–75. DOI: 10.2165/01312067-200801020-00001

Freedhoff, Y., & Hébert, P. C. (2011). Partnerships between health organizations and the food industry risk derailing public health nutrition. *Canadian Medical Association Journal*, *183*(3), 291–292. DOI: 10.1503/cmaj.110085

Frishammar, J., Essén, A., Bergström, F., & Ekman, T. (2023). Digital health platforms for the elderly? Key adoption and usage barriers and ways to address them. *Technological Forecasting and Social Change*, *189*, 122319. Advance online publication. DOI: 10.1016/j.techfore.2023.122319

Frost, E. K., Bosward, R., Aquino, Y. S., Braunack-Mayer, A., & Carter, S. M. (2022). Public views on ethical issues in healthcare artificial intelligence: Protocol for a scoping review. *Systematic Reviews*, *11*(1), 142. Advance online publication. DOI: 10.1186/s13643-022-02012-4 PMID: 35841073

Frost, L., & Reich, M. (1998). *Mectizan donation program: origins, experiences, and relationships with co-ordinating bodies for onchocerciasis control.* Harvard School of Public Health.

Fuentes, A. (2003). Remote interpretation of ultrasound images. *Clinical Obstetrics and Gynecology*, *46*(4), 878–881. DOI: 10.1097/00003081-200312000-00019 PMID: 14595230

Fu, M. L., Feng, Z. Y., & Chen, S. C. (2011). The enlightenment from health management experience in developed countries. *Chinese Health Service Management*, *3*(2), 233–236.

Galazzi, A., Fonda, F., Chiappinotto, S., Justi, L., Sønderskov Frydensberg, M., Lehmann Boesen, R., Macur, M., de San Pedro, M., Reixach Espaulella, E., & Palese, A. (2025). Recommendations to promote the digital healthcare transformation in the clinical practice: Findings from an international consensus development method. *BMC Health Services Research*, *25*(1). Advance online publication. DOI: 10.1186/s12913-025-13079-9

Ganguly, P., Jehan, K., de Costa, A., Mavalankar, D., & Smith, H. (2014). Considerations of private sector obstetricians on participation in the state led "Chiranjeevi Yojana" scheme to promote institutional delivery in Gujarat, India: A qualitative study. *BMC Pregnancy and Childbirth*, *14*(1), 1–13. DOI: 10.1186/1471-2393-14-352

Gaviria-Marin, M., Merigó, J. M., & Baier-Fuentes, H. (2019). Knowledge management: A global examination based on bibliometric analysis. *Technological Forecasting and Social Change*, *140*, 194–220. DOI: 10.1016/j.techfore.2018.07.006

Gbollie, E. F., Bantjes, J., Jarvis, L., Swandevelder, S., du Plessis, J., Shadwell, R., Davids, C., Gerber, R., Holland, N., & Hunt, X. (2023). Intention to use digital mental health solutions: A cross-sectional survey of university students attitudes and perceptions toward online therapy, mental health apps, and chatbots. *Digital Health*, *9*. Advance online publication. DOI: 10.1177/20552076231216559

Geng, Y. Q., Xiang, Q. J., Gao, J. A., Yan, Y., & Li, J. Y. (2024). Progress and framework of clean energy production: Bibliometric analysis from 2002 to 2022. *Energy Strategy Reviews*, *52*, 101270. Advance online publication. DOI: 10.1016/j.esr.2023.101270

Geracitano, J., Barron, L., McSwain, D., & Khairat, S. (2024). How is digital health suitability measured for communities? A systematic review. *Digital Health*, *10*, 20552076241288316. Advance online publication. DOI: 10.1177/20552076241288316 PMID: 39398896

Gerke, S., Yeung, S. R., & Cohen, I. G. (2020). Ethical and Legal Aspects of Ambient Intelligence in Hospitals. *Journal of the American Medical Association*, *323*(7), 601–602. DOI: 10.1001/jama.2019.21699 PMID: 31977033

Gervais, A., Karame, G. O., Wüst, K., Glykantzis, V., Ritzdorf, H., & Capkun, S. (2016, October). On the security and performance of proof of work blockchains. In *Proceedings of the 2016 ACM SIGSAC Conference on Computer and Communications Security* (pp. 3–16). DOI: 10.1145/2976749.2978341

Gidado, M., & Ejembi, C. (2009). Tuberculosis case management and treatment outcome: Assessment of the effectiveness of Public-Private Mix of tuberculosis programme in Kaduna State, Nigeria. *Annals of African Medicine*, *8*(1), 25–31. DOI: 10.4103/1596-3519.55760

Gikay, A. A. (2024). Risks, innovation, and adaptability in the UK's incrementalism versus the European Union's comprehensive artificial intelligence regulation. *International Journal of Law and Information Technology*, *32*(1), eaae013. https://ssrn.com/abstract=4700121. DOI: 10.1093/ijlit/eaae013

Giovanis, A., Pierrakos, G., Rizomyliotis, I., & Binioris, S. (2018). Assessing service quality and customer behavioral responses in hospital outpatient services: A formative measurement approach. *International Journal of Quality and Service Sciences*, *10*(2), 98–116. DOI: 10.1108/IJQSS-03-2017-0023

Glukhikh, I. N., Tolstolesova, L. A., & Arzikulov, O. A. U. (2021). Systems engineering methodology for designing digital public-private partnership platforms. *Applied System Innovation*, *4*(1), 1–13. DOI: 10.3390/asi4010004

Goirand, M., Austin, E., & Clay-Williams, R. (2021). Implementing Ethics in Healthcare AI-Based Applications: A Scoping Review. *Science and Engineering Ethics*, *27*(5), 61. Advance online publication. DOI: 10.1007/s11948-021-00336-3 PMID: 34480239

Gökalp, E., Gökalp, M. O., Çoban, S., & Eren, P. E. (2018). Analysing opportunities and challenges of integrated blockchain technologies in healthcare. In Eurosymposium on Systems Analysis and Design (pp. 174–183). DOI: 10.1007/978-3-030-00060-8_13

Goldacre, B., & Morley, J. (2022). Better, broader, safer: Using health data for research and analysis. Department of Health and Social Care. https://assets.publishing.service.gov.uk/government/uploads/system/uploads/attachment_data/file/1067058/summary-goldacre-review-using-health-data-for-research-and-analysis.pdf

Gonsalves, P. P., Ansari, S., Berry, C., Gonsalves, F., Iyengar, S., Kashyap, P., Mittal, D., Pal, S., Razdan, E., & Michelson, D. (2024). Co-designing digital mental health interventions with young people: 10 recommendations from lessons learned in low-and-middle-income countries. *Health Education Journal*, *84*(4), 373–384. DOI: 10.1177/00178969241297821

Gordon, W. J., & Catalini, C. (2018). Blockchain technology for healthcare: Facilitating the transition to patient-driven interoperability. *Computational and Structural Biotechnology Journal, 16*, 224–230. DOI: 10.1016/j.csbj.2018.06.003 PMID: 30069284

Goth Itoi, N. (2022). Could stable diffusion solve a gap in medical imaging data? Stanford University., https://hai.stanford.edu/news/could-stable-diffusion-solve-gap-medical-imaging-data, Retrieved November 29, 2022, from.

Gouveia, A. J., Ribeiro, J., Sousa, G., Barbosa, D., & Machado, M. (2025). Advancing Healthcare through Remote Patient Monitoring: A brief literature review. *Procedia Computer Science, 256*, 893–899. DOI: 10.1016/j.procs.2025.02.192

GOV.UK. (2025). *PM speech on AI opportunities action plan.* January 13.

Government of the United Arab Emirates. (2025, July 7). Data protection laws—UAE PDPL overview.

Greenhalgh, S., Guo, L., & Yeowell, G. (2025). 'In the midst of every crisis, lies great opportunity': Perceptions of the future use of artificial intelligence in the UK NHS primary care. *Musculoskeletal Care, 23*(2), e70092. DOI: 10.1002/msc.70092 PMID: 40238189

Greenhalgh, T., Wherton, J., Papoutsi, C., Lynch, J., Hughes, G., A'Court, C., Hinder, S., Procter, R., & Shaw, S. (2018). Analysing the role of complexity in explaining the fortunes of technology programmes: Empirical application of the NASSS framework. *BMC Medicine, 16*(1), 1–15. DOI: 10.1186/s12916-018-1050-6 PMID: 29754584

Groen, G., Jörns-Presentati, A., Dessauvagie, A., Seedat, S., van den Heuvel, L. L., Suliman, S., Grobler, G., Jansen, R., Mwape, L., Mukwato, P., Chapima, F., Korhonen, J., Stein, D. J., Jonker, D., Mudenda, J., Turunen, T., Valtiņš, K., Beinaroviča, A., Grada, L., & Lahti, M. (2022). Development of a Mobile Application for Detection of Adolescent Mental Health Problems and Feasibility Assessment with Primary Health Care Workers. *Issues in Mental Health Nursing, 43*(11), 1046–1055. DOI: 10.1080/01612840.2022.2124003

Groupe Speciale Mobile Association. (2021). Connected Women. The Mobile Gender Gap Report 2021. 65. https://www.gsma.com/r/wp-content/uploads/2021/07/The-Mobile-Gender-Gap-Report-2021.pdf

Guo, C., Ashrafian, H., Ghafur, S., Fontana, G., Gardner, C., & Prime, M. (2020). Challenges for the evaluation of digital health solutions—A call for innovative evidence generation approaches. npj. *Digital Medicine, 3*(1), 110. Advance online publication. DOI: 10.1038/s41746-020-00314-2 PMID: 32904379

Gusenbauer, M., & Haddaway, N. R. (2020). Which academic search systems are suitable for systematic reviews or meta-analyses? Evaluating retrieval qualities of Google Scholar, PubMed, and 26 other resources. *Research Synthesis Methods*, *11*(2), 181–217. DOI: 10.1002/jrsm.1378 PMID: 31614060

Haleem, A., Javaid, M., Singh, R. P., Suman, R., & Rab, S. (2021). Blockchain technology applications in healthcare: An overview. *International Journal of Intelligent Networks*, *2*, 130–139. DOI: 10.1016/j.ijin.2021.09.005

Halper, F. (2017). Advanced analytics: Moving toward AI, machine learning, and natural language processing (TDWI Best Practices Report).

Hamet, P., & Tremblay, J. (2017). Artificial intelligence in medicine. *Metabolism: Clinical and Experimental*, *69*, S36–S40. DOI: 10.1016/j.metabol.2017.01.011 PMID: 28126242

Hao, J., von Davier, A. A., Yaneva, V., Lottridge, S., von Davier, M., & Harris, D. J. (2024). Transforming assessment: The impacts and implications of large language models and generative AI. *Educational Measurement: Issues and Practice*, *43*(2), 16–29. DOI: 10.1111/emip.12602

Hardyman, W., Daunt, K. L., & Kitchener, M. (2015). Value co-creation through patient engagement in health care: A micro-level approach and research agenda. *Public Management Review*, *17*(1), 90–107. DOI: 10.1080/14719037.2014.881539

Harvey, J., & Powell, J. (2020). Factors influencing the implementation of self-management solutions in healthcare: An interview study with NHS managers. *British Journal of Health Care Management*, *26*(3), 61–70. DOI: 10.12968/bjhc.2019.0070

Hasselgren, A., Kralevska, K., Gligoroski, D., Pedersen, S. A., & Faxvaag, A. (2020). Blockchain in healthcare and health sciences—A scoping review. *International Journal of Medical Informatics*, *134*, 104040. DOI: 10.1016/j.ijmedinf.2019.104040 PMID: 31865055

Hassija, V., Chamola, V., Mahapatra, A., Singal, A., Goel, D., Huang, K., Scardapane, S., Spinelli, I., Mahmud, M., & Hussain, A. (2023). Interpreting black-box models: A review on explainable artificial intelligence. *Cognitive Computation*, *16*(1), 45–74. Advance online publication. DOI: 10.1007/s12559-023-10179-8

Health, U. V. A. (n.d.). International telehealth projects. https://uvahealth.com/services/telemedicine/international-health

Herington, J., McCradden, M. D., Creel, K., Boellaard, R., Jones, E. C., Jha, A. K., Rahmim, A., Scott, P. J. H., Sunderland, J. J., Wahl, R. L., Zuehlsdorff, S., & Saboury, B. (2023). Ethical Considerations for Artificial Intelligence in Medical Imaging: Deployment and Governance. *Journal of Nuclear Medicine, 64*(10), 1509–1515. DOI: 10.2967/jnumed.123.266110 PMID: 37620051

Herrmann, M., Wabro, A., & Winkler, E. (2024). Percentages and reasons: AI explainability and ultimate human responsibility within the medical field. *Ethics and Information Technology*, *26*(2), 26. Advance online publication. DOI: 10.1007/s10676-024-09764-8

Holland, J., Kingston, L., McCarthy, C., Armstrong, E., O'Dwyer, P., Merz, F., & McConnell, M. (2021). Service robots in the healthcare sector. *Robotics (Basel, Switzerland)*, *10*(1), 1–47. DOI: 10.3390/robotics10010047

Holtrop, J. S., Estabrooks, P. A., Gaglio, B., Harden, S. M., Kessler, R. S., King, D. K., Kwan, B. M., Ory, M. G., Rabin, B. A., Shelton, R. C., & Glasgow, R. E. (2021). Understanding and applying the RE-AIM framework: Clarifications and resources. *Journal of Clinical and Translational Science*, *5*(1). Advance online publication. DOI: 10.1017/cts.2021.789

Hoofnagle, C. J., van der Sloot, B., & Borgesius, F. Z. (2019). The European Union general data protection regulation: What it is and what it means. *Information & Communications Technology Law*, *28*(1), 65–98. DOI: 10.1080/13600834.2019.1573501

HOPS Healthcare. (2021, June 3). Introducing one of its kind EMR platform integrated with telemedicine patient app in Congo. https://hops.healthcare/blogs/introducing-one-of-its-kind-emr-platform-integrated-with-telemedicine-patient-app-in-kinshasa-d-r-congo

Horn, R., & Kerasidou, A. (2020). Sharing whilst caring: Solidarity and public trust in a data-driven healthcare system. *BMC Medical Ethics*, *21*(1), 1–7. DOI: 10.1186/s12910-020-00553-8 PMID: 33143692

Hou, X., Liu, L., & Cain, J. (2022). Can higher spending on primary healthcare mitigate the impact of ageing and non-communicable diseases on health expenditure? *BMJ Global Health*, *7*(12), e010513. Advance online publication. DOI: 10.1136/bmjgh-2022-010513 PMID: 36564087

Hu, R., Liao, Y., Du, Z., Hao, Y., Liang, H. and Sh,i L. (2016). Types of health care facilities and the quality of primary care: A study of characteristics and experiences of Chinese patients in Guangdong Province, China. *BMC Health Services Research*, 16(a):335. DOI: 10.1186/s12913-016-1604-2

Hu, L., Ding, H., Liu, S., Wang, Z., Hu, G., & Liu, Y. (2020). Influence of patient and hospital characteristics on inpatient satisfaction in China's tertiary hospitals: A cross-sectional study. *Health Expectations : An International Journal of Public Participation in Health Care and Health Policy*, *23*(1), 115–124. DOI: 10.1111/hex.12974

Hummel, P., & Braun, M. (2020). Just data? Solidarity and justice in data-driven medicine. *Life Sciences, Society and Policy*, *16*(1), 8. DOI: 10.1186/s40504-020-00101-7 PMID: 32839878

Husain, L., & Greenhalgh, T. (2025). Examining intersectionality and barriers to the uptake of video consultations among older adults from disadvantaged backgrounds with limited English proficiency: Qualitative narrative interview study. *Journal of Medical Internet Research*, *27*, e65690. Advance online publication. DOI: 10.2196/65690 PMID: 39761566

Hutchings, R. (2022). The impact of Covid-19 on the use of digital technology in the NHS. Nuffield Trust. https://www.nuffieldtrust.org.uk/sites/default/files/2020-08/the-impact-of-covid-19-on-the-use-of-digital-technology-in-the-nhs-web-2.pdf

Hutchings, R., & Morris, J. (2022). Digital health care across the UK: Where are we now? Nuffield Trust. https://www.nuffieldtrust.org.uk/resource/digital-health-care-across-the-uk-where-are-we-now

Ibrahim, H., Liu, X., Zariffa, N., Morris, A. D., & Denniston, A. K. (2021). Health data poverty: An assailable barrier to equitable digital health care. *The Lancet. Digital Health*, *3*(4), e260–e265. DOI: 10.1016/S2589-7500(20)30317-4 PMID: 33678589

Ichikawa, D., Kashiyama, M., & Ueno, T. (2017). Tamper-resistant mobile health using blockchain technology. *JMIR mHealth and uHealth*, *5*(7), e7938. DOI: 10.2196/mhealth.7938 PMID: 28747296

Idris-Umarfarouq, I., Afolabi, A. A., Olorunfemi, D. O., & Akinola, A. I. (2022). Systematic Overview of Remote Patient Monitoring in Nigeria (West Africa). *Telehealth and Medicine Today*, *7*(3), 359. DOI: 10.30953/tmt.v7.359

Ijiga, A. C., Peace, A. E., Idoko, I. P., Ezebuka, C. I., Harry, K. D., Ukatu, I. E., & Agbo, D. O. (2024). Technological innovations in mitigating winter health challenges in New York City, USA. *International Journal of Science and Research Archive*, *11*(1), 535–551. DOI: 10.30574/ijsra.2024.11.1.0078

Imtiaz, A., Farooq, G., Haq, Z. U., Ahmed, A., & Anwer, S. (2017). Public private partnership and utilization of maternal and child health services in district Abbottabad, Pakistan. *Journal of Ayub Medical College, Abbottabad*, *29*(2), 275–279.

Iniesta, R. (2023). The human role to guarantee an ethical AI in healthcare: A five-facts approach. *AI and Ethics*. Advance online publication. DOI: 10.1007/s43681-023-00353-x

Iyengar, K., Jain, V. K., & Vaishya, R. (2020). Pitfalls in telemedicine consultations in the era of COVID-19 and how to avoid them. *Diabetes & Metabolic Syndrome*, *14*(5), 797–799. DOI: 10.1016/j.dsx.2020.06.007

Jagarapu, J., & Savani, R. C. (2021). A brief history of telemedicine and the evolution of teleneonatology. *Seminars in Perinatology*, *45*(5), 151416. Advance online publication. DOI: 10.1016/j.semperi.2021.151416 PMID: 34006382

Jamali, D. (2004). Success and failure mechanisms of public private partnerships (PPPs) in developing countries: Insights from the Lebanese context. *International Journal of Public Sector Management*, *17*(5), 414–430. DOI: 10.1108/09513550410546598

Joiner, K. A., & Lusch, R. F. (2016). Evolving to a new service-dominant logic for health care. *Innovation and Entrepreneurship in Health*, *3*, 25–33. DOI: 10.2147/IEH.S93473

Joudyian, N., Doshmangir, L., Mahdavi, M., Tabrizi, J. S., & Gordeev, V. S. (2021). Public-private partnerships in primary health care: A scoping review. *BMC Health Services Research*, *21*(1), 1–18. DOI: 10.1186/s12913-020-05979-9

Joughin, A., Ibitoye, S., Cress, A., Shipway, D., & Braude, P. (2021). Developing a virtual geriatric perioperative medicine clinic: A mixed methods healthcare improvement study. *Age and Ageing*, *50*(4), 1391–1396. DOI: 10.1093/ageing/afab066 PMID: 33989380

Justinia, T. (2017). The UK's national programme for IT: Why was it dismantled? *Health Services Management Research*, *30*(1), 2–9. DOI: 10.1177/0951484816662492 PMID: 28166675

Kabukye, J. K., Nakku, J., Niwemuhwezi, J., Nsereko, J., Namagembe, R., Groen, I. D. E., Neumbe, R., Mubiru, D., Kisakye, C., Nanyonga, R., Sjölinder, M., Nilsson, S., & Wamala-Larsson, C. (2024). Assessing the Usage and Usability of a Mental Health Advice Telephone Service in Uganda: Mixed Methods Study. *Journal of Medical Internet Research*, *26*, e65692. DOI: 10.2196/65692

Kaigwa, L. C., Njenga, F., Ongeri, L., Nguithi, A., Mugane, M., Mbugua, G. M., Anundo, J., Kimari, M. Z., & Onono, M. (2022). Implementation of telepsychiatry in Kenya: Acceptability study. *BJPsych Open*, *8*(3), 1–6. DOI: 10.1192/bjo.2022.53

Kalenzi, C. (2022). Artificial intelligence and blockchain: How should emerging technologies be governed? *Frontiers in Research Metrics and Analytics*, *7*, 801549. Advance online publication. DOI: 10.3389/frma.2022.801549 PMID: 35224423

Kamya, C., Shearer, J., Asiimwe, G., Carnahan, E., Salisbury, N., Waiswa, P., Brinkerhoff, J., & Hozumi, D. (2017). Evaluating global health partnerships: A case study of a Gavi HPV vaccine application process in Uganda. *International Journal of Health Policy and Management*, *6*(6), 327–338. DOI: 10.15171/ijhpm.2016.137

Kanabar, V. (2023). *The AI revolution in project management: Elevating productivity with generative AI*. Sams Publishing.

Kanavos, P., Vogelsang, M., Haig, M., & Kolovou, V. (2022). Challenges for health systems seeking to embrace virtual health care for population health. *The European Journal of Health Economics : HEPAC : Health Economics in Prevention and Care*, *23*(7), 1079–1083. DOI: 10.1007/s10198-022-01503-4 PMID: 35921018

Kar, A. K., Varsha, P., & Rajan, S. (2023). Unravelling the impact of generative artificial intelligence (GAI) in industrial applications: A review of scientific and grey literature. *Global Journal of Flexible Systems Managment*, *24*(4), 659–689. DOI: 10.1007/s40171-023-00356-x

Karamagi, H. C., Muneene, D., Droti, B., Jepchumba, V., Okeibunor, J. C., Nabyonga, J., Asamani, J. A., Traore, M., & Kipruto, H. (2022). eHealth or e-Chaos: The use of Digital Health Interventions for Health Systems Strengthening in sub-Saharan Africa over the last 10 years: A scoping review. *Journal of Global Health*, *12*, 04090. DOI: 10.7189/jogh.12.04090

Karantias, K., Kiayias, A., & Zindros, D. (2020, February). *Proof-of-burn. In International Conference on Financial Cryptography and Data Security* (pp. 523–540). Springer.

Kasralikar, P., Polu, O. R., Chamarthi, B., Veer Samara Sihman Bharattej Rupavath, R., Patel, S., & Tumati, R. (2025). Blockchain for securing AI-driven healthcare systems: A systematic review and future research perspectives. *Cureus*. Advance online publication. DOI: 10.7759/cureus.83136 PMID: 40438823

Kasyapa, M. S. B., & Vanmathi, C. (2024). Blockchain integration in healthcare: A comprehensive investigation of use cases, performance issues, and mitigation strategies. *Frontiers in Digital Health*, *6*, 1359858. Advance online publication. DOI: 10.3389/fdgth.2024.1359858 PMID: 38736708

Katznelson, G., & Gerke, S. (2021). The need for health AI ethics in medical school education. *Advances in Health Sciences Education : Theory and Practice*, *26*(4), 1447–1458. DOI: 10.1007/s10459-021-10040-3 PMID: 33655433

Keelara, R., Sutherland, E., & Almyranti, M. (2025). Leading practices for the future of telemedicine: Implementing telemedicine post-pandemic. OECD Health Working Papers No. 173. DOI: 10.1787/18152015

Kelly, C. J., & Young, A. J. (2017). Promoting innovation in healthcare. *Future Healthcare Journal*, *4*(2), 121–125. DOI: 10.7861/futurehosp.4-2-121 PMID: 31098448

Kempt, H., Heilinger, J. C., & Nagel, S. K. (2022). Relative explainability and double standards in medical decision-making Should medical AI be subjected to higher standards in medical decision-making than doctors? *Ethics and Information Technology*, *24*(2), 20. Advance online publication. DOI: 10.1007/s10676-022-09646-x

Kerasidou, C., Kerasidou, A., Buscher, M., & Wilkinson, S. (2022). Before and beyond trust: Reliance in medical AI. *Journal of Medical Ethics*, *48*(11), 852–856. DOI: 10.1136/medethics-2020-107095 PMID: 34426519

Keskinbora, K. H. (2019). Medical ethics considerations on artificial intelligence. *Journal of Clinical Neuroscience : Official Journal of the Neurosurgical Society of Australasia*, *64*, 277–282. DOI: 10.1016/j.jocn.2019.03.001 PMID: 30878282

Kessem, L. (2022). *Healthcare breaches costliest for 12 years running, hit new $10.1M record high*. August 17. IBM.

Keyue, X., & Qiongfang, D. (2024). COVID-19 epidemic at low level but may rise during Spring Festival: National Health Commission. *Global Times (Beijing, China)*.

Khan, M. M., Ford, C., Dong, Y., & Afsarimanesh, N. (2024). *WIP: Impact of generative AI on learning: Foci and parameters for an assessment tool*. 2024 IEEE Frontiers in Education Conference (FIE), DOI: 10.1109/FIE61694.2024.10893560

Khan, M. M., Shah, N., Shaikh, N., Thabet, A., Alrabayah, T., & Belkhair, S. (2025). Towards secure and trusted AI in healthcare: A systematic review of emerging innovations and ethical challenges. *International Journal of Medical Informatics*, *195*, 105780. Advance online publication. DOI: 10.1016/j.ijmedinf.2024.105780 PMID: 39753062

Khemapech, I., Sansrimahachai, W., & Toahchoodee, M. (2019). Telemedicine – Meaning, Challenges, and Opportunities. *Siriraj Medical Journal*, *71*(3), 246–252. DOI: 10.33192/Smj.2019.38

Khezr, S., Moniruzzaman, M., Yassine, A., & Benlamri, R. (2019). Blockchain technology in healthcare: A comprehensive review and directions for future research. *Applied Sciences (Basel, Switzerland)*, *9*(9), 1736. Advance online publication. DOI: 10.3390/app9091736

Kiburi, S. K., Paruk, S., & Chiliza, B. (2022). Mobile phone ownership, digital technology use and acceptability of digital interventions among individuals on opioid use disorder treatment in Kenya. *Frontiers in Digital Health*, *4*. Advance online publication. DOI: 10.3389/fdgth.2022.975168

Kola, L., Abiona, D., Adefolarin, A. O., & Ben-Zeev, D. (2021). Mobile phone use and acceptability for the delivery of mental health information among perinatal adolescents in Nigeria: Survey study. In JMIR Mental Health (Vol. 8, Issue 1). JMIR Publications Inc. DOI: 10.2196/20314

Kontaxakis, G., Visvikis, D., Ohl, R., Sachpazidis, I., Suarez, J., Selby, P., Rest, C. C., Santos, A., Ortega, F., Diaz, J., & Pan, L. (2006). Integrated telemedicine applications and services for oncological positron emission tomography. *Oncology Reports*, *15*(4), 1091. DOI: 10.3892/or.15.4.1091 PMID: 16525707

Kowatsch, T., Otto, L., Harperink, S., Cotti, A., & Schlieter, H. (2019). A design and evaluation framework for digital health interventions. it - Information Technology, 61(5), 253–263. https://doi.org/DOI: 10.1515/itit-2019-0019

Kraus, S., Schiavone, F., Pluzhnikova, A., & Invernizzi, A. C. (2021). Digital transformation in healthcare: Analyzing the current state-of-research. *Journal of Business Research*, *123*, 557–567. DOI: 10.1016/j.jbusres.2020.10.030

Krick, T., Huter, K., Domhoff, D., Schmidt, A., Rothgang, H., & Wolf-Ostermann, K. (2019). Digital technology and nursing care: A scoping review on acceptance, effectiveness and efficiency studies of informal and formal care technologies. *BMC Health Services Research*, *19*(1), 400. Advance online publication. DOI: 10.1186/s12913-019-4238-3 PMID: 31221133

Krittanawong, C., Rogers, A. J., Aydar, M., Choi, E., Johnson, K. W., Wang, Z., & Narayan, S. M. (2019). Integrating blockchain technology with artificial intelligence for cardiovascular medicine. *Nature Reviews. Cardiology*, *17*(1), 1–3. DOI: 10.1038/s41569-019-0294-y PMID: 31605093

Krugmann, J. O., & Hartmann, J. (2024). Sentiment analysis in the age of generative AI. *Customer Needs and Solutions*, *11*(1), 3. DOI: 10.1007/s40547-024-00143-4

Kruse, C. S., Krowski, N., Rodriguez, B., Tran, L., Vela, J., & Brooks, M. (2018). Telehealth and patient satisfaction: A systematic review and narrative analysis. *BMJ Open*, *7*(8), e016242. Advance online publication. DOI: 10.1136/bmjopen-2017-016242 PMID: 28775188

Kumar, S., & Prasad, C. J. (2004). Public-private partnerships in urban infrastructure, *Kerala Calling*, 36-37.

Kumari, R., Singh, A. K., Verma, R., & Fetais, A. H. M. (2022). Enablers and challenges for e-health services: A systematic literature review. *International Journal of Electronic Government Research*, *18*(1), 1–17. DOI: 10.4018/IJEGR.298626

Kumar, M. S., & Ganesh, D. (2024). Improving telemedicine through IoT and cloud computing: Opportunities and challenges. *Advances in Engineering and Intelligence Systems*, *3*(3), 123–135. DOI: 10.22034/aeis.2024.474171.1217

Kunar, M. A., Montana, G., & Watson, D. G. (2024). Increasing transparency of computer-aided detection impairs decision-making in visual search. *Psychonomic Bulletin & Review*. Advance online publication. DOI: 10.3758/s13423-024-02601-5 PMID: 39448515

Kuznetsov, A., Sernani, P., Romeo, L., Frontoni, E., & Mancini, A. (2024). On the integration of artificial intelligence and blockchain technology: A perspective about security. *IEEE Access : Practical Innovations, Open Solutions*, *12*, 3881–3897. Advance online publication. DOI: 10.1109/ACCESS.2023.3349019

Kyrarini, M., Lygerakis, F., Rajavenkatanarayanan, A., Sevastopoulos, C., Nambiappan, H. R., Chaitanya, K. K., Babu, A. R., Mathew, J., & Makedon, F. (2021). A survey of robots in healthcare. *Technologies*, *9*(1), 8. DOI: 10.3390/technologies9010008

Lakmini, P. M., Naeem, R., & Keshav, D. (2019). Remote patient monitoring: A comprehensive study. *Journal of Ambient Intelligence and Humanized Computing*, *10*(1), 57–76. DOI: 10.1007/s12652-017-0598-x

Lam, S. S. (1997). SERVQUAL: A tool for measuring patients' opinions of hospital service quality in Hong Kong. *Total Quality Management*, *8*(4), 145–152. DOI: 10.1080/0954412979587

Larsen, A., Agorinya, J., Beaulieu, A., Sottie, E. Q., Buck, B., Obeng, K., Kyeremeh, B., Dogbe, F. K., Iddrisu, M. I., Dowuona, P. E. O., Tetteh, O. O. A., Emmanuel, O. B., Ofori-Atta, A., & Ben-Zeev, D. (2025). Digital health for early psychosis in Ghana: Patient and caregiver needs and preferences. *Schizophrenia*, *11*(1), 1–7. DOI: 10.1038/s41537-025-00554-9

Lawal, R. (2023).Transformative Potential of IoT on Smart Healthcare and Remote Patient Monitoring in Nigeria: A Literature MSC Internet of Things with Data Analytics. DOI: DOI: 10.13140/RG.2.2.24453.52966

Lawani-Luwaji, E., & Okafor, C. F. (2025). Perceptions of Telemedicine and Rural Healthcare Access in a Developing Country: A Case Study of Bayelsa State, Nigeria. *Barw Medical Journal*, *3*(4), 21–25. DOI: 10.58742/bmj.vi.187

Lee, D., & Yoon, S. N. (2021). Application of artificial intelligence-based technologies in the healthcare industry: Opportunities and challenges. *International Journal of Environmental Research and Public Health*, *18*(1), 271. DOI: 10.3390/ijerph18010271 PMID: 33401373

Leeming, G., Cunningham, J., & Ainsworth, J. (2019). A ledger of me: Personalizing healthcare using blockchain technology. *Frontiers in Medicine*, *6*, 171. DOI: 10.3389/fmed.2019.00171 PMID: 31396516

Leigh, S., Ashall-Payne, L., & Andrews, T. (2020). Barriers and facilitators to the adoption of mobile health among health care professionals from the United Kingdom: Discrete choice experiment. *JMIR mHealth and uHealth*, *8*(7), e17704. Advance online publication. DOI: 10.2196/17704 PMID: 32628118

Lennon, M. R., Bouamrane, M.-M., Devlin, A. M., O'Connor, S., O'Donnell, C., Chetty, U., Agbakoba, R., Bikker, A., Grieve, E., Finch, T., Watson, N., Wyke, S., & Mair, F. S. (2017). Readiness for delivering digital health at scale: Lessons from a longitudinal qualitative evaluation of a national digital health innovation program in the United Kingdom. *Journal of Medical Internet Research*, *19*(2), e6900. Advance online publication. DOI: 10.2196/jmir.6900 PMID: 28209558

LeRouge, C. M., Gupta, M., Corpart, G., & Arrieta, A. (2019). Health system approaches are needed to expand telemedicine use across nine latin american nations. *Health Affairs*, *38*(2), 212–221. DOI: 10.1377/hlthaff.2018.05274

Leung, L. (2015). Validity, reliability, and generalizability in qualitative research. *Journal of Family Medicine and Primary Care*, *4*(3), 324–327. DOI: 10.4103/2249-4863.161306 PMID: 26288766

Levac, D., Colquhoun, H., & O'Brien, K. K. (2010). Scoping studies: Advancing the methodology. *Implementation Science : IS*, *5*(1), 1–9. DOI: 10.1186/1748-5908-5-69

Levesque, J. F., Harris, M. F., & Russell, G. (2013). Patient-centred access to health care: Conceptualising access at the interface of health systems and populations. *International Journal for Equity in Health*, *12*(1), 1. DOI: 10.1186/1475-9276-12-18

Li, B., & Akintoye, A. (2003). An overview of public-private partnership. In Akintoye, A., Beck, M., & Hardcastle, C. (Eds.), *Public-private partnerships: managing risks and opportunities*. Blackwell Publishing Ltd., DOI: 10.1002/9780470690703.ch1

Li, L., Back, E., Lee, S., Shipley, R., Mapitse, N., Elbe, S., Smallman, M., Wilson, J., Yasin, I., Rees, G., Gordon, B., Murray, V., Roberts, S. L., Cupani, A., & Kostkova, P. (2025). Balancing risks and opportunities: Data-empowered-health ecosystems. *Journal of Medical Internet Research, 27*, e57237. DOI: 10.2196/57237 PMID: 40132190

Li, M., Lowrie, D. B., Huang, C.-Y., Lu, X.-C., Zhu, Y.-C., Wu, X.-H., Shayiti, M., Tan, Q.-Z., Yang, H.-L., Chen, S.-Y., Zhao, P., He, S.-H., Wang, X.-R., & Lu, H.-Z. (2015). Evaluating patients' perception of service quality at hospitals in nine Chinese cities by use of the SERVQUAL scale. *Asian Pacific Journal of Tropical Biomedicine*, *5*(6), 497–504. DOI: 10.1016/j.apjtb.2015.02.003

Limb, M. (2024). PM says NHS must "reform or die" following damning report into state of the service. *BMJ (Clinical Research Ed.)*, q2001. Advance online publication. DOI: 10.1136/bmj.q2001 PMID: 39266245

Limiri, D. M. (2025). The impact of long wait times on patient health outcomes: The growing NHS crisis. *Journal of Public Health, 3*. Advance online publication. DOI: 10.70389/PJPH.100020

Li, T., Long, Q., Chai, H., Zhang, S., Jiang, F., Liu, H., Huang, W., Jin, D., & Li, Y. (2025). Generative ai empowered network digital twins: Architecture, technologies, and applications. *ACM Computing Surveys*, *57*(6), 1–43. DOI: 10.1145/3711682

Liu, Q. Q. (2013). Discrimination of forest tourism concept based on ROST-CM analysis. [Social Sciences]. *Journal of Central South University of Forestry and Technology*, *7*(1), 20–23. DOI: 10.1007/s11771-000-0006-z

Liu, Y. F., & Wang, Z. (2016). The development model and its enlightenment of health management service industry in the United States. *Journal of the Asia Pacific Economy*, *3*, 75–81.

Liu, Y., Kong, Q., Yuan, S., & Klundert, J. (2018). Factors influencing choice of health system access level in China: A systematic review. *PLoS One*, *13*(8), e0201887. https://doi.org//. DOI: 10.1371/journal.pone.0201887

Li, W., Andreina, S., Bohli, J. M., & Karame, G. (2017, September). Securing proof-of-stake blockchain protocols. In *International Workshop on Data Privacy Management* (pp. 297–315). Springer.

Li, X., Krumholz, H. M., Yip, W., Cheng, K. K., De Maeseneer, J., Meng, Q., Mossialos, E., Li, C., Lu, J., Su, M., Zhang, Q., Xu, D. R., Li, L., Normand, S. T., Peto, R., Li, J., Wang, Z., Yan, H., Gao, R., & Hu, S. (2020). Quality of primary health care in China: Challenges and recommendations. *Lancet*, *395*(10239), 1802–1812. DOI: 10.1016/S0140-6736(20)30122-7

Li, X., Lu, J., Hu, S., Cheng, K. K., De Maeseneer, J., Meng, Q., Mossialos, E., Xu, D. R., Yip, W., Zhang, H., Krumholz, H. M., Jiang, L., & Hu, S. (2017). The primary health-care system in China. *Lancet*, *390*(10112), 2584–2594. DOI: 10.1016/S0140-6736(17)33109-4

Lloyds Bank. (2022). 2022 consumer digital index. https://www.lloydsbank.com/assets/media/pdfs/banking_with_us/whats-happening/221103-lloyds-consumer-digital-index-2022-report.pdf

Lönnroth, K., Uplekar, M., Arora, V. K., Juvekar, S., Lan, N. T., Mwaniki, D., & Pathania, V. (2004). Public-private mix for DOTS implementation: What makes it work? *Bulletin of the World Health Organization*, *82*(8), 580–586.

Low, S. T., Sakhardande, P. G., Lai, Y. F., Long, A. D., & Kaur-Gill, S. (2021). Attitudes and perceptions toward healthcare technology adoption among older adults in Singapore: A qualitative study. *Frontiers in Public Health*, *9*, 588590. Advance online publication. DOI: 10.3389/fpubh.2021.588590 PMID: 33659232

Lukas, H., Xu, C., Yu, Y., & Gao, W. (2020). Emerging telemedicine tools for remote COVID-19 diagnosis, monitoring, and management. *ACS Nano*, *14*(12), 16180–16193. DOI: 10.1021/acsnano.0c08494 PMID: 33314910

Lu, L., Xu, P., Wang, Y.-Y., & Wang, Y. (2023). Measuring service quality with text analytics: Considering both importance and performance of consumer opinions on social and non-social online platforms. *Journal of Business Research*, *169*, 114298. DOI: 10.1016/j.jbusres.2023.114298

Luo, H. (2016). The released program of 'Healthy China 2030'. *Science and Technology Daily*, *1*, 10–26.

Lupton, M. (2018). Some ethical and legal consequences of the application of artificial intelligence in the field of medicine. Trends in Medicine, 18(4), Article 100147.

MacIntyre, M. R., Cockerill, R. G., Mirza, O. F., & Appel, J. M. (2023). Ethical considerations for the use of artificial intelligence in medical decision-making capacity assessments. *Psychiatry Research*, *328*, 115466. Advance online publication. DOI: 10.1016/j.psychres.2023.115466 PMID: 37717548

Maghsoudi, M., Mohammadi, A., & Habibipour, S. (2024). Navigating and Addressing Public Concerns in AI: Insights From Social Media Analytics and Delphi. *IEEE Access : Practical Innovations, Open Solutions*, *12*, 126043–126062. DOI: 10.1109/ACCESS.2024.3440660

Mahajan, R., Lim, W. M., Sareen, M., Kumar, S., & Panwar, R. (2023). Stakeholder theory. *Journal of Business Research*, *166*, 114104. Advance online publication. DOI: 10.1016/j.jbusres.2023.114104

Maia, M. R., Castela, E., Pires, A., & Lapão, L. V. (2019). How to develop a sustainable telemedicine service? A pediatric telecardiology service 20 years on—An exploratory study. *BMC Health Services Research*, *19*(1), 681. Advance online publication. DOI: 10.1186/s12913-019-4511-5 PMID: 31547824

Maikomo, J. M., Targema, T. S., & Obun-Andy, M. K. (2021). COVID-19 and the new normal in developing societies: An appraisal of Nigerians' adaptation to digital life in public and private spheres. *Journal of Developing Societies*, *37*(3), 246–274. DOI: 10.1177/0169796X21996830

Malaria Consortium. (2019). How remote villages in Nigeria can beat malaria through community health. https://malariamustdie.com/nigeria-community-health

Malhotra, S., Chakrabarti, S., & Shah, R. (2013). Telepsychiatry: Promise, potential, and challenges. *Indian Journal of Psychiatry*, *55*(1), 3. DOI: 10.4103/0019-5545.105499 PMID: 23441027

Mamoshina, P., Ojomoko, L., Yanovich, Y., Ostrovski, A., Botezatu, A., Prikhodko, P., Izumchenko, E., Aliper, A., Romantsov, K., Zhebrak, A., Ogu, I. O., & Zhavoronkov, A. (2017). Converging blockchain and next-generation artificial intelligence technologies to decentralize and accelerate biomedical research and healthcare. *Oncotarget*, *9*(5), 5665–5690. DOI: 10.18632/oncotarget.22345 PMID: 29464026

Manja, V. (2023). The power of co-creating transformation. NHS Confederation. https://www.nhsconfed.org/articles/power-co-creating-transformation

Manyazewal, T., Woldeamanuel, Y., Blumberg, H. M., Fekadu, A., & Marconi, V. C. (2021). The potential use of digital health technologies in the African context: A systematic review of evidence from Ethiopia. *NPJ Digital Medicine*, *4*(1), 125. Advance online publication. DOI: 10.1038/s41746-021-00487-4 PMID: 34404895

Martin, G., Clarke, J., Liew, F., Arora, S., King, D., Aylin, P., & Darzi, A. (2019). Evaluating the impact of organisational digital maturity on clinical outcomes in secondary care in England. npj. *Digital Medicine*, *2*(1), 41. Advance online publication. DOI: 10.1038/s41746-019-0118-9 PMID: 31304387

Maynou Pujolràs, L., Pearson, G., McGuire, A., & Serra-Sastre, V. (2022). The diffusion of robotic surgery: Examining technology use in the English NHS. *Health Policy (Amsterdam)*, *126*(4), 325–336. DOI: 10.1016/j.healthpol.2022.02.007 PMID: 35307200

Mayorga-Ruiz, I., Jiménez-Pastor, A., Fos-Guarinos, B., López-González, R., García-Castro, F., & Alberich-Bayarri, Á. (2019). The role of AI in clinical trials. In *Artificial intelligence in medical imaging: Opportunities, applications and risks* (pp. 231–243). Springer. DOI: 10.1007/978-3-319-94878-2_16

Mbah, R. E., Hardgrave, C. M., Mbah, D. E., Nutt, A., & Russell, J. G. (2025). The impact of USAID budget cuts on global development initiatives: A review of challenges, responses, and implications. *Advances in Social Sciences Research Journal*, *12*(04), 219–232. Advance online publication. DOI: 10.14738/assrj.1204.18681

McLennan, S., Fiske, A., Tigard, D., Müller, R., Haddadin, S., & Buyx, A. (2022). Embedded ethics: A proposal for integrating ethics into the development of medical AI. *BMC Medical Ethics*, *23*(1), 6. Advance online publication. DOI: 10.1186/s12910-022-00746-3 PMID: 35081955

MediBloc Limited. (2025). Own your health data. It's rightfully yours. https://medibloc.com/

Meesala, A., & Paul, J. (2018). Service quality, consumer satisfaction and loyalty in hospitals: Thinking for the future. *Journal of Retailing and Consumer Services*, *40*, 261–269. DOI: 10.1016/j.jretconser.2016.10.011

Meffert, S., Mathai, M., Neylan, T., Mwai, D., Onyango, D. O., Rota, G., Otieno, A., Obura, R. R., Wangia, J., Opiyo, E., Muchembre, P., Oluoch, D., Wambura, R., Mbwayo, A., Kahn, J. G., Cohen, C. R., Bukusi, D., Aarons, G. A., Burger, R. L., & Ongeri, L. (2024). Preference of mHealth versus in-person treatment for depression and post-traumatic stress disorder in Kenya: Demographic and clinical characteristics. *BMJ Open*, *14*(11), 1–9. DOI: 10.1136/bmjopen-2023-083094

Mehta, A., da Silva Dias, L., Espinal, M., Jillellamudi, R., Mathew, R., Chauhan, A., Dhingra, K., & Verma, S. (2024). E-health implementation challenges: A comprehensive review of digital healthcare in the United States. *Journal of Knowledge Learning and Science Technology*, *3*(4), 233–246. DOI: 10.60087/jklst.v2.n3.p233

Mei, Z., Li, W., Chen, J., Yin, H., Song, Y., Tu, W., Ding, Z., Bai, Y., Jin, S., & Xu, G. (2024). The transformation of 20-year social participation policies of older people in China: Network analysis and text analysis. *PLoS One*, *19*(8), e0308401. DOI: 10.1371/journal.pone.0308401

Menage, J. (2020). Why Telemedicine Diminishes the Doctor-Patient Relationship. *British Medical Journal*. https://www.bmj.com/content/371/bmj.m4348

Mennella, C., Maniscalco, U., Di Pietro, G., & Esposito, M. (2024). Ethical and regulatory challenges of AI technologies in healthcare: A narrative review. *Heliyon, 10*(4), e26297. Advance online publication. DOI: 10.1016/j.heliyon.2024.e26297 PMID: 38384518

Merigó, J. M., & Yang, J. B. (2017). A bibliometric analysis of operations research and management science. *Omega, 73*, 37–48. DOI: 10.1016/j.omega.2016.12.004

Metta, C., Beretta, A., Pellungrini, R., Rinzivillo, S., & Giannotti, F. (2024). Towards Transparent Healthcare: Advancing Local Explanation Methods in Explainable Artificial Intelligence. *Bioengineering (Basel, Switzerland), 11*(4), 369. Advance online publication. DOI: 10.3390/bioengineering11040369 PMID: 38671790

Miao, R., Zhang, H., Wu, Q., Zhang, J., & Jiang, Z. (2019). Using structural equation modeling to analyze patient value, satisfaction, and loyalty: A case study of healthcare in China. *International Journal of Production Research, 58*(2), 577–596. DOI: 10.1080/00207543.2019.1598595

Michael, J., Cohn, A. L. A. N., & Butcher, J. R. (2018). Blockchain technology. *The Journal, 1*(7), 1–11.

Miller, T. E., & Derse, A. R. (2002). Between Strangers: The practice of medicine online. *Health Affairs (Project Hope), 21*(4), 168–179. DOI: 10.1377/hlthaff.21.4.168

Ministry of Economy, Trade and Industry. (Japan) & Personal Information Protection Commission (Japan). (2024, May 7). Global CBPR Forum.

Ministry of Health Saudi Arabia. (2024). To promote healthcare transformation... MOH calls for participation in the healthcare sandbox. https://www.moh.gov.sa/en/Ministry/MediaCenter/News/Pages/News-2024-08-20-001.aspx

Miranda, F. J., Chamorro, A., Murillo, L. R., & Vega, J. (2012). Primary health care services quality in Spain: A formative measurement approach using PLS path modeling. *International Journal of Quality and Service Sciences, 4*(4), 387–398. DOI: 10.1108/17566691211288368

Mittelstadt, B. (2019). Principles alone cannot guarantee ethical AI. *Nature Machine Intelligence, 1*(11), 501–507. DOI: 10.1038/s42256-019-0114-4

Moahi, K. H. (1999). Health Information Networks for Telehealth in Africa-Challenges and Prospects: A Review of the Literature. *Libri, 49*(1), 43–50. DOI: 10.1515/libr.1999.49.1.43

Moghadam, M. N., & Amiresmaili, M. (2009). Hospital services quality assessment—Hospitals of Kerman University of Medical Sciences as a tangible example of a developing country. *International Journal of Health Care Quality Assurance*, *24*(1), 57–66. DOI: 10.1108/09526861111098247

Moitra, M., Owens, S., Hailemariam, M., Wilson, K. S., Mensa-Kwao, A., Gonese, G., Kamamia, C. K., White, B., Young, D. M., & Collins, P. Y. (2023). Global Mental Health: Where We Are and Where We Are Going. *Current Psychiatry Reports*, *25*(7), 301–311. DOI: 10.1007/s11920-023-01426-8

Molefi, D. M. (2015).The status of telemedicine in Africa. https://nuviun.com/content/the-status-of-telemedicine-in-africa

Molinari, G., Molinari, M., Di Biase, M., & Brunetti, N. D. (2017). Telecardiology and its settings of application: An update. *Journal of Telemedicine and Telecare*, *24*(5), 373–381. DOI: 10.1177/1357633X16689432 PMID: 28084886

Moodley, K. (2024). Artificial intelligence (AI) or augmented intelligence? How big data and AI are transforming healthcare: Challenges and opportunities. *Samj South African Medical Journal*, *114*(1), 16–20. DOI: 10.7196/SAMJ.2024.v114i2.1631 PMID: 38525617

Moody, L., Wood, E., Needham, A., Booth, A., Aranda, A. J., & Tindale, W. (2022). Identifying individual enablers and barriers to the use of digital technology for the self-management of long term conditions by older adults. *Journal of Medical Engineering & Technology*, *46*(6), 448–461. DOI: 10.1080/03091902.2022.2089249 PMID: 35748238

Morley, J., DeVito, N. J., & Zhang, J. (2023). Generative AI for medical research. *BMJ (Clinical Research Ed.)*, *382*, 1551. DOI: 10.1136/bmj.p1551

Moulaei, K., Akhlaghpour, S., & Fatehi, F. (2025). Patient consent for the secondary use of health data in artificial intelligence (AI) models: A scoping review. *International Journal of Medical Informatics*, *198*, 105872. Advance online publication. DOI: 10.1016/j.ijmedinf.2025.105872 PMID: 40107041

Mudiyanselage, K. W. W., De Santis, K. K., Jörg, F., Saleem, M., Stewart, R., Zeeb, H., & Busse, H. (2024). The effectiveness of mental health interventions involving non-specialists and digital technology in low-and middle-income countries – a systematic review. *BMC Public Health*, *24*(1). Advance online publication. DOI: 10.1186/s12889-023-17417-6

Mudyarabikwa, O., & Regmi, K. (2016). Public-private partnerships and efficiency in public procurement of primary healthcare infrastructure: A qualitative research in the NHS UK. *Journal of Public Health (Berlin)*, *24*(2), 91–100. DOI: 10.1007/s10389-015-0701-8

Mühlensiepen, F., Kurkowski, S., Krusche, M., Mucke, J., Prill, R., Heinze, M., Welcker, M., Schulze-Koops, H., Vuillerme, N., Schett, G., & Knitza, J. (2021). Digital health transition in rheumatology: A qualitative study. *International Journal of Environmental Research and Public Health*, *18*(5), 2636. Advance online publication. DOI: 10.3390/ijerph18052636 PMID: 33807952

Muhos, M., Saarela, M., Foit, D.Jr, & Rasochova, L. (2019). Management priorities of digital health service start-ups in California. *The International Entrepreneurship and Management Journal*, *15*(1), 43–62. DOI: 10.1007/s11365-018-0546-z

Muinga, N., Magare, S., Monda, J., English, M., Fraser, H., Powell, J., & Paton, C. (2020). Digital health systems in Kenyan Public Hospitals: A mixed-methods survey. *BMC Medical Informatics and Decision Making*, *20*(1), 1–14. DOI: 10.1186/s12911-019-1005-7

Munishi, C., Ndumwa, H. P., Massawe, J. E., Njiro, B. J., Ngowi, J., Suhartono, S., Busse, A., Campello, G., Garofalo, G., Cipolla, P., Nyandindi, C., Ubuguyu, O., & Sunguya, B. (2023). Acceptability of using mobile Health (mHealth) as an intervention tool for people with drug use disorders in Tanga, Tanzania. PLOS Digital Health, 2(9 September). DOI: 10.1371/journal.pdig.0000257

Munn, Z., Peters, M. D. J., Stern, C., Tufanaru, C., McArthur, A., & Aromataris, E. (2018). Systematic review or scoping review? Guidance for authors when choosing between a systematic or scoping review approach. *BMC Medical Research Methodology*, *18*(1), 143. Advance online publication. DOI: 10.1186/s12874-018-0611-x PMID: 30453902

Musa, S., Ramatu, A., Haliru, L., Abigail, D., & Gumbi, S. (2023). Establishing a paediatric telemedicine centre in a low-resource setting: Experience and challenges from a teaching hospital in Kaduna, Nigeria. *Sri Lanka Journal of Child Health*, *52*(2), 155–160. DOI: 10.4038/sljch.v52i2.10548

Mustafa, S. H., Mohammed, E. A., Makkawi, S. T., & Mohammed, Y. Y. (2024). Attitudes of university students in Sudan towards digital mental health. *South Sudan Medical Journal*, *17*(4), 185–189. DOI: 10.4314/ssmj.v17i4.6

Musyoka, C. M., Mbwayo, A., Donovan, D. M., & Mathai, M. (2023). Student peer mentoring: Feasibility and acceptability of mHealth-based tool for alcohol and substance abuse prevention by peer mentors at a university in Kenya. *PLOS Digital Health*, *2*(1). Advance online publication. DOI: 10.1371/journal.pdig.0000177

Muula, A. S. (2006). Will Africa achieve the millennium development goals? *Croatian Medical Journal*, *47*(1), 194–196.

Mwaka, E. S., Bazzeketa, D., Mirembe, J., Emoru, R. D., Twimukye, A., & Kivumbi, A. (2025). Barriers to and enhancement of the utilization of digital mental health interventions in low-resource settings: Perceptions of young people in Uganda. *Digital Health*, *11*, 20552076251321696. DOI: 10.1177/20552076251321698

My Doctor Medical Group. (2021). Bitcoin and cryptocurrency. https://mydoctorsf.com/bitcoin/

Nadia, J., Kalvin, B., Abi, G., Simran, J., Boraiba, K., Rosie, L., Dominca, L., Jakub, Z., & Claire, S. (2025). GSMA - The Mobile Gender Gap Report 2025. 1–72. www.gsmaintelligence.com

Naslund, J. A., Aschbrenner, K. A., Araya, R., Marsch, L. A., Unützer, J., Patel, V., & Bartels, S. J. (2017). Digital technology for treating and preventing mental disorders in low-income and middle-income countries: A narrative review of the literature. *The Lancet. Psychiatry*, *4*(6), 486–500. DOI: 10.1016/S2215-0366(17)30096-2

National Audit Office. (2020). Digital transformation in the NHS. https://www.nao.org.uk/wp-content/uploads/2019/05/Digital-transformation-in-the-NHS.pdf

National Audit Office. (2022). Introducing integrated care systems: Joining up local services to improve health outcomes. https://www.nao.org.uk/wp-content/uploads/2022/10/Integrated-Care-Systems-Funding-and-accountability-for-local-health-and-care.pdf

National Health and Family Planning Commission of the People's Republic of China. (2015). *Further improving the action plan for medical services*. http://www.nhfpc.gov.cn/yzygj/ylfwjh/gxyg_index.shtml

National Health Service. (2019). The NHS Long Term Plan. https://www.longtermplan.nhs.uk/wp-content/uploads/2019/08/nhs-long-term-plan-version-1.2.pdf

National Information Technology Development Agency. (2007). ACT 2007 ACT NO. 28. Federal Republic of Nigeria Official Gazette No. 99, Vol. 94 Lagos. https://nitda.gov.ng/wp-content/uploads/2020/11/NITDA-ACT-2007-2019-Edition1.pdf

National Institute of Standards and Technology (NIST). (2023). *Artificial Intelligence Risk Management Framework (AI RMF 1.0)*. U.S. Department of Commerce., DOI: 10.6028/NIST.AI.100-1

National Legislative Bodies. (2011). Nigeria: Evidence Act, 2011. https://www.refworld.org/legal/legislation/natlegbod/2011/en/104226

Ncube, B., Mars, M., & Scott, R. E. (2023). Perceptions and attitudes of patients and healthcare workers towards the use of telemedicine in Botswana: An exploratory study. *PLoS One*, *18*(2), e0281754. Advance online publication. DOI: 10.1371/journal.pone.0281754 PMID: 36795740

Ncube, B., Mars, M., & Scott, R. E. (2023). Recommendations for developing a telemedicine strategy for Botswana: A meta-synthesis. *International Journal of Environmental Research and Public Health*, *20*(18), 6718. Advance online publication. DOI: 10.3390/ijerph20186718 PMID: 37754578

Neal, D., Engelsma, T., Tan, J., Craven, M. P., Marcilly, R., Peute, L., Dening, T., Jaspers, M., & Dröes, R. (2022). Limitations of the new ISO standard for health and wellness apps. *The Lancet. Digital Health*, *4*(2), e80–e82. DOI: 10.1016/S2589-7500(21)00273-9 PMID: 35090677

Nelson, D., Inghels, M., Kenny, A., Skinner, S., McCranor, T., Wyatt, S., Phull, J., Nanyonjo, A., Yusuff, O., & Gussy, M. (2023). Mental health professionals and telehealth in a rural setting: A cross sectional survey. *BMC Health Services Research*, *23*(1), 9083. Advance online publication. DOI: 10.1186/s12913-023-09083-6 PMID: 36849933

Newell, J. N., Pande, S., Baral, S., Bam, D., & Malla, P. (2005). Leadership, management and technical lessons learnt from a successful public-private partnership for TB control in Nepal. *The International Journal of Tuberculosis and Lung Disease : The Official Journal of the International Union against Tuberculosis and Lung Disease*, *9*(9), 1013–1017.

Nguyen, D. C., Pathirana, P. N., Ding, M., & Seneviratne, A. (2021). BEdgeHealth: A decentralized architecture for edge-based IoMT networks using blockchain. *IEEE Internet of Things Journal*, *8*(14), 11743–11757. DOI: 10.1109/JIOT.2021.3058953

NHS Confederation. (2022). Data and research transformation in the NHS: What must be addressed? https://www.nhsconfed.org/publications/data-and-research-transformation-nhs-what-must-be-addressed

NHS England. (2021a). Resources for integrated care: Case studies. https://www.england.nhs.uk/integratedcare/resources/case-studies/army-of-tech-angels-to-help-people-with-shopping-and-virtual-life/

NHS England. (2021b). Building strong integrated care systems everywhere. https://www.england.nhs.uk/wp-content/uploads/2021/06/B0905-vcse-and-ics-partnerships.pdf

NHS England. (2022). Digital transformation. https://www.england.nhs.uk/digitaltechnology/

NHS England. (2023). *Delivery plan for recovering access to primary care*. NHS England.

NHS England. (2025). *GP practices embrace technology to improve patient access and provide choice*. April 24.

Nigeria Data Protection Act. (2023). Explanatory Memorandum. https://placng.org/i/wp-content/uploads/2023/06/Nigeria-Data-Protection-Act-2023.pdf

Nigeria Data Protection Commission. (2023). Nigeria Data Protection Act (NDPA) 2023.

Noel, N. B., Maryam, N. B., Yila, E., Nkala, C. A., & Banwat, M. E. (2024). Knowledge and Perception of Telemedicine among Medical Students of the University of Jos, Plateau State, Nigeria. *Nigerian Medical Journal : Journal of the Nigeria Medical Association*, *64*(6), 816–824.

Nora, G. A. M., Alberton, A., & Ayala, D. H. F. (2023). Stakeholder theory and actor-network theory: The stakeholder engagement in energy transitions. *Business Strategy and the Environment*, *32*(1), 673–685. DOI: 10.1002/bse.3168

Nortje, G., Oladeji, B., Gureje, O., & Seedat, S. (2016). Effectiveness of traditional healers in treating mental disorders: A systematic review. *The Lancet. Psychiatry*, *3*(2), 154–170. DOI: 10.1016/S2215-0366(15)00515-5

Novelli, C., Taddeo, M., & Floridi, L. (2023). Accountability in artificial intelligence: What it is and how it works. *AI & Society*, *39*(1), 1871–1882. Advance online publication. DOI: 10.1007/s00146-023-01635-y

Nyende, H. (2018). The role of technology in value co-creation of maternal healthcare: A service-dominant logic perspective [Doctoral dissertation, University of Agder]. CORE. https://core.ac.uk/download/pdf/301378486.pdf

O'Cathail, M., Sivanandan, A. M., Diver, C., Patel, P., & Christian, J. (2020). The use of patient-facing teleconsultations in the National Health Service: Scoping review. *JMIR Medical Informatics*, *8*(3), e15380. Advance online publication. DOI: 10.2196/15380 PMID: 32175911

O'Grady, M. A., Mootz, J., Suleman, A., Sweetland, A., Teodoro, E., Anube, A., Feliciano, P., Bezuidenhout, C., Dos Santos, P. F., Fumo, W., Gouveia, L., Pinsky, I., Mello, M., Kann, B., & Wainberg, M. L. (2022). Mobile technology and task shifting to improve access to alcohol treatment services in Mozambique. *Journal of Substance Abuse Treatment*, *134*. Advance online publication. DOI: 10.1016/j.jsat.2021.108549

Obermeyer, Z., Powers, B., Vogeli, C., & Mullainathan, S. (2019). Dissecting racial bias in an algorithm used to manage the health of populations. *Science*, *366*(6464), 447–453. DOI: 10.1126/science.aax2342 PMID: 31649194

Obotu, A. S. (2019). Perceived Effect of Telemedicine on Medical Service Delivery by Federal Medical Centers in North Central Zone of Nigeria. *Library Philosophy and Practice* (e-journal). 3051. https://digitalcommons.unl.edu/libphilprac/3051

Odhiambo, R., & Mars, M. (2018). Patients' understanding of telemedicine terms required for informed consent when translated into Kiswahili. *BMC Public Health*, *18*(1), 588. Advance online publication. DOI: 10.1186/s12889-018-5499-1 PMID: 29720139

Odunuga, K. V., Owoicho, O. E., Oredipe, F. B., Oke, O. E., Okogu, S. I., Anipole, O., Sunmola, M. A., Bamgbose, O. A., & Adebanjo, A. O. (2024). Artificial Intelligence in Nigeria's Health Sector, *Scholar. Journal of Computational Science*, *1*(8), 15–19. DOI: 10.5281/zenodo.13226114

OECD. (2022). Going digital guide to data governance policy making. OECD Publishing. https://www.oecd.org/en/publications/going-digital-guide-to-data-governance-policy-making_40d53904-en.html

OECD. (2024a). *Regulatory approaches to artificial intelligence in finance (OECD Artificial Intelligence Papers, No. 24)*. OECD Publishing.

OECD. (2024b). Collective action for responsible AI in health (OECD Artificial Intelligence Papers, No. 10). OECD Publishing. https://www.oecd.org/en/publications/collective-action-for-responsible-ai-in-health_f2050177-en.html

Office of the National Coordinator for Health IT. (2024, January 9). Health Data, Technology, and Interoperability (HTO-1) Final Rule. *Federal Register*, *89*, 1192.

Ogundipe, R. O., Omotosho, O. E., & John-Akinola, Y. O. (2025). Perception, attitude and use of digital health platforms for mental health promotion among students in a national university in the south-western part of Nigeria: A cross-sectional study. *Digital Health, 11*. Advance online publication. DOI: 10.1177/20552076251331841

Okamoto, S., Kataoka, M., Itano, M., & Sawai, T. (2025). AI-based medical ethics education: Examining the potential of large language models as a tool for virtue cultivation. *BMC Medical Education, 25*(1), 185. Advance online publication. DOI: 10.1186/s12909-025-06801-y PMID: 39910559

Olliario, P. (1997). Will the fight against tropical diseases benefit from orphan drug status? *Tropical Medicine & International Health : TM & IH, 2*(2), 113–115. DOI: 10.1046/j.1365-3156.1997.d01-234.x

Omboni, S., Padwal, R. S., Alessa, T., Benczúr, B., Green, B. B., Hubbard, I., Kario, K., Khan, N. A., Konradi, A., Logan, A. G., Lu, Y., Mars, M., McManus, R. J., Melville, S., Neumann, C. L., Parati, G., Renna, N. F., Ryvlin, P., Saner, H., & Wang, J. (2022). The worldwide impact of telemedicine during COVID-19: Current evidence and recommendations for the future. *Connected Health*. Advance online publication. DOI: 10.20517/ch.2021.03 PMID: 35233563

Omidian, H. (2024). Synergizing blockchain and artificial intelligence to enhance healthcare. *Drug Discovery Today, 29*(9), 104111. DOI: 10.1016/j.drudis.2024.104111 PMID: 39034026

Onireti, O., Zhang, L., & Imran, M. A. (2019, December). On the viable area of wireless practical Byzantine fault tolerance (PBFT) blockchain networks. In *2019 IEEE Global Communications Conference (GLOBECOM)* (pp. 1–6). IEEE. DOI: 10.1109/GLOBECOM38437.2019.9013778

Onsongo, S., Kamotho, C., Rinke de Wit, T. F., & Lowrie, K. (2023). Experiences on the utility and barriers of telemedicine in healthcare delivery in Kenya. *International Journal of Telemedicine and Applications, 2023*, 1487245. Advance online publication. DOI: 10.1155/2023/1487245 PMID: 37180825

Onyeabor, U. S., Okenwa, W. S., Onwuasoigwe, O., Lasebikan, O. A., Schaaf, T., Pinkwart, N., & Balzer, F. (2024). Telemedicine in the age of the pandemics: The prospects of web-based remote patient monitoring systems for orthopaedic ambulatory care management in the developing economies. *Digital Health, 10*, 1–16. DOI: 10.1177/20552076241226964

Organization for Economic Cooperation and Development. (2023). *Health at a Glance 2023: OECD Indicators*. OECD Publishing., DOI: 10.1787/7a7afb35-

Orife, I., Kreutzer, J., Sibanda, B., Whitenack, D., Siminyu, K., Martinus, L., Ali, J. T., Abbott, J., Marivate, V., Kabongo, S., Meressa, M., Murhabazi, E., Ahia, O., van Biljon, E., Ramkilowan, A., Akinfaderin, A., Öktem, A., Akin, W., Kioko, G., & Bashir, A. (2020). Masakhane — Machine Translation For Africa. 1–4. https://arxiv.org/abs/2003.11529

Osborn, T. L., Wasanga, C. M., & Ndetei, D. M. (2022). Transforming mental health for all. In The BMJ. DOI: 10.1136/bmj.o1593

Ossa, L. A., Lorenzini, G., Milford, S. R., Shaw, D., Elger, B. S., & Rost, M. (2024). Integrating ethics in AI development: A qualitative study. *BMC Medical Ethics, 25*(1), 10. Advance online publication. DOI: 10.1186/s12910-023-01000-0 PMID: 38262986

Ossa, L. A., Milford, S. R., Rost, M., Leist, A. K., Shaw, D. M., & Elger, B. S. (2024). AI Through Ethical Lenses: A Discourse Analysis of Guidelines for AI in Healthcare. *Science and Engineering Ethics, 30*(3), 24. Advance online publication. DOI: 10.1007/s11948-024-00486-0 PMID: 38833207

Ouzzani, M., Hammady, H., Fedorowicz, Z., & Elmagarmid, A. (2016). Rayyan-a web and mobile app for systematic reviews. *Systematic Reviews, 5*(1), 1–10. DOI: 10.1186/s13643-016-0384-4

Oyeyemi, S. O., & Wynn, R. (2014). Giving cell phones to pregnant women and improving services may increase primary health facility utilization: A case-control study of a Nigerian project. *Reproductive Health, 11*(1), 8. DOI: 10.1186/1742-4755-11-8

Oyinlola, A. (2024). Redefining healthcare delivery in rural areas through telemedicine.https://www.africanchangestories.org/2024/03/23/redefining-healthcare-delivery-in-rural-areas-through-telrmedicine/

Page, M. J., McKenzie, J. E., Bossuyt, P. M., Boutron, I., Hoffmann, T. C., Mulrow, C. D., Shamseer, L., Tetzlaff, J. M., Akl, E. A., Brennan, S. E., Chou, R., Glanville, J., Grimshaw, J. M., Hróbjartsson, A., Lalu, M. M., Li, T., Loder, E. W., Mayo-Wilson, E., McDonald, S., & Moher, D. (2021). The PRISMA 2020 statement: An updated guideline for reporting systematic reviews. *BMJ (Clinical Research Ed.), 372*. Advance online publication. DOI: 10.1136/bmj.n71

Palmer, A., & Schwan, D. (2024). More Process, Less Principles: The Ethics of Deploying AI and Robotics in Medicine. *Cambridge Quarterly of Healthcare Ethics, 33*(1), 121-134, Article Pii s0963180123000087. https://doi.org/DOI: 10.1017/S0963180123000087

Pandian, P. S. (2016). An Overview of Telemedicine Technologies for Healthcare Applications. *International Journal of Biomedical and Clinical Engineering*, *5*(2), 29–52. DOI: 10.4018/IJBCE.2016070103

Papadopoulos, I., Koulouglioti, C., Lazzarino, R., & Ali, S. (2020). Enablers and barriers to the implementation of socially assistive humanoid robots in health and social care: A systematic review. *BMJ Open*, *10*(1), e033096. DOI: 10.1136/bmjopen-2019-033096 PMID: 31924639

Papathanasiou, D. (2024). Utilization of generative AI for enabling knowledge contextualization among stakeholders for enhancing circularity in the construction industry.

Papoutsi, C., & Greenhalgh, T. (2024). Innovation, improvement, and implementation–conceptual frameworks for thinking through complex change. In *eHealth research theory and development* (pp. 220–236). Routledge. DOI: 10.4324/9781003302049-15

Paramesha, M., Rane, N., & Rane, J. (2024). Enhancing resilience through generative artificial intelligence such as ChatGPT. DOI: 10.2139/ssrn.4832533

Parasuraman, A., Berry, L. L., & Zeithaml, V. A. (1988). SERVQUAL: A multiple-item scale for measuring consumer perceptions of service quality. *Journal of Retailing*, *64*(1), 12–40.

Paris Declaration. (2005). Paris declaration on aid effectiveness: ownership, harmonisation, alignment, results and mutual accountability, *High level forum on joint progress toward enhanced aid effectiveness: harmonization, alignment and results. 2nd high level forum on aid effectiveness*. Paris, 28 February-2 March. Paris: OECD Publishing.

Parker, V. J., Economou, N. J., Health, D., & Silcox, C. (2024.). *White Paper. AI governance in health systems. Aligning innovation, accountability, and trust*. Margolis Institute for Health Policy, Duke Health.

Patel, R., Loraine, E., & Gréaux, M. (2022). Impact of COVID-19 on digital practice in UK paediatric speech and language therapy and implication for the future: A national survey. *International Journal of Language & Communication Disorders*, *57*(5), 1112–1119. DOI: 10.1111/1460-6984.12750 PMID: 35925005

Patel, V., Saxena, S., Lund, C., Thornicroft, G., Baingana, F., Bolton, P., Chisholm, D., Collins, P. Y., Cooper, J. L., Eaton, J., Herrman, H., Herzallah, M. M., Huang, Y., Jordans, M. J. D., Kleinman, A., Medina-Mora, M. E., Morgan, E., Niaz, U., & Omigbodun, O. UnÜtzer, Jü. (2018). The Lancet Commission on global mental health and sustainable development. *Lancet*, *392*(10157), 1553–1598. DOI: 10.1016/S0140-6736(18)31612-X

Peifer, Y., Jeske, T., & Hille, S. (2022). Artificial intelligence and its impact on leaders and leadership. *Procedia Computer Science, 200*, 1024–1030. https://doi.org/ rights and contentDOI: 10.1016/j.procs.2022.01.301Get

Penchansky, R., & Thomas, J. W. (1981). The Concept of Access: Definition and Relationship to Consumer Satisfaction. *Medical Care*, *19*(2). https://journals.lww.com/lww-medicalcare/fulltext/1981/02000/the_concept_of_access__definition_and_relationship.1.aspx

Peng, J. M., & Lin, Y. (2009). The blend of Confucianism, Taoism and Buddhism in Sun Simiao medical ethics thought. *Medical Philosophy*, *30*(17), 23–24.

Pennic, J. (2019). Healthcare blockchain startup BurstIQ nabs $5.5M for HIPAA-compliant blockchain platform. HIT Consultant. https://hitconsultant.net/2019/10/01/burstiq-hipaa-compliant-blockchain-platform-funding/

Peter, I. D., Danjuma-Karau, K. J., Omokhuale, E. M., & Yakubu, J. C. (2025). A Mixed Methods Study of the Challenges and Prospects of Utilizing Telemedicine in the Delivery of Healthcare to Nigerian Children. *International Journal of Public Health*, *70*, 1607790. DOI: 10.3389/ijph.2025.1607790

Petersson, L., Vincent, K., Svedberg, P., Nygren, J. M., & Larsson, I. (2023). Ethical considerations in implementing AI for mortality prediction in the emergency department: Linking theory and practice. *Digital Health*, *9*, 20552076231206588. Advance online publication. DOI: 10.1177/20552076231206588 PMID: 37829612

Philippe, T. J., Sikder, N., Jackson, A., Koblanski, M. E., Liow, E., Pilarinos, A., & Vasarhelyi, K. (2022). Digital Health Interventions for Delivery of Mental Health Care: Systematic and Comprehensive Meta-Review. *JMIR Mental Health*, *9*(5). Advance online publication. DOI: 10.2196/35159

Ploug, T., & Holm, S. (2020). The four dimensions of contestable AI diagnostics - A patient-centric approach to explainable AI. *Artificial Intelligence in Medicine*, *107*, 101901. Advance online publication. DOI: 10.1016/j.artmed.2020.101901 PMID: 32828448

Polevikov, S. (2023). Advancing AI in healthcare: A comprehensive review of best practices. *Clinica Chimica Acta; International Journal of Clinical Chemistry, 548*, 117519. Advance online publication. DOI: 10.1016/j.cca.2023.117519 PMID: 37595864

Popay, J., Roberts, H., Sowden, A., Petticrew, M., Arai, L., Rodgers, M., & Britten, N. (2006). Narrative Synthesis in Systematic Reviews: A Product from the ESRC Methods Programme. ESRC Methods Programme, 2006, 93. DOI: 10.13140/2.1.1018.4643

Pote, H., Rees, A., Holloway-Biddle, C., & Griffith, E. (2021). Workforce challenges in digital health implementation: How are clinical psychology training programmes developing digital competences? *Digital Health, 7*, 1–11. DOI: 10.1177/2055207620985396 PMID: 33628457

Prabu, A. (2021). SmartScope: An AI-powered digital auscultation device to detect cardiopulmonary diseases. *Authorea Preprints.*

PRISMA. (2021). PRISMA_2020_expanded_checklist.pdf.

PwC. (2024). *Essential eight technologies for health services: AI leads investment priorities*. PwC, August 19.

Qureshi, M. O., & Syed, R. S. (2014). The impact of robotics on employment and motivation of employees in the service sector, with special reference to health care. *Safety and Health at Work, 5*(4), 198–202. DOI: 10.1016/j.shaw.2014.07.003 PMID: 25516812

Rajkomar, A., Hardt, M., Howell, M. D., Corrado, G., & Chin, M. H. (2018). Ensuring Fairness in Machine Learning to Advance Health Equity. *Annals of Internal Medicine, 169*(12), 866-+. https://doi.org/DOI: 10.7326/M18-1990

Ramiah, I., & Reich, M. R. (2006). Building effective public-private partnerships: Experiences and lessons from the African Comprehensive HIV/AIDS Partnerships (ACHAP). *Social Science & Medicine, 63*(2), 397–408. DOI: 10.1016/j.socscimed.2006.01.007

Rangan, S., Juvekar, S., Rasalpurkar, S., Morankar, S., Joshi, A., & Porter, J. (2004). Tuberculosis control in rural India: Lessons from public-private collaboration. *The International Journal of Tuberculosis and Lung Disease : The Official Journal of the International Union against Tuberculosis and Lung Disease, 8*(5), 552–559.

Rao, K. Q., Yin, L., & Liu, Y. L. (2000). The effect on the development of social economy from the health transition of Chinese residents and the change of the demand for health services. *Zhongguo Weisheng Jingji, 9*, 5–11.

Raposo, M. L., Alves, H. M., & Duarte, P. A. (2009). Dimensions of service quality and satisfaction in healthcare: A patient's satisfaction index. *Service Business*, *3*(1), 85–100. DOI: 10.1007/s11628-008-0055-1

Rashid, W. E. W., & Jusoff, H. K. (2009). Service quality in health care setting. *International Journal of Health Care Quality Assurance*, *22*(5), 471–482. DOI: 10.1108/09526860910975580

Rasid, M. F., & Woodward, B. (2005). Bluetooth telemedicine processor for multichannel biomedical signal transmission via mobile cellular networks. *IEEE Transactions on Information Technology in Biomedicine*, *9*(1), 35–43. DOI: 10.1109/TITB.2004.840070

Raskin, M. (2016). Law and legality of smart contracts. *Georgetown Law Technology Review*, *1*, 305.

Rathore, N., Kumari, A., Patel, M., Chudasama, A., Bhalani, D., Tanwar, S., & Alabdulatif, A. (2025). Synergy of AI and blockchain to secure electronic healthcare records. *Security and Privacy*, *8*(1), e463. DOI: 10.1002/spy2.463

Ray, P. P., Dash, D., Salah, K., & Kumar, N. (2020). Blockchain for IoT-based healthcare: Background, consensus, platforms, and use cases. *IEEE Systems Journal*, *15*(1), 85–94. DOI: 10.1109/JSYST.2020.2963840

Reddy, S., Allan, S., Coghlan, S., & Cooper, P. (2020). A governance model for the application of AI in health care. *Journal of the American Medical Informatics Association : JAMIA*, *27*(3), 491–497. DOI: 10.1093/jamia/ocz192 PMID: 31682262

Richardson, J. P., Smith, C., Curtis, S., Watson, S., Zhu, X., Barry, B., & Sharp, R. R. (2021). Patient apprehensions about the use of artificial intelligence in healthcare. *NPJ Digital Medicine*, *4*(1), 140. Advance online publication. DOI: 10.1038/s41746-021-00509-1 PMID: 34548621

Richter, M., & Dragano, N. (2018). Micro, macro, but what about meso? The institutional context of health inequalities. *International Journal of Public Health*, *63*(2), 163–164. DOI: 10.1007/s00038-017-1064-4 PMID: 29250722

Roehrs, A., Da Costa, C. A., & da Rosa Righi, R. (2017). OmniPHR: A distributed architecture model to integrate personal health records. *Journal of Biomedical Informatics*, *71*, 70–81. DOI: 10.1016/j.jbi.2017.05.012 PMID: 28545835

Rogers, E. M. (2003). *Diffusion of Innovations* (5th ed.). Free Press.

Roski, J., Maier, E. J., Vigilante, K., Kane, E. A., & Matheny, M. E. (2021). Enhancing trust in AI through industry self-governance. *Journal of the American Medical Informatics Association : JAMIA*, *28*(7), 1582–1590. DOI: 10.1093/jamia/ocab065 PMID: 33895824

Ross, J., Stevenson, F., Dack, C., Pal, K., May, C., Michie, S., Barnard, M., & Murray, E. (2018). Developing an implementation strategy for a digital health intervention: An example in routine healthcare. *BMC Health Services Research*, *18*(1), 794. Advance online publication. DOI: 10.1186/s12913-018-3615-7 PMID: 30340639

Ross, T. W., & Yan, J. (2020). Comparing public-private partnerships and traditional public procurement: efficiency vs. flexibility. In Geva-May, I., Guy Peters, B., & Muhleisen, J. (Eds.), *Institutions and Governance in Comparative Policy Analysis Studies*. Routledge., DOI: 10.4324/9780429441622-9

Rubeis, G., Dubbala, K., & Metzler, I. (2022). "Democratizing" artificial intelligence in medicine and healthcare: Mapping the uses of an elusive term. *Frontiers in Genetics*, *13*, 902542. Advance online publication. DOI: 10.3389/fgene.2022.902542 PMID: 36046243

Ruckert, A., & Labonté, R. (2014). Public-private partnerships (PPPs) in global health: The good, the bad and the ugly. *Third World Quarterly*, *35*(9), 1598–1614. DOI: 10.1080/01436597.2014.970870

Ruger, J. P. (2007). Global health governance and the World Bank. *Lancet*, *370*(9597), 1471–1474. DOI: 10.1016/S0140-6736(07)61619-5

Ryu, S. (2012). Telemedicine: Opportunities and developments in member States: Report on the second Global Survey on eHealth 2009 (Global Observatory for eHealth Series, Volume 2). *Healthcare Informatics Research*, *18*(2), 153. DOI: 10.4258/hir.2012.18.2.153

Sabiri, K., Sousa, F., & Rocha, T. (2025). A systematic review of privacy-preserving blockchain applications in healthcare. *Multimedia Tools and Applications*, *84*(32), 39925–39980. Advance online publication. DOI: 10.1007/s11042-024-20541-z

Saeed, H., Malik, H., Bashir, U., Ahmad, A., Riaz, S., Ilyas, M., Bukhari, W. A., & Khan, M. I. A. (2022). Blockchain technology in healthcare: A systematic review. *PLoS One*, *17*(4), e0266462. DOI: 10.1371/journal.pone.0266462 PMID: 35404955

Safavi, K., & Kalis, B. (2019). How AI can change the future of healthcare. *Harvard Business Review*.

Saheb, T., Saheb, T., & Carpenter, D. O. (2021). Mapping research strands of ethics of artificial intelligence in healthcare: A bibliometric and content analysis. *Computers in Biology and Medicine, 135*, 104660. Advance online publication. DOI: 10.1016/j.compbiomed.2021.104660 PMID: 34346319

Sandbox Dubai. (2025). We are Sandbox Dubai—Healthcare Sandbox. https://www.sandboxdubai.gov.ae/sandboxes/health-care-sandbox

Sand, M., Durán, J. M., & Jongsma, K. R. (2022). Responsibility beyond design: Physicians' requirements for ethical medical AI. *Bioethics, 36*(2), 162–169. DOI: 10.1111/bioe.12887 PMID: 34089625

Sankar, B. S., Gilliland, D., Rincon, J., Hermjakob, H., Yan, Y., Adam, I., Lemaster, G., Wang, D., Watson, K., Bui, A., Wang, W., & Ping, P. P. (2024). Building an Ethical and Trustworthy Biomedical AI Ecosystem for the Translational and Clinical Integration of Foundation Models. *Bioengineering (Basel, Switzerland), 11*(10), 984. Advance online publication. DOI: 10.3390/bioengineering11100984 PMID: 39451360

Santandrea, M., Bailey, S., & Giorgino, M. (2016). Value for money in UK healthcare public-private partnerships: A fragility perspective. *Public Policy and Administration, 31*(3), 260–279. DOI: 10.1177/0952076715618003

Santra, S., Kukreja, P., Saxena, K., Gandhi, S., & Singh, O. V. (2024). Navigating regulatory and policy challenges for AI enabled combination devices. *Frontiers in Medical Technology, 6*, 1473350. Advance online publication. DOI: 10.3389/fmedt.2024.1473350 PMID: 39669903

Sasseville, M., Ouellet, S., Rhéaume, C., Sahlia, M., Couture, V., Després, P., Paquette, J.-S., Darmon, D., Bergeron, F., & Gagnon, M. P. (2025). Bias Mitigation in Primary Health Care Artificial Intelligence Models: Scoping Review. *Journal of Medical Internet Research, 27*, e60269. Advance online publication. DOI: 10.2196/60269 PMID: 39773888

Saudi Data & AI Authority (SDAIA). (2023). Implementing regulations of the Personal Data Protection Law.

Saudi Data & AI Authority (SDAIA). (2023, April 23). Personal Data Protection Law (PDPL).

Savirimuthu, J. (2020). The GDPR, AI and the NHS code of conduct for data-driven health and care technology. In *Health data privacy under the GDPR* (pp. 133–156). Routledge., DOI: 10.4324/9780429022241-10

Saw, S. N., & Ng, K. H. (2022). Current challenges of implementing artificial intelligence in medical imaging. *Physica Medica : PM : An International Journal Devoted to the Applications of Physics to Medicine and Biology : Official Journal of the Italian Association of Biomedical Physics (AIFB)*, *100*, 12–17. DOI: 10.1016/j.ejmp.2022.06.003 PMID: 35714523

Sawyer, C., Hassan, L., Sainsbury, J., Carney, R., Bucci, S., Burgess, H., Lovell, K., Torous, J., & Firth, J. (2023). Using digital technology to promote physical health in mental healthcare: A sequential mixed-methods study of clinicians' views. *Early Intervention in Psychiatry*. Advance online publication. DOI: 10.1111/eip.13441 PMID: 37318221

Schank, R. C., & Abelson, R. P. (1977). *Scripts, plans, goals, and understanding: An inquiry into human knowledge structures*. Lawrence Erlbaum.

ScienceDirect. (2023). Cochrane Library. https://www.sciencedirect.com/topics/nursing-and-health-professions/cochrane-library

Scipion, C. E., Manchester, M. A., Federman, A., Wang, Y., & Arias, J. J. (2025). Barriers to and facilitators of clinician acceptance and use of artificial intelligence in healthcare settings: A scoping review. *BMJ Open*, *15*(4), e092624. DOI: 10.1136/bmjopen-2024-092624 PMID: 40233955

Scott, R. E., Ndumbe, P., & Wootton, R. (2005). An e-health needs assessment of medical residents in Cameroon. *Journal of Telemedicine and Telecare*, *11*(2_suppl, Suppl 2), S78–S80. DOI: 10.1258/135763305775124911 PMID: 16375807

Sebastiani, R., & Anzivino, A. (2022). The long and winding road of eHealth: The service ecosystem perspective. *Journal of Business and Industrial Marketing*, *37*(10), 2036–2049. DOI: 10.1108/JBIM-02-2021-0107

Selvadurai, N., & Matulionyte, R. (2020). Reconsidering creativity: Copyright protection for works generated using artificial intelligence. *Journal of Intellectual Property Law & Practice*, *15*(7), 536–543. DOI: 10.1093/jiplp/jpaa062

Sendek Anteneh, D., Kelkay, J. M., Wubneh, H. D., Beshir, M. A., & Gashu, K. D. (2025). Intention to use digital-based psychosocial counseling and its predictors among students in University of Gondar, Northwest Ethiopia, 2023: Using modified unified theory of acceptance and use of technology model. *SAGE Open Medicine*, *13*. Advance online publication. DOI: 10.1177/20503121241307136

Shabbir, A., Malik, S. A., & Malik, S. A. (2016). Measuring patients' healthcare service quality perceptions, satisfaction, and loyalty in public and private sector hospitals in Pakistan. *International Journal of Quality & Reliability Management, 33*(5), 538–557. DOI: 10.1108/IJQRM-06-2014-0074

Shafei, I., Walburg, J., & Taher, A. (2019). Verifying alternative measures of healthcare service quality. *International Journal of Health Care Quality Assurance, 32*(2), 516–533. DOI: 10.1108/IJHCQA-05-2016-0069

Shah, P., Thornton, I., Kopitnik, N. L., & Hipskind, J. E. (2023). Informed Consent. National Library of Medicine. https://www.ncbi.nlm.nih.gov/books/NBK430827/

Shaheen, M. Y. (2021). Applications of artificial intelligence (AI) in healthcare: A review. ScienceOpen *Preprints*.

Shaikh, M., Memon, S. A., Ebrahimi, A., & Wiil, U. K. (2025). A systematic literature review for blockchain-based healthcare implementations. *Health Care, 13*(9), 1087. Advance online publication. DOI: 10.3390/healthcare13091087 PMID: 40361865

Sharma-Misra, S., Maru, M., Tomita, A., & Paruk, S. (2023). Access and use of digital technology by patients with psychosis at a hospital in South Africa. *South African Journal of Psychiatry, 29*. Advance online publication. DOI: 10.4102/sajpsychiatry.v29i0.2151

Sharma, S. (2024). Benefits or concerns of AI: A multistakeholder responsibility. *Futures, 157*, 103328. DOI: 10.1016/j.futures.2024.103328

Shaw, J., Ali, J., Atuire, C. A., Cheah, P. Y., Español, A. G., Gichoya, J. W., Hunt, A., Jjingo, D., Littler, K., Paolotti, D., & Vayena, E. (2024). Research ethics and artificial intelligence for global health: Perspectives from the global forum on bioethics in research. *BMC Medical Ethics, 25*(1), 46. Advance online publication. DOI: 10.1186/s12910-024-01044-w PMID: 38637857

Shefchek, K. A., Harris, N. L., Gargano, M., Matentzoglu, N., Unni, D., Brush, M., Keith, D., Conlin, T., Vasilevsky, N., Zhang, X. A., Balhoff, J. P., Babb, L., Bello, S. M., Blau, H., Bradford, Y., Carbon, S., Carmody, L., Chan, L. E., Cipriani, V., & Osumi-Sutherland, D. (2020). The Monarch Initiative in 2019: An integrative data and analytic platform connecting phenotypes to genotypes across species. *Nucleic Acids Research, 48*(D1), D704–D715. DOI: 10.1093/nar/gkz997

Sheikh, K., Porter, J., Kielmann, K., & Rangan, S. (2006). Public-private partnerships for equity of access to care for tuberculosis and HIV/AIDS: Lessons from Pune, India. *Transactions of the Royal Society of Tropical Medicine and Hygiene, 100*(4), 312–320. DOI: 10.1016/j.trstmh.2005.04.023

Shekoni, O., Iversen, S., Diaz, G. J., Aune, A., Ubuane, P. O., Imam, Z., & André, B. (2024). Healthcare workers' perceptions about the use of mobile health technologies in public health facilities in Lagos, Nigeria. *SAGE Open Medicine*, *12*, 20503121231224568. DOI: 10.1177/20503121231224568 PMID: 38347851

Shen, N., Kassam, I., Chen, S., Ma, C., Wang, W., Boparai, N., Jankowicz, D., & Strudwick, G. (2022). Canadian perspectives of digital mental health supports: Findings from a national survey conducted during the COVID-19 pandemic. *Digital Health*, *8*. Advance online publication. DOI: 10.1177/20552076221102253

Shi, D., Zhang, W., Zhang, W., & Ding, X. (2019). A review on lower limb rehabilitation exoskeleton robots. *Chinese Journal of Mechanical Engineering*, *32*(1), 1–11. DOI: 10.1186/s10033-019-0389-8

Shigekawa, E., Fix, M., Corbett, G., Roby, D. H., & Coffman, J. (2018). The current state of telehealth evidence: A rapid review. *Health Affairs*, *37*(12), 1975–1982. DOI: 10.1377/hlthaff.2018.05132

Shojaei, P., Gjorgievska, E. V., & Chow, Y.-W. (2024). Security and privacy of technologies in health information systems: A systematic literature review. *Computers*, *13*(2), 41. Advance online publication. DOI: 10.3390/computers13020041

Shore, J. H., Schneck, C. D., & Mishkind, M. C. (2020). Telepsychiatry and the coronavirus disease 2019 pandemic—Current and future outcomes of the rapid virtualization of psychiatric care. *JAMA Psychiatry*, *77*(12), 1211–1212. DOI: 10.1001/jamapsychiatry.2020.1643 PMID: 32391861

Shuaib, M., Alam, S., Shabbir Alam, M., & Shahnawaz Nasir, M. (2021). Compliance with HIPAA and GDPR in blockchain-based electronic health record. *Materials Today: Proceedings*. Advance online publication. DOI: 10.1016/j.matpr.2021.03.059

Siala, H., & Wang, Y. C. (2022). SHIFTing artificial intelligence to be responsible in healthcare: A systematic review. *Social Science & Medicine*, *296*, 114782. Advance online publication. DOI: 10.1016/j.socscimed.2022.114782 PMID: 35152047

Sibeko, G., Temmingh, H., Mall, S., Williams-Ashman, P., Thornicroft, G., Susser, E. S., Lund, C., Stein, D. J., & Milligan, P. D. (2017). Improving adherence in mental health service users with severe mental illness in South Africa: A pilot randomized controlled trial of a treatment partner and text message intervention vs. treatment as usual PACTR201610001830190 PACTR. *BMC Research Notes*, *10*(1). Advance online publication. DOI: 10.1186/s13104-017-2915-z

Silow-Carroll, S. (2008). *Iowa's 1st five initiative: Improving early childhood developmental services through public-private partnerships*. Commonwealth Fund.

Simcik Arese, N. (2018). Seeing like a city-state: Behavioural planning and governance in Egypt's first affordable gated community. *International Journal of Urban and Regional Research*, *42*(3), 461–482. DOI: 10.1111/1468-2427.12601

Sindakis, S., & Showkat, G. (2024). The digital revolution in India: Bridging the gap in rural technology adoption. *Journal of Innovation and Entrepreneurship*, *13*(1), 29. DOI: 10.1186/s13731-024-00380-w

Singh, V., Johnson, K. R., Jacob, A. G., & John, O. (2025). The potential of digital health interventions to address health system challenges in Southeast Asia: A scoping review. *Digital Health*, *11*. Advance online publication. DOI: 10.1177/20552076241311062

Solaiman, E., & Awad, C. (2025). Trust and dependability in blockchain & AI based MedIoT applications: Research challenges and future directions. https://doi.org// arXiv.2501.02647DOI: 10.48550

Soni, P. K., & Kumari, U. (2025). Revitalizing Health Governance: Charting a Resilient Path for India's Future. In *Intersecting realities of health resilience and governance in India: Emerging domestic and global perspectives* (pp. 55–73). Springer Nature Singapore.

Sophia. (2023, August 28). The future of healthcare in Congo: The era of telemedicine. SYNWELL. https://www.synwell-sante.com/en/post/the-future-of-healthcare-in-congo-the-era-of-telemedicine

Sorsdahl, K., Stein, D. J., Grimsrud, A., Seedat, S., Flisher, A. J., Williams, D. R., & Myer, L. (2009). Traditional Healers in the Treatment of Common Mental Disorders in South Africa. *The Journal of Nervous and Mental Disease*, *197*(6). https://journals.lww.com/jonmd/fulltext/2009/06000/traditional_healers_in_the_treatment_of_common.9.aspx

Spena, T. R., & Cristina, M. (2020). Practising innovation in health ecosystem: The agency of third-party actors. *Journal of Business and Industrial Marketing*, *35*(3), 390–403. DOI: 10.1108/JBIM-01-2019-0048

Spence, M. (1973). Job market signaling. *The Quarterly Journal of Economics*, *87*(3), 355–374. DOI: 10.2307/1882010

Steel, Z., Marnane, C., Iranpour, C., Chey, T., Jackson, J. W., Patel, V., & Silove, D. (2014). The global prevalence of common mental disorders: A systematic review and meta-analysis 1980-2013. *International Journal of Epidemiology*, *43*(2), 476–493. DOI: 10.1093/ije/dyu038

Steijn, B., Klijn, E. H., & Edelenbos, J. (2011). Public private partnerships: Added value by organizational form or management? *Public Administration, 89*(4), 1235–1252. DOI: 10.1111/j.1467-9299.2010.01877.x

Steil, J., Finas, D., Beck, S., Manzeschke, A., & Haux, R. (2019). Robotic systems in operating theaters: New forms of team–machine interaction in health care. *Methods of Information in Medicine, 58*(1), E14–E25. DOI: 10.1055/s-0039-1692465 PMID: 31342471

Stoumpos, A. I., Kitsios, F., & Talias, M. A. (2023). Digital transformation in healthcare: Technology acceptance and its applications. *International Journal of Environmental Research and Public Health, 20*(4), 3407. DOI: 10.3390/ijerph20043407 PMID: 36834105

Stuckler, D., Basu, S., & McKee, M. (2011). Global health philanthropy and institutional relationships: How should conflicts of interest be addressed? *PLoS Medicine, 8*(4), e1001020. DOI: 10.1371/journal.pmed.1001020

Su, X., Li, X., & Kang, Y. (2019). A Bibliometric Analysis of Research on Intangible Cultural Heritage Using CiteSpace. *SAGE Open, 2019*(4). https://doi.org/doi: DOI: 10.1177/2158244019840119

Subbe, C. P., Øvretveit, J., Quinn, N., & Wyatt, J. C. (2019). Opportunities and barriers for usage of personal health records in hospital: Report from a workshop of the Health Informatics Unit at Royal College of Physicians. *Future Healthcare Journal, 6*(1), 52–55. DOI: 10.7861/futurehosp.6-1-52 PMID: 31098587

Sultana, S., & Pagán, J. A. (2023). Use of Telehealth to Address Depression and Anxiety in Low-income US Populations: A Narrative Review. *Journal of Primary Care & Community Health, 14*. Advance online publication. DOI: 10.1177/21501319231168036

Sun, Z., Han, D., Li, D., Wang, X., Chang, C.-C., & Wu, Z. (2022). A blockchain-based secure storage scheme for medical information. EURASIP Journal on Wireless Communications and Networking, 2022(1). DOI: 10.1186/s13638-022-02122-6

Swain, S., & Kar, N. C. (2018). Hospital service quality as antecedent of patient satisfaction—A conceptual framework. *International Journal of Pharmaceutical and Healthcare Marketing, 12*(3), 251–269. DOI: 10.1108/IJPHM-06-2016-0028

Taeihagh, A. (2025). Governance of generative AI. *Policy and Society, 44*(1), 1–22. DOI: 10.1093/polsoc/puaf001

Tagde, P., Tagde, S., Bhattacharya, T., Tagde, P., Chopra, H., Akter, R., Kaushik, D., & Rahman, M. (2021). Blockchain and artificial intelligence technology in e-Health. *Environmental Science and Pollution Research International, 28*(38), 52810–52831. DOI: 10.1007/s11356-021-16223-0 PMID: 34476701

Tahir, U. A., Barber, J. L., Cruz, D. E., Kars, M. E., Deng, S., Tuftin, B., Gillman, M. G., Benson, M. D., Robbins, J. M., Chen, Z. Z., Rao, P., Katz, D. H., Farrell, L., Sofer, T., Hall, M. E., Ekunwe, L., Tracy, R. P., Durda, P., Taylor, K. D., & Gerszten, R. E. (2024). Proteogenomic analysis integrated with electronic health records data reveals disease-associated variants in Black Americans. *The Journal of Clinical Investigation, 134*(21), e181802. DOI: 10.1172/JCI181802 PMID: 39316441

Tam, J. L. M. (2019). Examining the role of customer self-efficacy in service encounters. *Services Marketing Quarterly, 40*(4), 269–284. DOI: 10.1080/15332969.2019.1666534

Tandon, A., Dhir, A., Islam, N., & Mäntymäki, M. (2020). Blockchain in healthcare: A systematic literature review, synthesizing framework and future research agenda. *Computers in Industry, 122*, 103290. Advance online publication. DOI: 10.1016/j.compind.2020.103290

Tang, L., Li, J. X., & Fantus, S. (2023). Medical artificial intelligence ethics: A systematic review of empirical studies. *Digital Health, 9*, 20552076231186064. Advance online publication. DOI: 10.1177/20552076231186064 PMID: 37434728

Tan, T. F., Thirunavukarasu, A. J., Jin, L., Lim, J., Poh, S., Teo, Z. L., Ang, M., Chan, R. P., Ong, J., Turner, A., Karlström, J., Wong, T. Y., Stern, J., & Ting, D. S.-W. (2023). Artificial intelligence and digital health in global eye health: Opportunities and challenges. *The Lancet. Global Health, 11*(9), e1432–e1443. DOI: 10.1016/S2214-109X(23)00323-6

Taquette, S. R., & Borges da Matta Souza, L. M. (2022). Ethical dilemmas in qualitative research: A critical literature review. *International Journal of Qualitative Methods, 21*, 1–15. DOI: 10.1177/16094069221078731

Tarabusi, C. C., & Vickery, G. (1998a). Globalization in the pharmaceutical industry, part I. *International Journal of Health Services, 28*(1), 67–105. DOI: 10.2190/7JDR-2TFN-2B3X-TYF5

Tarabusi, C. C., & Vickery, G. (1998b). Globalization in the pharmaceutical industry, part II. *International Journal of Health Services, 28*(2), 281–303. DOI: 10.2190/B6VR-NND7-46BL-PY5G

Taylor, K., Hall, B., & Siegel, S. (2019). Closing the digital gap: Shaping the future of UK healthcare. Deloitte. https://www2.deloitte.com/content/dam/Deloitte/uk/Documents/life-sciences-health-care/deloitte-uk-life-sciences-health-care-closing-the-digital-gap.pdf

Tchao, E. T., Acquah, I., Kotey, S. D., Aggor, C. S., & Kponyo, J. J. (2019). On telemedicine implementations in Ghana. *International Journal of Advanced Computer Science and Applications*, *10*(3). Advance online publication. DOI: 10.14569/IJACSA.2019.0100325

te Marvelde, K. (2025). Designing LLM driven tools to support collaboration in complex multi-stakeholder systems, MS Thesis, Delft University of Technology, Delft, Netherlands, 2025.

Terkelsen, C. J., Nørgaard, B. L., Lassen, J. F., Gerdes, J. C., Ankersen, J. P., Rømer, F., Nielsen, T. T., & Andersen, H. R. (2002). Telemedicine is used for remote pre-hospital diagnosing in patients suspected of acute myocardial infarction. *Journal of Internal Medicine*, *252*(5), 412–420. DOI: 10.1046/j.1365-2796.2002.01051.x PMID: 12528759

Terry, A. L., Kueper, J. K., Beleno, R., Brown, J. B., Cejic, S., Dang, J., Leger, D., McKay, S., Meredith, L., Pinto, A. D., Ryan, B. L., Stewart, M., Zwarenstein, M., & Lizotte, D. J. (2022). Is primary health care ready for artificial intelligence? What do primary health care stakeholders say? *BMC Medical Informatics and Decision Making*, *22*(1), 237. DOI: 10.1186/s12911-022-01984-6 PMID: 36085203

Thangaraj, P. M., Benson, S. H., Oikonomou, E. K., Asselbergs, F. W., & Khera, R. (2024). Cardiovascular care with digital twin technology in the era of generative artificial intelligence. *European Heart Journal*, *45*(45), 4808–4821. DOI: 10.1093/eurheartj/ehae619

The American Telemedicine Association. (2017). ATA 2017 Telehealth 2.0 Conference abstracts. *Telemedicine Journal and e-Health : The Official Journal of the American Telemedicine Association*, *23*(4), A-78. DOI: 10.1089/tmj.2017.29005-A.abstracts PMID: 28410061

The General Office of the State Council of the People's Republic of China. (2015). *Notice of the General Office of the State Council on issuing several policies and measures for promoting the accelerated development of private medical institutions.* https://www.gov.cn/zhengce/content/2015-06/15/content_9845.htm

The Health Foundation. (2018). Cost pressures on the NHS will only grow. https://www.health.org.uk/news-and-comment/news/cost-pressures-on-the-nhs-will-only-grow-it-needs-a-long-term-funding-solution-and-that-is

The Hewitt Review. (2023). An independent review of integrated care systems. https://assets.publishing.service.gov.uk/government/uploads/system/uploads/attachment_data/file/1148568/the-hewitt-review.pdf

The King's Fund. (2023a). Actions to support partnership: Addressing barriers to working with the VCSE sector in integrated care systems. https://www.kingsfund.org.uk/sites/default/files/2023-04/Addressing_barriers_to_working_with_the_VCSE_sector_in_integrated_care_systems_0.pdf

The King's Fund. (2023b). Key facts and figures about the NHS. https://www.kingsfund.org.uk/audio-video/key-facts-figures-nhs

The King's Fund. (2024). *Key facts and figures about the NHS*. The King's Fund, June 25.

The Topol Review. (2019). Preparing the healthcare workforce to deliver the digital future. https://topol.hee.nhs.uk/wp-content/uploads/HEE-Topol-Review-2019.pdf

Thrall, J. H., Boland, G., & Larson, D. B. (2020). Teleradiology: Expanding the reach of radiology. *Radiology*, *295*(3), 636–641. DOI: 10.1148/radiol.2020192652

Thurzo, A. (2025). Provable AI Ethics and Explainability in Medical and Educational AI Agents: Trustworthy Ethical Firewall. *Electronics (Basel)*, *14*(7), 1294. Advance online publication. DOI: 10.3390/electronics14071294

Tolley, C., Seymour, H., Watson, N., Nazar, H., Heed, J., & Belshaw, D. (2023). Barriers and opportunities for the use of digital tools in medicines optimization across the interfaces of care: Stakeholder interviews in the United Kingdom. *JMIR Medical Informatics*, *11*, e42458. Advance online publication. DOI: 10.2196/42458 PMID: 36897631

Topol, E. J. (2019). High-performance medicine: The convergence of human and artificial intelligence. *Nature Medicine*, *25*(1), 44–56. DOI: 10.1038/s41591-018-0300-7 PMID: 30617339

Torous, J., Bucci, S., Bell, I. H., Kessing, L. V., Faurholt-Jepsen, M., Whelan, P., Carvalho, A. F., Keshavan, M., Linardon, J., & Firth, J. (2021). The growing field of digital psychiatry: Current evidence and the future of apps, social media, chatbots, and virtual reality. *World Psychiatry; Official Journal of the World Psychiatric Association (WPA)*, *20*(3), 318–335. DOI: 10.1002/wps.20883

Torous, J., Myrick, K. J., Rauseo-Ricupero, N., & Firth, J. (2020). Digital mental health and COVID-19: Using technology today to accelerate the curve on access and quality tomorrow. *JMIR Mental Health*, *7*(3), 1–6. DOI: 10.2196/18848

Trappl, R. (Ed.). (1986). *Impacts of artificial intelligence: Scientific, technological, military, economic, societal, cultural, and political* (2nd ed.). Elsevier Science.

Tredinnick, L., & Laybats, C. (2023). The dangers of generative artificial intelligence. *Business Information Review, 40*(2), 46–48. DOI: 10.1177/02663821231183756

Trivedi, R., & Jagani, K. (2018). Perceived service quality, repeat use of healthcare services and inpatient satisfaction in emerging economy: Empirical evidences from India. *International Journal of Pharmaceutical and Healthcare Marketing, 12*(3), 288–306. DOI: 10.1108/IJPHM-11-2017-0065

Tun, H. M., Rahman, H. A., Naing, L., & Malik, O. A. (2025). Trust in artificial intelligence–based clinical decision support systems among healthcare workers: Systematic review. *Journal of Medical Internet Research, 27*, e69678. DOI: 10.2196/69678 PMID: 40772775

Turnbull, S., Lucas, P. J., Hay, A. D., & Cabral, C. (2021). The role of economic, educational and social resources in supporting the use of digital health technologies by people with T2D: A qualitative study. *BMC Public Health, 21*(1), 10325. Advance online publication. DOI: 10.1186/s12889-021-10325-7 PMID: 33546661

Tuzov, V., & Lin, F. (2024). Two paths of balancing technology and ethics: A comparative study on AI governance in China and Germany. *Telecommunications Policy, 48*(10), 102850. Advance online publication. DOI: 10.1016/j.telpol.2024.102850

Twamley, J., Hamer, O., Hill, J., Kenyon, R., Twamley, H., Casey, R., Zhang, J., Williams, A., & Clegg, A. (2022). Exploring the perceptions of former ICU patients and clinical staff on barriers and facilitators to the implementation of virtual reality exposure therapy: A qualitative study. *Nursing in Critical Care*. Advance online publication. DOI: 10.1111/nicc.12868 PMID: 36458458

Ubalaeze, S. (2025). The impact of digital transformation on healthcare delivery in Nigeria: Challenges and recommendations. *International Journal of Research and Scientific Innovation, 11*(15), 498–509.

Ueda, D., Kakinuma, T., Fujita, S., Kamagata, K., Fushimi, Y., Ito, R., Matsui, Y., Nozaki, T., Nakaura, T., Fujima, N., Tatsugami, F., Yanagawa, M., Hirata, K., Yamada, A., Tsuboyama, T., Kawamura, M., Fujioka, T., & Naganawa, S. (2024). Fairness of artificial intelligence in healthcare: Review and recommendations. *Japanese Journal of Radiology, 42*(1), 3–15. DOI: 10.1007/s11604-023-01474-3 PMID: 37540463

Ukaoha, K. C., & Egbokhare, F. A. (2012). Prospects and Challenges of Telemedicine in Nigeria. *Journal of Medical and Biomedical Sciences*, *3*(1), 65–70. DOI: 10.7813/jmbs.2012/3-1/10

Ukpe, E. (2025). Transforming Healthcare: Telemedicine's Role and Impact in Nigeria. *IOSR Journal of Humanities and Social Science*, *30*(2), 20–26. DOI: 10.9790/0837-3002072026

Ullah, A. N. Z., Huque, R., Husain, A., Akter, S., Islam, A., & Newell, J. N. (2012). Effectiveness of involving the private medical sector in the National TB Control Programme in Bangladesh: Evidence from mixed methods. *BMJ Open*, *2*(6), e001534. DOI: 10.1136/bmjopen-2012-001534

Ulnicane, I. (2025). Governance fix? Power and politics in controversies about governing generative AI. *Policy and Society*, *44*(1), 70–84. DOI: 10.1093/polsoc/puae022

Um, K. H., & Lau, A. K. W. (2018). Healthcare service failure: How dissatisfied patients respond to poor service quality. *International Journal of Operations & Production Management*, *38*(5), 1245–1270. DOI: 10.1108/IJOPM-11-2016-0669

Ungureanu, A. M., Matei, S. C., & Malita, D. (2025). Controversies in the Application of AI in Radiology-Is There Medico-Legal Support? Aspects from Romanian Practice. *Diagnostics (Basel)*, *15*(2), 230. Advance online publication. DOI: 10.3390/diagnostics15020230 PMID: 39857113

Unsworth, H., Dillon, B., Collinson, L., Powell, H., Salmon, M., Oladapo, T., Ayiku, L., Shield, G., Holden, J., Patel, N., Campbell, M., Greaves, F., Joshi, I., Powell, J., & Tonnel, A. (2021). The NICE Evidence Standards Framework for digital health and care technologies—Developing and maintaining an innovative evidence framework with global impact. *Digital Health*, *7*, 1–20. DOI: 10.1177/20552076211018617 PMID: 34249371

Uplekar, M. (2016). Public-private mix for tuberculosis care and prevention. What progress? What prospects? *The International Journal of Tuberculosis and Lung Disease : The Official Journal of the International Union against Tuberculosis and Lung Disease*, *20*(11), 1424–1429. DOI: 10.5588/ijtld.15.0536

Vakaniaki, E. H., Kacita, C., Kinganda-Lusamaki, E., O'Toole, Á., Wawina-Bokalanga, T., Mukadi-Bamuleka, D., Amuri-Aziza, A., Malyamungu-Bubala, N., Mweshi-Kumbana, F., Mutimbwa-Mambo, L., Belesi-Siangoli, F., Mujula, Y., Parker, E., Muswamba-Kayembe, P.-C., Nundu, S. S., Lushima, R. S., Makangara-Cigolo, J.-C., Mulopo-Mukanya, N., Pukuta-Simbu, E., & Mbala-Kingebeni, P. (2024). Sustained human outbreak of a new MPXV clade I lineage in eastern Democratic Republic of Congo. *Nature Medicine*, *30*(10), 2791–2795. DOI: 10.1038/s41591-024-03130-3 PMID: 38871006

Valencia-Arias, A., Piedrahita, L. B., Zapata, A. B., & Arias, M. L. B. (2018). Mapping the healthcare service quality domain: A bibliometric analysis. *Journal of Clinical and Diagnostic Research : JCDR*, *12*(8), IC01–IC05. DOI: 10.7860/JCDR/2018/30361.11863

Valentinov, V., & Roth, S. (2024). Relationality in transaction cost economics and stakeholder theory: A new conceptual framework. *Business Ethics, the Environment & Responsibility*, *33*(3), 535–546. DOI: 10.1111/beer.12652

Vallès-Peris, N., Barat-Auleda, O., & Domènech, M. (2021). Robots in healthcare? What patients say. *International Journal of Environmental Research and Public Health*, *18*(18), 9933. Advance online publication. DOI: 10.3390/ijerph18189933 PMID: 34574861

Vallverdú, J. (2024). Generative AI and causality. In *Causality for Artificial Intelligence: From a Philosophical Perspective* (pp. 55–61). Springer., DOI: 10.1007/978-981-97-3187-9_6

van Breugel, B., Liu, T., Oglic, D., & van der Schaar, M. (2024). Synthetic data in biomedicine via generative artificial intelligence. *Nature Reviews Bioengineering*, *2*(12), 991–1004. DOI: 10.1038/s44222-024-00245-7

Van Daalen, O. L. (2023). The right to encryption: Privacy as preventing unlawful access. *Computer Law & Security Review*, *49*, 105804. DOI: 10.1016/j.clsr.2023.105804

van Heerden, A. C., Pozuelo, J. R., & Kohrt, B. A. (2023). Global mental health services and the impact of artificial intelligence-powered large language models. *JAMA Psychiatry*, *80*(7), 662–664. DOI: 10.1001/jamapsychiatry.2023.1253

van Kolfschooten, H., & van Oirschot, J. (2024). The EU Artificial Intelligence Act (2024): Implications for healthcare. *Health Policy (Amsterdam)*, *149*, 105152. Advance online publication. DOI: 10.1016/j.healthpol.2024.105152 PMID: 39244818

Vargo, S. L., & Lusch, R. F. (2017). Service-dominant logic 2025. *International Journal of Research in Marketing*, *34*(1), 46–67. DOI: 10.1016/j.ijresmar.2016.11.001

Varnosfaderani, S. M., & Forouzanfar, M. (2024). The Role of AI in Hospitals and Clinics: Transforming Healthcare in the 21st Century. *Bioengineering (Basel, Switzerland), 11*(4), 337. Advance online publication. DOI: 10.3390/bioengineering11040337 PMID: 38671759

Vasilevsky, N., Essaid, S., Matentzoglu, N., Harris, N. L., Haendel, M., Robinson, P., & Mungall, C. J. (2020). Mondo Disease Ontology: Harmonizing disease concepts across the world. *CEUR Workshop Proceedings*, *2807*, 1–2.

Vera San Juan, N., Martin, S., Barnett, P., Chandrasekar, A., Makhmud, A., & Palacios, J. (2024). Digital Mental Health Landscaping in Low-and Middle-Income Countries Rapid Research Evaluation and Appraisal Lab (Rreal). *Wellcome Open Research*, *9*(383). https://www.rapidresearchandevaluation.com/

VFMatch. (n.d.). VFMatch. https://vfmatch.org/explore/facilities/5e5d6ecfaf007f0082810279

Vogus, T. J., & McClelland, L. C. (2016). When the customer is the patient: Lessons from healthcare research on patient satisfaction and service quality ratings. *Human Resource Management Review*, *26*(1), 37–49. DOI: 10.1016/j.hrmr.2015.09.005

Vo, V., Chen, G., Aquino, Y. S., Carter, S. M., Do, Q. N., & Woode, M. E. (2023). Multi-stakeholder preferences for the use of artificial intelligence in healthcare: A systematic review and thematic analysis. *Social Science & Medicine*, *338*, 116357. Advance online publication. DOI: 10.1016/j.socscimed.2023.116357 PMID: 37949020

Vukoli, M., (2017). *Rethinking Permissioned Blockchains*. In the ACM Workshop.

Wagstaff, A., Yip, W., Lindelow, M., & Hsiao, W. C. (2009). China's health system and its reform: A review of recent studies. *Health Economics*, *18*(S2), S7–S23. DOI: 10.1002/hec.1518

Wang, Y., Li, Y., Chen, Y., Lu, S., & Yu, P. (2024). The Role of Emerging Technologies in Modernizing the Healthcare Industry: Case Studies from China. *European Academic Journal - II CHINA, 1*(1). https://eaj.ebujournals.lu/index.php/EAJ_II/article/view/112

Wang, B. J., Asan, O., & Zhang, Y. Q. (2024). Shaping the future of chronic disease management: Insights into patient needs for AI-based homecare systems. *International Journal of Medical Informatics*, *181*, 105301. Advance online publication. DOI: 10.1016/j.ijmedinf.2023.105301 PMID: 38029700

Wang, B. T. (2024). Prompts and large language models: A new tool for drafting, reviewing and interpreting contracts? *Law. Technology and Humans*, *6*(2), 88–106. DOI: 10.5204/lthj.3483

Wang, C. Y., Liu, S. R., Yang, H., Guo, J. L., Wu, Y. X., & Liu, J. L. (2023). Ethical Considerations of Using ChatGPT in Health Care. *Journal of Medical Internet Research, 25*, e48009. Advance online publication. DOI: 10.2196/48009 PMID: 37566454

Wang, H., Xiong, W., Wu, G., & Zhu, D. (2018). Public-private partnership in public administration discipline: A literature review. *Public Management Review*, *20*(2), 293–316. DOI: 10.1080/14719037.2017.1313445

Wang, X., Geng, N., Jiang, S., Zhou, L., & Jiang, Z. (2021). Optimal design of health-care services after the separation of prescribing and dispensing. *International Journal of Production Research*, *60*(9), 2918–2941. DOI: 10.1080/00207543.2021.1906459

Watson, A., Mellotte, H., Hardy, A., Peters, E., Keen, N., & Kane, F. (2022). The digital divide: Factors impacting on uptake of remote therapy in a South London psychological therapy service for people with psychosis. *Journal of Mental Health*, *31*(6), 825–832. DOI: 10.1080/09638237.2021.1952955 PMID: 34319202

Watson, G. J., Desouza, K. C., Ribiere, V. M., & Lindič, J. (2021). Will AI ever sit at the C-suite table? The future of senior leadership. *Business Horizons*, *64*(4), 465–474. DOI: 10.1016/j.bushor.2021.02.011

Wells, R. A., Gallarza, M. G., Andreu, L., & Calero, R. (2015). Application of service dominant logic to the medical device industry. *International Review on Public and Nonprofit Marketing*, *12*(3), 207–235. DOI: 10.1007/s12208-015-0126-7

WHO. (2024). Digital Health and Innovation Achieving health for all through innovation and digital transformation. www.who.int/teams/digital-health-and-innovation/digital-channels/fides

Wibowo, M. F., Pyle, A., Lim, E., Ohde, J. W., Liu, N., & Karlström, J. (2025). Insights Into the Current and Future State of AI Adoption Within Health Systems in Southeast Asia: Cross-Sectional Qualitative Study. *Journal of Medical Internet Research, 27*. Advance online publication. 10.2196/71591

Wijk, J., Zietsma, C., Dorado, S., Bakker, F. G. A., & Martí, I. (2019). Social innovation: Integrating micro, meso, and macro level insights from institutional theory. *Business & Society*, *58*(5), 887–918. DOI: 10.1177/0007650318789104

Wildlife Conservation Society. (2004). *One World, One Health: building interdisciplinary bridges to health in a globalized world, One World One Health. The Rockefeller University, 29 September*. Wildlife Conservation Society.

Willem, T., Fritzsche, M. C., Zimmermann, B. M., Sierawska, A., Breuer, S., Braun, M., Ruess, A. K., Bak, M., Schönweitz, F. B., Meier, L. J., Fiske, A., Tigard, D., Müller, R., McLennan, S., & Buyx, A. (2024). Embedded Ethics in Practice: A Toolbox for Integrating the Analysis of Ethical and Social Issues into Healthcare AI Research. *Science and Engineering Ethics*, *31*(1), 3. Advance online publication. DOI: 10.1007/s11948-024-00523-y PMID: 39718728

Williams, M. G., Stott, R., Bromwich, N., Oblak, S. K., Espir, C. A., & Rose, J. B. (2020). Determinants of and barriers to adoption of digital therapeutics for mental health at scale in the NHS. *BMJ Innovations*, *6*(3), 92–98. DOI: 10.1136/bmjinnov-2019-000384

Williamson, S. M., & Prybutok, V. (2024). Balancing privacy and progress: A review of privacy challenges, systemic oversight, and patient perceptions in AI-driven healthcare. *Applied Sciences (Basel, Switzerland)*, *14*(2), 675. Advance online publication. DOI: 10.3390/app14020675

Winter, A., Ammenwerth, E., Haux, R., Marschollek, M., Steiner, B., & Jahn, F. (2023). *Health Informatics: Health Information Systems Technological and Management Perspectives* (3rd ed.). Springer., DOI: 10.1007/978-3-031-12310-8

Wolff, K. (2024). Preparing future lawyers to draft contracts and communicate with clients in the era of generative AI. *Transactions: The Tennessee Journal of Business Law*, *25*(3), 8.

World Bank Group. (2023). *Structuring PPP projects*. Public-Private Partnership Legal Resource Center. https://ppp.worldbank.org/public-private-partnership/structuring-ppp-projects (Accessed 23 May 2023).

World Bank. (2023). *Digital-in-health: unlocking the value for everyone*. Washington, DC: World Bank Publications. https://openknowledge.worldbank.org/handle/10986/40212 (Accessed 18 August 2023).

World Bank. (2025). Regulatory sandboxes for digital health. https://documents.worldbank.org/en/publication/documents-reports/documentdetail/099011825011040830

World Economic Forum. (2023). *Scaling smart solutions with AI in health: unlocking impact on high potential use cases*. Geneva: World Economic Forum. https://www.weforum.org/reports/scaling-smart-solutions-with-ai-in-health-unlocking-impact-on-high-potential-use-cases/#:~:text=26%20June%202023-,Scaling%20Smart%20Solutions%20with%20AI%20in%20Health%3A%20Unlocking,on%20High%20potential%20use%20cases&text=The%20healthcare%20sector%20is%20grappling,potential%20to%20tackle%20these%20issues (Accessed 26 June 2023).

World Health Organization. (1978). Declaration of Alma-Ata, *primary health care: report of the International Conference on Primary Health Care*. Alma-Ata, 6-12 September. Geneva: WHO Press.

World Health Organization. (1997). *Health-for-all Policy for the 21st Century, HQ (document EB101/8)*. WHO.

World Health Organization. (1999). *WHO guidelines on collaboration and partnerships with commercial enterprises*. WHO Press.

World Health Organization. (2006). *Quality of care: A process for making strategic choices in health systems*. WHO Press.

World Health Organization. (2016). Global diffusion of eHealth: Making universal health coverage achievable. https://apps.who.int/iris/handle/10665/252529

World Health Organization. (2021). Global strategy on digital health 2020–2025. Geneva. https://www.who.int/publications/i/item/9789240020924

World Health Organization. (2021). Global strategy on digital health 2020–2025. https://apps.who.int/iris/bitstream/handle/10665/344249/9789240020924-eng.pdf

World Health Organization. (2021). Global strategy on digital health 2020–2025. https://www.who.int/publications/i/item/9789240020924

World Health Organization. (2023). Health system governance. https://www.who.int/health-topics/health-systems-governance#tab=tab_1

World Health Organization. (2025, March 13). Telemedicine: Opportunities and developments in Member State. WHO Regional Office for Africa. https://www.afro.who.int/publications/telemedicine-opportunities-and-developments-member-state

World Medical Assembly. (1999). Statement on Accountability, Responsibilities and Ethical Practice of Telemedicine 1999. https://www.wma.net/e/press/1999_5

Wronka, C. (2024). Crypto-asset regulatory landscape: A comparative analysis of the crypto-asset regulation in the UK and Germany. *Journal of Asset Management, 25*(4), 417–426. Advance online publication. DOI: 10.1057/s41260-024-00358-z

Wu, H., Deng, Z., Wang, B., & Wu, T. (2020). Online service qualities in the multi-stage process and patients' compliments: A transaction cycle perspective. *Information & Management, 57*(5), 103230. DOI: 10.1016/j.im.2019.103230

Xie, Y., Lu, L., Gao, F., He, S., Zhao, H., Fang, Y., Yang, J., An, Y., Ye, Z., & Dong, Z. (2021). Integration of artificial intelligence, blockchain, and wearable technology for chronic disease management: A new paradigm in smart healthcare. *Current Medical Science*, *41*(6), 1123–1133. DOI: 10.1007/s11596-021-2485-0 PMID: 34950987

Xu, X. P., Ke, D. G., Deng, D. N., Houser, S. H., Li, X. N., Wang, Q., & Shan, N. C. (2019). An innovative medical consultation model in mainland China: Acceptance and perceptions. *International Journal of Health Care Quality Assurance*, *32*(7), 1057. DOI: 10.1108/IJHCQA-02-2017-0033

Yaeger, K., Martini, M., Rasouli, J., & Costa, A. (2019). Emerging blockchain technology solutions for modern healthcare infrastructure. *Journal of Scientific Innovation in Medicine*, *2*(1), 1. DOI: 10.29024/jsim.7

Yang, G., Ye, Q. H., & Xia, J. (2022). Unbox the black-box for the medical explainable AI via multi-modal and multi-centre data fusion: A mini-review, two showcases and beyond. *Information Fusion*, *77*, 29–52. DOI: 10.1016/j.inffus.2021.07.016 PMID: 34980946

Yang, L., Ene, I. C., Belaghi, R. A., Koff, D., Stein, N., & Santaguida, P. (2022). Stakeholders' perspectives on the future of artificial intelligence in radiology: A scoping review. *European Radiology*, *32*(3), 1477–1495. DOI: 10.1007/s00330-021-08214-z PMID: 34545445

Yellowlees, P., Shore, J., & Roberts, L. (2010). Practice guidelines for videoconferencing-based telemental health—October 2009. *Telemedicine Journal and e-Health : The Official Journal of the American Telemedicine Association*, *16*(10), 1074–1089. DOI: 10.1089/tmj.2010.0148 PMID: 21186991

Yip, W., & Hsiao, W. C. (2015). What drove the cycles of Chinese health system reforms? *Health Systems and Reform*, *1*(1), 52–61. DOI: 10.4161/23288604.2014.995005

Yufeng, X. (2018). *Consumer experience and satisfaction of private health management service enterprises in China* [Doctoral dissertation, Iscte – Instituto Universitário de Lisboa]. Iscte Repository. http://hdl.handle.net/10071/17314

Yu, P., Lu, S., Long, Z., Chen, Y., Qian, J., & Shah, Z. A. (2024). Exploring Ethical Considerations in Utilizing Generative AI for Global Knowledge Sharing in Higher Education. In Yu, P., Mulli, J., Syed, Z. A. S., & Umme, L. (Eds.), *Facilitating Global Collaboration and Knowledge Sharing in Higher Education With Generative AI* (pp. 1–27). IGI Global., DOI: 10.4018/979-8-3693-0487-7.ch001

Yu, P., Xue, W., & Mahendran, R. (2022). The Development and Impact of China's Digital Transformation in the Medical Industry. In Rodrigues, M. A., & Proença, J. F. (Eds.), *Impact of Digital Transformation on the Development of New Business Models and Consumer Experience* (pp. 97–128). IGI Global., DOI: 10.4018/978-1-7998-9179-6.ch006

Yu, P., & Xu, Y. (2022). Public-Private Partnership for Healthcare in China: The Effectiveness on the Regional Cities of Healthcare Service. In Akkaya, B., Jermsittiparsert, K., & Gunsel, A. (Eds.), *Handbook of Research on Current Trends in Asian Economics, Business, and Administration* (pp. 328–348). IGI Global., DOI: 10.4018/978-1-7998-8486-6.ch018

Zafar Ullah, A., Newell, J. N., Ahmed, J. U., Hyder, M., & Islam, A. (2006). Government-NGO collaboration: The case of tuberculosis control in Bangladesh. *Health Policy and Planning*, *21*(2), 143–155. DOI: 10.1093/heapol/czj014

Zahidi, S. (2023). *Future of jobs report*, April 30. World Economic Forum. https://www.weforum.org/publications/the-future-of-jobs-report-2023/digest/

Zakarneh, S. K., Qaroush, Z., & Dawabsheh, A. (2022). Cryptocurrencies advantages and disadvantages: A review. *International Journal of Applied Sciences and Smart Technologies*, *4*(1), 1–20. DOI: 10.24071/ijasst.v5i1.4611

Zarei, E. (2015). Service Quality of Hospital Outpatient Departments: Patients' Perspective. *International Journal of Health Care Quality Assurance*, *28*(8), 778–790. DOI: 10.1108/IJHCQA-09-2014-0097

Zeng, X. H., Zheng, Y. X., & Zhang, Q. (2015). Study on definition of smart tourism based on content analysis. *Resources Development & Market*, *10*, 1246–1249.

Zhang, J., & Zhang, Z. M. (2023). Ethics and governance of trustworthy medical artificial intelligence. *BMC Medical Informatics and Decision Making*, *23*(1), 7. Advance online publication. DOI: 10.1186/s12911-023-02103-9 PMID: 36639799

Zhang, M., Guo, X., & Wu, T. (2019). Impact of free contributions on private benefits in online healthcare communities. *International Journal of Electronic Commerce*, *23*(4), 492–523. DOI: 10.1080/10864415.2019.1655208

Zhang, W., Deng, Z., Hong, Z., Evans, R., Ma, J., & Zhang, H. (2018). Unhappy patients are not alike: Content analysis of the negative comments from China's Good Doctor Website. *Journal of Medical Internet Research*, *20*(1), e35. DOI: 10.2196/jmir.8223

Zhang, Y., Zhang, L., Zhang, X., Yang, M. M., Zhang, S., Li, S.-J., & Huang, Y.-Y. (2018). Hospital service quality and patient loyalty: The mediation effect of empathy. *Journal of Business and Industrial Marketing, 33*(8), 1176–1186. DOI: 10.1108/JBIM-02-2018-0072

Zheng, Z., Xie, S., Dai, H., Chen, X., & Wang, H. (2017, June). An overview of blockchain technology: Architecture, consensus, and future trends. In 2017 IEEE International Congress on Big Data (BigData Congress) (pp. 557–564). IEEE.

Zheng, Y., Zeng, M., Deng, B., Bin, H., Liu, F., & Lin, X. (2024). Topic mining and sentiment analysis based on the online review from MOOC platform's logistics course. *SAGE Open, 14*(4), 21582440241303486. Advance online publication. DOI: 10.1177/21582440241303486

Zhou, A. Y., Zghebi, S. S., Hodkinson, A., Hann, M., Grigoroglou, C., Ashcroft, D. M., Esmail, A., Chew-Graham, C. A., Payne, R., Little, P., Lusignan, S., Cherachi-Sohi, S., Spooner, S., Zhou, A. K., Kontopantelis, E., & Panagioti, M. (2022). Investigating the links between diagnostic uncertainty, emotional exhaustion, and turnover intention in General Practitioners working in the United Kingdom. *Frontiers in Psychiatry, 13*, 936067. DOI: 10.3389/fpsyt.2022.936067 PMID: 35958644

Zhou, K. R., & Gattinger, G. (2024). The Evolving Regulatory Paradigm of AI in MedTech: A Review of Perspectives and Where We Are Today. *Therapeutic Innovation & Regulatory Science, 58*(3), 456–464. DOI: 10.1007/s43441-024-00628-3 PMID: 38528278

Zhuang, Q. D., Hussein, M. K., Ariffin, N. F. M., & Yunos, M. Y. M. (2022). Landscape character: A knowledge mapping analysis using CiteSpace. *International Journal of Environmental Science and Technology, 19*(10), 10477–10492. DOI: 10.1007/s13762-022-04279-5

Zhuk, A. (2025). Beyond the blockchain hype: Addressing legal and regulatory challenges. *SN Social Sciences, 5*(2), 11. Advance online publication. DOI: 10.1007/s43545-024-01044-y

About the Contributors

Cong Sui is a HealthTech innovator and consultant with dual PhDs and an MBA. He is currently working in West Midlands Health Tech Innovation Accelerator supported by West Midlands Combined Authority. He devotes himself to the whole innovation journey, including the initial innovation, commercialising innovations, investing innovations and the final adoption into global health system. He aims to accelerate innovations and apply entrepreneurial skills to deliver quality healthcare services and address the global health challenges, e.g. sustainability, health equity, universal health coverage, etc. He was invited as an Investment Mentor at the Asian Financial Forum (AFF). He participated in a consulting project aimed at developing an innovative national health system for the Saudi Arabia Ministry of Health. Additionally, he acts as a contributor to establish the Global Health & Digital Innovation Foundation. Dr Sui is also a research fellow in the Healthcare Technologies Institute based at the University of Birmingham. As a biomaterial scientist and chemical engineer, his extensive research backgrounds encompass orthopedic wound, biomaterial, nanotechnology, imaging and microencapsulation. Dr. Sui has published 12 papers, 1 book chapter and has filed 2 patents. One of his patented technology has addressed a critical challenge in the FMCG sector, garnering attention from more than 20 national and international companies. This work has been published in Chemical Engineering Science, invited by an executive editor of the journal. In addition, he conducted several industrial R&D projects for FMCG companies, including Unilever, Firmenich and Philips UK. Dr Sui was awarded an MBA in Global Health (with distinction) from the Global Business School for Health at University College London in 2024. He completed his first PhD in Biomaterials at Hefei National Laboratory for Physical Sciences at the Microscale, University of Science and Technology of China in 2017, followed by a second PhD in Chemical Engineering from the University of Birmingham in 2018. In addition to his academic achievements, Dr Sui also attended executive courses in Venture Capital Fundamentals at London Business School, Leading Digital Transformation in Health

Care at Harvard University and Business, International Relations and the Political Economy at London School of Economics and Political Science.

Poshan (Sam) Yu is a Chinese-Australian professional with an astonishingly diverse background and an extensive collection of remarkable accomplishments. In the academic sphere, he currently teaches at the University of Victoria Program at Soochow University. Previously, he held the position of an external professor of financial technology and finance at SKEMA Business School. He also serves as a visiting researcher at the Australian Studies Centre of Shanghai University, a guest professor at emlyon business school China, and an adjunct faculty member at George Washington University's master (finance) program at Renmin University of China. As a visiting professor at Krirk University in Thailand and an EU-Asia research coordinator at the European Business Institute in Luxembourg, he brings a truly global perspective to his teaching and research activities. He is a member of the IP & Innovation Researchers of Asia (IPIRA) Network and the Global South Dialogue on Economic Crime (GSDEC), further enriching his academic engagement. His prior role as a casual academic at the University of South Australia Business School has significantly enhanced and diversified his academic portfolio. From September 2020 to February 2021, he held the position of visiting scholar at The Chinese University of Hong Kong on two occasions. His scholarly pursuits are extensive and multifaceted. As an editor for the European Academic Journal (Special Issue) - European Business Institute in Luxembourg, an editor for Humanities & Social Sciences Communications (an SSCI-indexed journal), and an associate editor for the International Journal of Interdisciplinary Research in Social Science, he plays a crucial role in the dissemination of knowledge. He is an ad hoc reviewer for a number of prestigious journals and academic presses, including Applied Economics, Applied Artificial Intelligence, Cogent Economics & Finance, Humanities and Social Sciences Communications, Journal of Chinese Economic and Business Studies, Journal of Digital Learning and Education, The Singapore Economic Review, ILMA Journal of Social Sciences & Economics, Journal of Environmental Issues and Climate Change, Advances in Global Economic and Business Journal, The Interdisciplinary Social Sciences Journal Collection, Common Ground Research Networks, Imprint - Xi'an Jiaotong-Liverpool University, Innovative Teaching and Learning, IBT Journal of Business Studies, Journal of Infrastructure Policy and Development, and Innovative Informatics and Artificial Intelligence Research. Moreover, he is an international editorial advisory board member for several edited books such as Advancing STEM Education and Innovation in a Time of Distance Learning (Scopus-indexed), Multidisciplinary Perspectives Towards Building a Digitally Competent Society (Scopus-indexed), Handbook of Research on SDGs for Economic Development, Social Development, and Environmental Protection, and Implications for Entrepreneurship and Enterprise Development in the Blue Economy. He has released more than 12 journal articles, among which 6 are listed as ABDC: B/SSCI. He has also contributed over 70 peer-reviewed book chapters imprinted by renowned publishers like IGI Global, Routledge, and Springer. He has edited 22 books, with 14 English-edited books indexed by Scopus and 6 Chinese-edited books. Notably, the book about Innovation & Exploration: The Development of FinTech in Jiangsu China has received the 14th Outstanding Achievement Award of Philosophy and Social Sciences in Suzhou and the 3rd prize of the 2018 Jiangsu Provincial Education Science Research Achievement Award by Jiangsu Provincial Department of Education. His receipt of four Xi'an Jiaotong-Liverpool University (XJTLU) National University Teaching Innovation Awards from 2016 to 2020 and being recognized as a top contender in the same national competition in 2016 led to his appointment as the Institute of Leadership and Education Advanced Development (ILEAD) Research Fellow by XJTLU. In 2021, he received The Outstanding Contribution Award for Industrial Research Development in China, CIE100 issued by Wisdom China Magazine: Beijing. Beyond academia, he is actively involved in various industries. He is an entrepreneur and venture capitalist, collaborating with alumni and senior faculty members from Cambridge University. Additionally, he is a guest financial news commentator on over 30 media platforms in China. In the business world, he holds significant positions. He is a regional partner in China for FasterCapital based in Dubai, United Arab Emirates. He also serves as vice president at Tinbowah Investment in Beijing and as an honorary vice president of the Belt and Road Blockchain Association. Furthermore, he mentors businesses for AIC RAISE in Coimbatore, India, the Griffith Industry Mentoring Program in Australia, and University College London Innovation & Enterprise. In 2023, he was invited to act as a venture capital panel judge and mentor at 'Y&Archer A Stream 2023' conference in Jeju, South Korea. His research interests are broad and encompass financial technology, regulatory technology, blockchain, web 3.0 in financial services, generative AI, public-private partnerships, mergers and acquisitions, private equity, venture capital, startups, family offices, IoTs, supply chain finance, intellectual property, art finance, wine, back-door listing, intangible cultural heritage, and Chinese economy & policy. His extensive experience in international fintech, edtech, startup, social media, and cleantech companies across India, the UK, Australia, Hong Kong, and China is truly remarkable. His three-year tenure in significant leadership positions within the Chinese-Australian media marketing and public relations sector, along with his role as an OzAsia Festival Ambassador in Australia, has exerted a profound influence on his current modus operandi as an academic and business consultant. Additionally, it has considerably broadened his perspective within the international multicultural arts community and enlarged his business network. This multifaceted experience has furnished him with a more comprehensive and inclusive outlook on academia, industry, and research. He is fully dedicated to making substantial contributions in these areas and is keen on furthering his development in the future. Incidentally, Sam has an inclination towards wine, arts, and reading.

***

Sharadhi A.K is a graduate student researcher currently pursuing her Master of Science in Information Science (MSIS) from the College of Information Science, University of Arizona, Tucson, USA. She completed her B.Tech in Computer Science and Engineering from MS Ramaiah University of Applied Sciences in Bangalore, Karnataka, India. She has published several research papers in prestigious IEEE and Elsevier journals, as well as at international conferences, covering topics such as crowd simulation, cardiovascular disease detection, software defect prediction, and computer vision applications. Her research interests include human-centered computing, Human-Computer Interaction (HCI), simulation, cyber psychology, healthcare informatics, and digital health interventions—particularly at the intersection of human well-being and technology. With interdisciplinary expertise spanning computer science, information systems, and healthcare applications, she actively contributes to academic literature as a reviewer for Elsevier journals, including Intelligent Systems with Applications and the Journal of Information and Intelligence.

Esther Anaiye is a graduate of the National Open University of Nigeria. She is a practicing Nurse with years of experience in several medical health sectors in Nigeria. She has passion for medical excellence.

Ana Brochado is a Full Professor at Universidade Aberta and a researcher at DINAMIA'CET – Centre for Socioeconomic and Territorial Studies. She holds a BSc in Economics, an MSc in Quantitative Methods, and a PhD in Management. She has authored or co-authored over 100 publications in leading international journalsand delivered over 200 presentations at international conferences worldwide. Her work has been cited over 4,700 times. She is listed in the Stanford/Elsevier Top 2% Scientists List for the years 2022, 2023, and 2024.

Yiheng Chen is an independent researcher. Her research interests encompass fintech, banking, and business analysis.

Basil Daudu holds a PhD in Social and Political Philosophy and specializes in AI and African Studies (society, politics, and culture). He is a licensed instructor and a seasoned Microsoft innovative facilitator. He has contributed to various academic journals and book chapters. Currently, he is a staff of Kogi State University, Anyigba, Nigeria, serving as a senior lecturer and a researcher in the Department of Philosophy.

Julie Davies is Professor of Healthcare Management and Leadership Development and Head of Business School Accreditations, Rankings and Branding at Brunel Business School in London. Her research interests include qualitative research, healthcare workforce, hybrid strategic leadership development, management education, micro-entrepreneurship and workplace inclusion in the UK, India and Saudi Arabia. Julie is an associate editor of Long Range Planning. She is a practitioner Fellow of the Chartered Institute of Personnel and Development and hospice trustee. Previously she led an Erasmus Plus project in the UK on HRM in regional SMEs. julie.davies@brunel.ac.uk @juliedaviesUK

Sheikh Mateen Ellahi is an experienced GP partner in the northeast of England, healthcare consultant and keynote speaker. His main interests involve consulting with GP practice partners to manage their practice effectively to improve patient care and the patient experience aligned with business objectives. Mateen has a keen interest in exploring the impact of changes and technology within primary care in the UK on a larger scale, and the implications that this has for patient safety. He completed an MBA Health with distinction at University College London in 2022.

Xinyuan Jiang as Independent Researcher her research interests include health economics, business finance and HealthTech

Dimitrios Kalogeropoulos is Chief Executive at the Global Health Digital Innovation Foundation, UK, and Health Executive in Residence at the UCL Global Business School for Health. A recognised leader in global health, he brings over three decades of experience in health governance and digital innovation. With a PhD in Artificial Intelligence in Medicine since the 1990s, he has pioneered the application of AI to systems medicine and advised global organisations—including the World Bank, WHO, PAHO, the European Commission, and the Bill & Melinda Gates Foundation—on health, technology, and governance. He has advanced global health by fostering open innovation ecosystems and systems capital across Asia, Europe, and the Americas. His policy contributions include pivotal roles in the Healthy China 2030 initiative, jointly led by the Chinese government, the World Bank Group, and WHO, and in shaping the EU AI Act. As a member of the EU AI Office's Plenary Forum, he supports the development of the first General-Purpose AI Code of Practice. He contributes to initiatives ensuring AI delivers societal value and mitigates systemic inequities, including his role on the Stakeholders Advisory Group of the International Observatory on Information and Democracy.

Dr. Kalogeropoulos is a member of the IEEE European Public Policy Committee and Global Policy Caucus, and a founding member of the International Advisory Committee for the IEEE Global Standardised Registry for Medical Mobile Health Applications, where he chairs the Ethics Subcommittee. His participation in the WHO-led Health Data Collaborative's Working Group on Digital Health and Climate Policy highlights his commitment to evidence-based solutions for global challenges. He founded and chairs the IEEE SA Industry Connections program IC24-015 on AI for Public Health and Climate-Resilient Health Systems and leads the P3493.1™ Working Group to develop a Standard Framework for Secure, Compliant, Coordinated, and Inclusive Healthcare Data Recycling, with an initial focus on cancer care. This initiative bridges policy and innovation to enable ethical, sustainable secondary use of healthcare data. With extensive experience, including his tenure at IBM, Dr. Kalogeropoulos advises start-ups and organisations globally, offering strategic insights into digital transformation and policy alignment. A sought-after speaker, he champions innovation, equity, and sustainability, collaborating with accelerator programs like CancerX and the WHO/Europe Strategic Partnership Initiative for Data and Digital Health.

Dede Latey is a medical doctor, health financing and policy professional as well as a digital health innovator who founded MindITGH, Ghana's first toll-free mental healthcare helpline. He holds a bachelors degree in medical sciences, a bachelors degree in medicine and surgery and a masters in Heath Policy Planning and Financing. His works in digital mental health innovation have been featured by the BBC, World Bank Group and WHO.

Han Liew, BSN, RN, MBA (Health) is a Registered Nurse with extensive experience across acute hospital settings and population health, specializing in medical and surgical domains. He has supported the deployment of digital health technologies to enhance clinical safety, workforce capability, and care delivery. Currently, Han serves as an Engagement Lead at National University Hospital (Singapore), where he plays a key role in driving an innovation culture within the hospital. Han establishes and nurtures strategic partnerships across industry, academia, and the broader healthcare ecosystem, actively identifying collaboration opportunities to translate ideas into impactful innovations. He works closely with clinicians, technology partners, startups, and researchers to accelerate innovation, validate use cases, and enable scalable implementation within real-world clinical settings.

Robert Lubajo is a Technical Officer at WHO Regional Office for Africa, leading efforts to strengthen diagnostic systems across the 47 member states. With a background in medical laboratory science and dual master's degrees in Public Healthy and Health Policy Planning and Financing, he has worked with UNDP and several NGOs on epidemic and pandemic preparedness and response, advancing health systems, policy and research across Africa and MENA region.

Chandra Lukita is an educational pioneer with a scientific focus in the field of Management and Entrepreneurship, he has successfully published 29 Scopus-indexed journals and is actively involved as a reviewer for various national and international journals. In his academic career, he is also recognized as a book author, keynote speaker at numerous national and international conferences, and an active contributor to public leadership initiatives. In addition, he is known as a skilled entrepreneur with strategic capabilities in managing and developing various business lines. The integration of academic insight and practical business experience makes him a figure capable of bringing academic values into the industrial world, creating new opportunities, and inspiring many entrepreneurs to grow and adapt in an ever-changing era.

Mohan Mishra is an international technology and corporate lawyer (18+ yrs) specialising in AI, blockchain, and virtual-asset–enabled business models, with a focus on regulatory design, AML/CFT controls, and cross-border licensing across the UAE, India, Europe and Singapore. Experienced in multi-jurisdictional virtual-asset frameworks and FATF-aligned compliance for high-risk digital businesses (crypto, forex/CFD, iGaming), with additional depth in data, cyber, and AI governance. Completed the Oxford Artificial Intelligence Programme (Saïd, 2025), linking legal/regulatory analysis with AI capabilities.

Marzena Nieroda is a person-centred health-services scholar whose grounding in commercial market research keeps consumer and patient voices central and fuels interdisciplinary collaboration. Rooted in marketing science—consumer behaviour, service design and innovation—she maps and refines well-being journeys across organisations and systems, coupling them with digital technologies to deliver efficient, resource-conscious care. Her current work has two strands. First, she uses systems thinking and journey-mapping to explore how the places people live, work and age shape health behaviours and outcomes, then redesigns lifestyle and ageing experiences accordingly developing behaviour-change programmes and service pathways illustrated by cases in women's health and menopause, weight management and cancer risk. Second, she advances Open Health, a global federated-data platform that interconnects partners from research, public agencies, industry and the third sector. By enriching its privacy-preserving analytics with behavioural and contextual variables, she ensures tools—from risk-prediction engines to service-planning dashboards—mirror lived realities while safeguarding data. Marzena blends qualitative, quantitative and mixed methods approaches and convenes clinicians, technologists, policymakers and patient groups to co-create actionable solutions. Her work has attracted support from Cancer Research UK, Greater Manchester Cancer Vanguard, the European Commission, Digitally Enhanced Advanced Services (DEAS), EPSRC, University College London and the University of Manchester.

Rajan Punitharajah is a Senior Director, Data and Analytics, at Ipsen, a mid-sized global biopharmaceutical company which improves patients' lives through research, innovation and the development of transformative medicines in oncology, rare disease and neuroscience. Rajan has over 20 years' experience in implementing data governance, data management, ownership and stewardship with executive teams globally. Previously, he worked in firms such as PepsiCo, O2, Johnson Matthey, and Unilever. He earned an MSc in AI Strategy at Brunel University of London.

Abdul Seckam, PhD, is the Head of Research and Academia at Healthcare Business Solutions UK (HBSUK) who leads in-house research and grant applications and generate, publish and present papers and presentations working with clinical leads in various Virtual Lucy specialities. Abdul facilitates external research/ evaluation projects through project stakeholder groups and engages. with external agencies such as patient and other stakeholder groups and compiling reports and recommendations for clinical and product strategy. He also lead on digital analysis for product evaluation, governance and machine learning at HBSUK. Abdul is also an Associate Tutor at Cardiff Metropolitan University. His research focuses on digital healthcare interventions with a focus on patient and stakeholder engagement in the creation of innovative healthcare solutions. Abdul also is the co-creator of two Public and Patient Involvement (PPI) Committees; Stroke Hub Wales (SHW) and HBSUK and involves committee member insights and co-production in various national and international research projects. Abdul has contributed to various research projects funded by Stroke Research, Innovation and Education Fund (SRIEF) Welsh Government, Arts Council Wales, Biovici Limited and Zenzium Limited, SMARTExpertise, Welsh Government and Cardiff Metropolitan University. Abdul has presented and published at various local, national and international conference proceedings and in journals respectively. (ORCHID ID: 0000-0002-4516-9366),

Samuel Tshikuta ws born in the Democratic Republic of Congo (DR Congo), Sam K is a dedicated health science professional with a global academic and research footprint. He earned his undergraduate degree from Rajiv Gandhi University of Health Sciences in India, where he also presented groundbreaking research at a public health conference in Bengaluru on the prevention of cholera and Ebola in the

DR Congo. While back home in Kolwezi, he shared insights on the psychological stress experienced by international students, reflecting his deep concern for student well-being. Driven by a passion for community health, he collaborated with local NGOs to support HIV/AIDS prevention initiatives and sanitation efforts across Congo. His academic journey continued in the United States at Coppin State University, where he pursued his master's degree. In 2024, he presented research on the challenges of the Internet of Things (IoT) in health data management at the MdHIMA Annual Conference, followed by a 2025 presentation on telemedicine in Central Africa, spotlighting the DR Congo. His core passions lie in research, medical science, and music disciplines through which he seeks to impact both local and global communities.

Index

A

Adoption 1, 2, 4, 5, 6, 10, 12, 13, 18, 19, 21, 22, 23, 28, 31, 32, 34, 36, 75, 76, 77, 78, 89, 91, 92, 93, 95, 98, 104, 105, 107, 114, 115, 116, 123, 124, 125, 132, 134, 135, 136, 137, 138, 150, 151, 152, 153, 155, 156, 158, 162, 166, 171, 180, 184, 185, 187, 195, 274, 275, 316, 317, 320, 324, 325, 332, 333, 334
Africa 21, 69, 75, 78, 81, 82, 83, 88, 89, 90, 91, 92, 93, 94, 95, 96, 97, 98, 101, 104, 107, 109, 114, 115, 116, 126, 127, 128, 129, 131, 169, 172, 175, 178, 179, 180, 181, 185, 187, 188, 189, 191, 193, 194, 195, 202, 204, 205, 274, 324, 350
AI-Blockchain Convergence 328, 332
Artificial Intelligence 2, 16, 22, 31, 32, 35, 36, 41, 49, 54, 55, 64, 65, 66, 68, 69, 71, 72, 103, 116, 123, 126, 127, 129, 131, 132, 140, 154, 183, 184, 241, 242, 243, 244, 245, 247, 248, 249, 250, 251, 252, 253, 254, 256, 257, 258, 259, 260, 261, 264, 265, 266, 267, 268, 269, 270, 271, 274, 275, 276, 283, 289, 293, 294, 301, 302, 303, 304, 307, 308, 337, 338, 340, 341, 342, 343, 344, 346, 347, 348

B

Barrier 22, 41, 89, 92, 140, 141, 145, 147, 150, 153, 154, 161, 178, 181, 182, 211, 327
Barriers 1, 3, 5, 6, 12, 18, 21, 23, 26, 28, 31, 32, 33, 34, 35, 77, 82, 83, 88, 90, 95, 97, 100, 107, 114, 115, 116, 127, 133, 134, 137, 138, 140, 142, 144, 145, 146, 147, 148, 149, 150, 152, 153, 155, 157, 162, 165, 166, 171, 182, 183, 184, 192, 275, 300, 332, 338, 346
Blockchain 274, 275, 296, 300, 307, 308, 309, 310, 311, 314, 315, 316, 320, 321, 322, 323, 324, 326, 327, 328, 329, 330, 331, 332, 333, 334, 335, 336, 337, 338, 339, 340, 341, 342, 343, 344, 345, 346, 347, 348
BurstIQ 307, 309, 310, 329, 330, 331, 333, 334, 335, 336, 338, 345

C

China 15, 33, 207, 208, 209, 210, 211, 214, 215, 216, 230, 231, 232, 233, 234, 235, 236, 237, 238, 239, 241, 273, 274, 275, 276, 280, 283, 286, 287, 289, 304, 305
Content Analysis 155, 207, 210, 216, 230, 231, 239, 303

D

Data Governance 158, 183, 249, 257, 308, 324, 326, 337, 344, 349
Data Privacy 19, 25, 35, 44, 45, 62, 80, 85, 111, 113, 148, 153, 185, 244, 249, 254, 260, 274, 282, 292, 293, 300, 329, 332, 343
Digital Health 2, 3, 4, 7, 10, 12, 18, 19, 20, 22, 23, 28, 29, 31, 32, 48, 53, 69, 71, 91, 93, 94, 112, 116, 130, 131, 133, 134, 135, 136, 137, 138, 139, 140, 141, 142, 145, 147, 149, 150, 151, 152, 153, 154, 155, 156, 157, 158, 159, 160, 161, 162, 163, 164, 166, 167, 171, 172, 178, 179, 180, 182, 183, 184, 185, 186, 188, 189, 190, 191, 192, 193, 194, 195, 202, 203, 204, 230, 268, 269, 303, 307, 308, 309, 324, 338, 342, 347
Digital Innovation 39, 42, 48, 135
Digital Transformation 1, 6, 9, 10, 12, 36, 133, 134, 135, 137, 138, 139, 140, 141, 142, 149, 151, 152, 154, 155, 156, 157, 158, 162, 163, 164, 188, 195, 305, 346
DR Congo 75, 76, 77, 79, 80, 81, 83, 85, 86, 87, 88, 89, 94, 95, 96

E

Efficiency 3, 5, 8, 9, 11, 13, 15, 17, 18, 19, 20, 44, 53, 54, 59, 60, 61, 68, 70, 98, 106, 107, 114, 123, 124, 131, 134, 136, 147, 210, 213, 221, 226, 227, 228, 229, 232, 242, 243, 252, 274, 276, 294, 297, 298, 315, 333, 341
eHealth 35, 97, 100, 101, 159, 164, 191, 202, 203, 204
Enabler 55, 137, 138, 140, 141, 145, 151, 152
Ethical Compliance 260, 276, 291, 297
Ethical Issues 3, 13, 15, 241, 242, 243, 244, 245, 247, 248, 249, 250, 253, 254, 255, 256, 260, 261, 262, 266, 275, 283
Ethics 6, 33, 110, 112, 113, 126, 188, 237, 244, 245, 247, 248, 251, 252, 254, 255, 257, 260, 262, 263, 264, 265, 266, 267, 268, 269, 270, 271, 273, 274, 275, 276, 277, 279, 280, 282, 283, 284, 286, 287, 289, 290, 291, 292, 293, 294, 295, 296, 297, 299, 301, 302, 303, 304, 309, 322, 339, 342

G

Generative AI 39, 42, 48, 51, 54, 55, 56, 65, 66, 67, 68, 69, 70, 71, 72, 275, 282, 291, 292, 295, 296, 299, 304, 337
Global Health 31, 33, 39, 40, 41, 42, 43, 44, 46, 47, 48, 49, 50, 51, 52, 53, 56, 57, 58, 59, 60, 61, 62, 63, 64, 65, 66, 68, 70, 71, 97, 167, 172, 187, 191, 204, 241, 242, 269, 274, 275, 297
Global Health Challenges 241, 242, 274, 275
Governance 2, 5, 12, 17, 19, 23, 25, 27, 29, 35, 36, 45, 52, 53, 56, 58, 59, 60, 61, 65, 70, 71, 110, 127, 144, 151, 158, 166, 183, 184, 241, 242, 249, 252, 253, 254, 255, 256, 257, 260, 261, 262, 266, 268, 269, 271, 273, 274, 275, 276, 284, 287, 290, 291, 295, 298, 299, 300, 301, 303, 304, 308, 310, 311, 314, 320, 322, 324, 325, 326, 327, 328, 332, 333, 334, 335, 336, 337, 339, 344, 349
GPS 5, 7, 8, 17

H

Healthcare 1, 2, 3, 4, 5, 6, 7, 8, 9, 10, 11, 12, 13, 14, 15, 16, 17, 18, 19, 20, 21, 22, 23, 24, 25, 26, 27, 28, 29, 30, 31, 32, 33, 34, 35, 36, 40, 41, 42, 44, 45, 46, 53, 54, 55, 56, 57, 59, 60, 62, 63, 65, 68, 70, 75, 76, 77, 78, 79, 81, 82, 83, 84, 85, 86, 87, 88, 89, 90, 91, 92, 93, 94, 95, 96, 97, 98, 99, 100, 103, 104, 105, 106, 107, 108, 109, 110, 111, 112, 113, 114, 115, 116, 117, 118, 119, 120, 121, 122, 123, 124, 125, 126, 127, 128, 130, 131, 132, 133, 134, 135, 136, 137, 138, 139, 140, 142, 144, 145, 146, 147, 150, 151, 152, 153, 154, 156, 157, 159, 161, 162, 164, 165, 167, 169, 171, 173, 176, 178, 184, 185, 186, 187, 189, 190, 207, 208, 209, 210, 211, 212, 213, 214, 215, 216, 226, 228, 229, 230, 231, 232, 233, 234, 236, 237, 238, 239, 243, 244, 249, 250, 251, 254, 256, 257, 258, 259, 260, 262, 264, 265, 266, 267, 268, 269, 270, 273, 274, 275, 276, 277, 283, 286, 287, 291, 293, 294, 295, 296, 297, 298, 299, 300, 301, 302, 303, 304, 307, 308, 309, 310, 311, 314, 315, 316, 317, 318, 319, 320, 321, 322, 323, 324, 325, 326, 327, 328, 329, 330, 331, 332, 333, 334, 335, 336, 337, 338, 339, 340, 341, 342, 343, 344, 345, 346, 347, 348, 349
Healthcare Equity 276
Healthcare Provider 40, 81, 93, 112, 113, 132, 145
Health Technologies 7, 10, 29, 31, 35, 94, 104, 133, 166, 167, 169, 171, 172, 184, 185, 186, 297, 303, 338

I

Implementation 1, 2, 4, 5, 9, 10, 11, 12, 14, 17, 21, 22, 28, 30, 34, 35, 54, 59, 60, 68, 76, 77, 78, 89, 90, 91, 92, 95, 97, 99, 103, 114, 127, 131, 133, 134, 137, 138, 139, 140, 142, 147, 148, 151, 156, 157, 158, 161, 164, 166, 167, 185, 189, 191, 251, 261, 262, 276, 290, 294, 295, 297, 300, 302, 310, 329, 333, 336

Informatics 31, 36, 61, 69, 98, 100, 104, 126, 127, 131, 132, 139, 157, 164, 165, 264, 267, 268, 269, 270, 271, 303, 341, 345

Innovation 2, 5, 10, 12, 18, 19, 20, 25, 32, 35, 36, 39, 42, 48, 55, 59, 62, 65, 66, 67, 77, 85, 96, 97, 113, 114, 124, 135, 137, 140, 158, 159, 161, 162, 165, 166, 183, 184, 195, 254, 255, 257, 261, 271, 273, 276, 290, 293, 296, 297, 298, 299, 308, 309, 320, 322, 323, 324, 325, 326, 327, 328, 329, 333, 335, 336, 339, 348

L

Liability Definition 251, 260

M

Medical Decision-Making 241, 242, 243, 244, 245, 247, 248, 250, 266, 267, 275, 282, 292

Medical Technology 242, 243, 345

N

NASSS Framework 1, 4, 5, 30, 32

NHS England 6, 15, 29, 32, 34, 133, 134, 135, 137, 138, 140, 144, 149, 150, 151, 153, 155, 156, 157, 163, 164

Nigeria 18, 19, 20, 23, 29, 31, 35, 36, 67, 94, 95, 103, 104, 105, 107, 109, 110, 111, 112, 114, 115, 116, 117, 118, 119, 123, 124, 125, 126, 127, 128, 129, 130, 131, 175, 178, 179, 180, 187, 188, 191, 193, 202, 204, 205, 324, 341, 344

P

Partnership Analysis Framework 39, 42, 48, 51, 63

Patient 2, 3, 4, 5, 6, 7, 8, 9, 10, 11, 13, 14, 16, 18, 19, 23, 24, 25, 26, 27, 28, 29, 30, 34, 55, 79, 81, 84, 85, 87, 88, 93, 98, 103, 105, 106, 107, 108, 109, 110, 112, 113, 116, 117, 118, 120, 121, 123, 124, 125, 126, 127, 128, 129, 130, 132, 134, 136, 139, 140, 144, 145, 146, 152, 153, 154, 157, 161, 164, 167, 191, 207, 208, 209, 210, 212, 213, 214, 215, 218, 219, 221, 223, 225, 226, 227, 229, 230, 231, 232, 233, 234, 235, 236, 237, 238, 239, 243, 250, 251, 253, 257, 258, 259, 260, 267, 268, 270, 273, 274, 275, 276, 277, 283, 284, 286, 287, 289, 290, 291, 292, 293, 294, 295, 296, 297, 298, 300, 302, 303, 307, 308, 309, 310, 311, 315, 316, 318, 319, 320, 321, 323, 324, 327, 328, 329, 332, 333, 334, 336, 340, 341, 347, 350

Patient Satisfaction 6, 98, 106, 208, 209, 227, 229, 234, 237, 238, 291

Patient Welfare 273, 274, 275, 276, 277, 287, 290, 296, 300

Primary Healthcare 1, 2, 4, 5, 7, 28, 29, 30, 33, 68, 81, 86, 208, 209, 231

Private Hospital 207

Public-Private Partnership 40, 51, 53, 54, 64, 67, 68, 69, 72, 275, 304

R

Remote Area 132

Remote Monitoring 8, 11, 17, 22, 77, 78, 79, 103, 105, 106, 107, 114, 119, 120, 123, 137, 139, 140

S

Service Quality 20, 207, 208, 209, 210, 211, 212, 213, 214, 215, 219, 226, 229, 230, 231, 233, 234, 235, 236, 237, 238, 239

T

Telemedicine 15, 18, 33, 75, 76, 77, 78, 79, 80, 81, 82, 83, 84, 86, 87, 88, 89, 90, 91, 92, 93, 94, 95, 96, 97, 98, 99, 100, 101, 103, 104, 105, 106, 107, 109, 110, 111, 112, 114, 115, 116, 117, 118, 119, 120, 121, 122, 123, 124, 125, 126, 127, 128, 129, 130, 131, 132, 136, 139, 140, 160, 170, 187, 189, 191, 202, 203, 204, 274, 309

Transparency 5, 19, 25, 45, 154, 243, 244, 249, 250, 252, 254, 258, 259, 267, 275, 282, 286, 289, 292, 293, 294, 295, 296, 297, 298, 300, 311, 314, 315, 316, 320, 325, 326, 333, 339

U

UK 1, 2, 7, 8, 10, 12, 16, 17, 18, 19, 20, 22, 23, 29, 31, 32, 39, 53, 68, 70, 127, 133, 137, 142, 159, 160, 161, 163, 164, 165, 167, 169, 265, 277, 293, 294, 295, 296, 298, 307, 347

www.ingramcontent.com/pod-product-compliance
Lightning Source LLC
LaVergne TN
LVHW062327300926
849161LV00007B/1601